MEG: An Introduction to Methods

MEG: An Introduction to Methods

Edited by

Peter C. Hansen
Morten L. Kringelbach
Riitta Salmelin

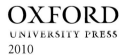

OXFORD

UNIVERSITY PRESS

2010

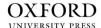

Oxford University Press, Inc., publishes works that further
Oxford University's objective of excellence
in research, scholarship, and education.

Oxford   New York
Auckland   Cape Town   Dar es Salaam   Hong Kong   Karachi
Kuala Lumpur   Madrid   Melbourne   Mexico City   Nairobi
New Delhi   Shanghai   Taipei   Toronto

With offices in
Argentina   Austria   Brazil   Chile   Czech Republic   France   Greece
Guatemala   Hungary   Italy   Japan Poland   Portugal   Singapore
South Korea   Switzerland   Thailand   Turkey   Ukraine   Vietnam

Published by Oxford University Press, Inc.
198 Madison Avenue, New York, New York 10016

www.oup.com

Oxford is a registered trademark of Oxford University Press, Inc.

Library of Congress Cataloging-in-Publication Data

MEG : an introduction to methods / [edited by] Peter C. Hansen, Morten L. Kringelbach, and Riitta Salmelin.
p. ; cm.
Includes bibliographical references and index.
ISBN 978-0-19-530723-8
1. Magnetoencephalography. I. Hansen, Peter C., 1963- II. Kringelbach, Morten L. III. Salmelin, Riitta.
[DNLM: 1. Magnetoencephalography—methods. 2. Nervous System Diseases—diagnosis.
WL 141 M496 2010]
RC386.6.M36M44 2010
616.8'047547—dc22
2010002216

9   8   7   6   5   4   3

Printed in the United States of America
on acid-free paper

Contents

Introduction

Magnetoencephalography (MEG) is a neuroimaging technique that uses an array of sensors positioned over the scalp that are extremely sensitive to minuscule changes in the magnetic fields produced by small changes in the electrical activity within the brain. It is, therefore, a direct measurement of neural activity. MEG as technique for investigating neural function in the brain is not new but was originally pioneered in the late 1960's. However, it is only since the early 1990's, with the introduction of high-density (200+) detector grids covering the whole head, that the full potential of MEG has begun to be realized. At the present time, MEG has grown to be a significant neuroimaging technique, with an increasing number of users and with the number of scientific papers utilizing MEG increasing year on year.

The casual reader of this book may well be wondering what the great attraction of MEG is. Why bother with MEG when alternative neuroimaging techniques, particularly functional magnetic resonance imaging (fMRI) and electroencephalography (EEG), exist and seem to be attractive? To begin to answer this question, let us consider an example of what the amazingly complicated human brain is actually capable of achieving in a real world situation. Imagine driving home from work in your car and suddenly experiencing a car in the opposite lane swerving into your lane. You somehow manage to avoid a crash but are left wondering how your brain made this possible.

Consider all of the complex sensory processing, object recognition, evaluation, executive planning, cognitive decisions, motor events and strong emotions evinced in the previous sequence of events that have occurred in a time window of perhaps 750 ms or less. With MEG, the sequence of neural events can be readily tracked with at least 750 snapshots of sensor data, from which one can reconstruct 750 three-dimensional plots of current distribution in the brain. In fMRI, neural activation in this same time window, indirectly measured via local changes in the level of blood oxygenation, is typically compressed to one measured brain volume. Although fMRI localizes the active areas with high spatial accuracy, it provides no real-time information of neural involvement and is therefore not ideal to track brain activity related to the kind of rapid decision-making that made it possible for you to survive the near crash.

This book is aimed at everyone interested in MEG. The reader may wish to use MEG because there is a specific neuroscience question which they think could best be answered with MEG, or because MEG happens to be the functional neuroimaging method that is available. Either way, one needs to be aware of the possibilities and limitations of the method in order to produce reliable and meaningful results. This book is intended to provide the reader with some basic tools for planning and executing MEG experiments and for analyzing and interpreting the data. The reader will appreciate this is a rapidly evolving field, and the chapters presented here are by no means exhaustive. Nevertheless, we hope that the practical approach we have sought in these chapters will be helpful when pursuing MEG studies.

The great strength of all neurophysiological methods, EEG as well as MEG, is that the detected signal directly reflects real-time information transfer between neurons. Neural activation induces an electric current that generates in turn corresponding electric and magnetic fields which are measured. Analysis of EEG data has traditionally been limited to dealing with the timing information available to the electrodes stuck to the scalp as the electric field changes at each electrode. However, MEG analysis has, from the onset, sought instead to localize the neural sources of electric current within the brain by using the time courses of the changes in the magnetic field recorded by an array of detectors. The reason for this difference of approach is straightforward. Electric fields (and therefore EEG) are strongly influenced by large changes of electric conductivity between the brain, skull and scalp, creating marked distortion. Currently, it is not feasible to noninvasively determine the geometry and conductivity of these different structures accurately and efficiently in individual subjects. The magnetic field (and therefore MEG) are affected significantly less by the same structures, causing far less distortion. Because of the concentric organization of these physiological structures, conductivity varies primarily along the radial direction. As a result, the magnetic field recorded outside of the head is essentially the same as the one that would be recorded on the exposed brain surface, making reconstruction far more accurate. As always, benefits come with cost. MEG is most sensitive to tangentially oriented currents that are located close to the sensors, i.e., in the cortex, whereas EEG is equally sensitive to signals from neural sources in any orientation and potentially can reach to deeper structures. In practice, though, the heightened sensitivity of MEG to tangential currents is a great asset in source localization, as it markedly simplifies the 'inverse problem', i.e., the complex relationship between current sources and electromagnetic fields. The electrophysiological basis of MEG and the basic mathematical formulation are described in Chapter 1 (Lopes da Silva).

Knowledge of instrumentation is essential for understanding what is actually being measured in MEG and how it is done. For example, one needs to be aware of the different types of detection coils that can be used for recording the MEG data, as this influences the appearance of the signals at the sensor level. If conclusions are drawn solely based on the sensor signals, without proceeding to some form of source reconstruction, it is crucial to know the structure of the detector coils. Chapter 2 (Parkkonen) describes the principles of MEG hardware, and Chapter 3 (Parkkonen & Salmelin) provides guidelines for performing successful measurements. These chapters also discuss the important steps involved in preprocessing MEG data, including evaluation of possible artifacts and the effects of filtering. Chapter 4 (Salmelin & Parkkonen) focuses on the design of MEG experiments and considers the selection of parameters also with respect to that in behavioral and fMRI neuroimaging studies.

The unique power of MEG is that it combines the localization of active brain areas with reasonable spatial accuracy, together with the extraction of the time courses of activation in those areas with excellent temporal accuracy. Source analysis and reconstruction is now usually an integral part of the analysis of MEG data. Indeed, decomposition of the MEG sensor signals into activity of specific neural sources enhances and clarifies stimulus and task effects. Sources of early cortical somatosensory responses, for example, may be localized very precisely because of the lack of simultaneous activation from elsewhere in the cortex. Relative locations of sources within subjects can also be determined fairly accurately, such as the distance between areas in the somatosensory cortex that are activated by electrical stimulation of the thumb versus little finger. It is important to keep in mind that MEG (or EEG) data allow estimation of the centre of an active brain area but do not provide detailed information about its shape. The precise appearance of the resulting activity map is determined by the specific analysis method employed.

Chapter 5 (Baillet) outlines the general concepts and assumptions for the various approaches that are currently used in MEG source analysis. Many of those methods are applicable to EEG data as well or were initially developed in that domain. Because of the inverse problem, some constraints are needed in order to proceed from the distribution of magnetic field to configuration of neural sources. A widely used and robust approach is to represent the neural sources by a physiologically plausible and mathematically simple model, an equivalent current dipole. Chapter 6 (Salmelin) discusses the practical application of this method to analysis of both evoked responses and oscillatory background activity. Chapter 7 (Jensen & Hesse) focuses on another approach in which constraints are set to the solution of the inverse problem by accepting the result that accounts for the measured signals with the smallest overall amount of electric current. Chapter 8 (Hämäläinen et al.) illustrates a conceptually similar approach, but with minimization of the overall power, in which the activity is additionally constrained to the cortex based on individual structural magnetic resonance images (MRIs) and the process may be further guided by functional MRI (fMRI) activation maps. Chapter 9 (Gross et al.) details the use of spatial filters ('beamformers') in the detection of interconnected neural networks. Chapter 10 (Pantazis & Leahy) outlines recent advances in performing fMRI-type statistical analysis on distributed MEG maps (cf. Chapters 7 to 9) keeping in mind, however, that time courses of activity in different brain areas determined from MEG signals are highly correlated with each other, which is not the case for the voxel time courses in fMRI data. Chapter 11 (Poline et al.) addresses the combined use of different neuroimaging techniques.

Most analysis approaches are initially tested on very simple sensory or motor paradigms, with one or maximally two experimental conditions, and typically on a single subject. In reality, neuroscience questions can be far more complex, usually with multiple experimental conditions in multiple subjects. Chapters 5 through 10 touch upon these issues as well. The reader will appreciate that all approaches have their advantages and disadvantages, and the choice between different analysis methods in the end should best be determined by the particular research question of interest. Modeling the sources as focal equivalent current dipoles is a mathematically transparent approach, with the minimum number of assumptions, but it generally requires manual intervention and benefits from expertise. Distributed source reconstruction approaches tend to be more automated and require less manual intervention and may, therefore, be freer from potential analyst bias. Their possible risk lies in their mathematical complexity and hidden assumptions. However, it should be realized that no method is inherently better than the others and none of them can truly circumvent the inverse problem. Ideally, and certainly when in doubt, the reader would be well advised to use more than one method to analyze MEG data and to compare between them.

Chapters 12 through 15 (Kakigi & Forss; Salmelin; Mäkelä; Kringelbach et al.) provide a set of examples of MEG studies ranging from basic sensory processing to cognitive tasks, and to the use of MEG in a clinical setting. The topics we chose to describe here obviously reflect only a very small part of the various research questions that MEG has been applied to. Nevertheless, we hope they will give a general idea of the possibilities of the MEG method.

To conclude, the reader should appreciate that the whole field of MEG research is very much a dynamic and growing one. In this book, a selection of scientists with long experience in MEG, each with their own view and voice, seek to provide some seasoned practical tools for the recording and analysis of MEG data and to offer their insights into various conceptual and technical issues that continue to be discussed and developed. We hope this will be helpful and informative to new MEG users.

Happy MEG recordings!

Peter Hansen
Morten Kringelbach
Riitta Salmelin

Helsinki and Oxford

Contributors

Tipu Z. Aziz, Department of Physiology, Anatomy and Genetics, University of Oxford, Oxford, UK

Sylvain Baillet, COGIMAGE laboratory, Centre de Recherche sur le Cerveau et la Moelle, CNRS, INSERM, University Pierre & Marie Curie, Paris and Department of Neurology, Medical College of Wisconsin/Froedtert Hospital, Milwaukee, USA

Nina Forss, Brain Research Unit, Low Temperature Laboratory, Aalto University, Helsinki, Finland

Line Garnero, Inserm, Paris, France

Alex L. Green, Department of Physiology, Anatomy and Genetics, University of Oxford, Oxford, UK

Joachim Gross, Centre for Cognitive Neuroimaging, Department of Psychology, University of Glasgow, Scotland

Matti S. Hämäläinen, Athinoula A. Martinos Center for Biomedical Imaging, Massachusetts General Hospital, Charlestown, MA, USA

Peter C. Hansen, Department of Physiology, Anatomy and Genetics, University of Oxford, Oxford, UK

Christian Hesse, Donders Institute for Brain, Cognition and Behavior, Radboud University Nijmegen

Ole Jensen, Donders Institute for Brain, Cognition and Behavior, Radboud University Nijmegen

Ryusuke Kakigi, National Institute for Physiological Sciences, Okazaki, Japan

Morten L. Kringelbach, Dept. of Psychiatry, University of Oxford, UK and Aarhus University, Denmark.

Jan Kujala, Brain Research Unit, Low Temperature Laboratory, Aalto University, Helsinki, Finland

Pierre-Jean Lahaye, Inserm, Paris, France

Richard M. Leahy, Signal and Image Processing Institute, University of Southern California, CA, USA

Fa-Hsuan Lin, Athinoula A. Martinos Center for Biomedical Imaging, Massachusetts General Hospital, Charlestown, MA, USA

Fernando H. Lopes da Silva, Centre of Neurosciences, Swammerdam Institute for Life Sciences, University of Amsterdam, The Netherlands

Jyrki P. Mäkelä, BioMag laboratory, HUSLAB, Helsinki University Central Hospital

John C. Mosher, Los Alamos National Laboratory, NM, USA

Dimitrios Pantazis, Signal and Image Processing Institute, University of Southern California, CA, USA

Lauri Parkkonen, Brain Research Unit, Low Temperature Laboratory, Aalto University, Helsinki, Finland

Jean-Baptiste Poline, Inserm, Paris, France

Riitta Salmelin, Brain Research Unit, Low Temperature Laboratory, Aalto University, Helsinki, Finland

Alfons Schnitzler, Department of Neurology, Heinrich Heine University, Dusseldorf, Germany

1

Electrophysiological Basis of MEG Signals

Fernando H. Lopes da Silva

- MEG signals recorded at the scalp are generated by synchronous activity of tens of thousands of neurons
- Mainly postsynaptic currents in apical dendrites contribute to MEG signals
- MEG signals are highly sensitive to currents tangential to the skull, originating in the cortical sulci
- MEG fields reflect the primary neuronal currents directly, with minimum distortion from different layers – brain tissue, skull, scalp – with different electric conductivities
- Estimation of MEG sources implies the construction of computational models of the biophysical sources and of the volume conductor

Magnetoencephalography (MEG) is the technique of measuring the magnetic fields generated by brain activity, and was pioneered by Cohen (1968). An important feature of MEG/EEG is the ability to record varying signals generated by the brain in relation to states of activity, whether determined by intrinsic processes—e.g., different states of sleep and alertness—or in relation to motor acts and sensory events (Hari, 2005). In this overview, we will focus on the basic physiological and biophysical aspects of how magnetic signals are generated in the brain. We start, however, with a brief description of the main features of MEG as a method to study brain functions in man.

Main Features of MEG

MEG provides information about the dynamics of the activities of populations of neurons of the cerebral cortex. The time resolution capabilities of MEG and EEG are unrivalled. Nevertheless, MEG, like EEG, has a basic limitation in that the neuronal signals are only recorded from the scalp. Consequently, there is no unique solution to the problem of reconstructing where exactly the sources of these signals are localized within the brain. This problem is commonly referred to as *the inverse problem*. The standard approach to overcome the non-uniqueness of the inverse problem in MEG/EEG is to introduce constraints on the possible solutions, in order to exclude all solutions except the one that is most suitable to describe the data. Thus, the functional localization of brain sources of MEG/EEG signals depends to some degree on the models used and on the corresponding assumptions, and therefore will have some degree of uncertainty.

This contrasts with the spatial accuracy of MRI brain images, where the MRI technology affords a truer 3-dimensional reconstruction. It explains partly why the development of clinical applications of MEG has been slow, since the research on how to optimize estimates of the solutions of the inverse problem has been arduous, and has only recently reached a stage where consensual strategies are emerging. These inherent difficulties, along with the fact that MEG needs rather costly facilities, account for the restraint of medical specialists in promoting this new methodology, and the hesitation of hospital administrators in supporting the necessary investments in material and human resources. Nonetheless, MEG has proven a most valuable tool in research, not only of neurocognitive processes (Salmelin et al., 1994) but also in clinical settings (Van 't Ent et al., 2003), as presented further in this volume.

Some Basic Notions of Cellular Neurophysiology

Neurons generate time-varying electrical currents when activated. These are ionic currents generated at the level of cellular membranes; i.e, they consist of transmembrane currents. We can distinguish two main forms of neuronal activation (Lopes da Silva & van Rotterdam, 2005): the fast depolarization of the neuronal membranes that results in the action potential mediated by sodium and potassium voltage-dependent ionic conductances g_{Na} and $g_{K(DR)}$, and the more protracted change of membrane potential due to synaptic activation mediated by several neurotransmitter systems. The action potential consists of a rapid change of membrane potential, such that the intracellular potential jumps suddenly from negative to positive, and quickly, in 1 or 2 milliseconds, returns to the resting intracellular negativity. In this way, a nerve impulse is generated that has the remarkable property of propagating along axons and dendrites without loss of amplitude. The contribution of other ionic conductances to the magnetic field is discussed below, in relation to new insights obtained using computer models.

Regarding the slower postsynaptic potentials, two main kinds have to be distinguished: the excitatory (EPSPs) and the inhibitory (IPSPs) potentials, which depend on the type of neurotransmitter and corresponding receptor, and their interaction with specific ionic channels and/or intracellular second messengers.

Generally speaking, at the level of a synapse in the case of the EPSP, the transmembrane current is carried by positive ions inwards. In the case of the IPSP, it is carried by negative ions inwards or positive ions outwards. Thus the positive electric current is directed to the extracellular medium in the case of an EPSP, and it is directed from the inside of the neuron to the outside in the case of an IPSP (Figure 1–1).

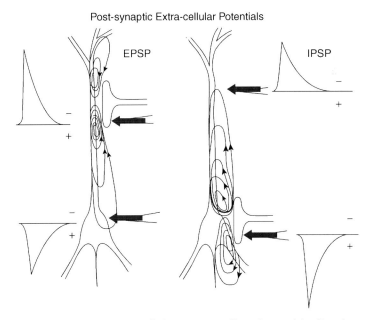

Figure 1–1. Intra- and extracellular current flow in an idealized pyramidal neuron due to different types of synaptic activation. EPSP: excitatory synapse at the level of the apical dendrite; the generated current of positive ions flows inwards, causing depolarization of the cell. This results in an active sink at the level of synapse. The extracellularly measured EPSP has a negative polarity at the level of the synapse. At the soma there is a passive source, and the potential has a reversed polarity. IPSP: inhibitory synapse at the level of the soma. A current of negative ions flows inwards causing hyperpolarization of the cell; this results in an active source at the level of the synapse. The extracellularly measured IPSP has a positive polarity at the level of the soma. At the level of the distal apical dendrite there is a passive sink, and the potential has a reversed polarity. (Adapted from Niedermeyer & Lopes da Silva, 2005).

As a consequence of these currents in the extracellular medium, an active sink is generated at the level of an excitatory synapse, whereas an active source occurs in the case of an inhibitory synapse. The flow of these compensating extracellular currents depends on the electrical properties of the local tissue. Glial cells occupy an important part of the space between neurons, and are coupled to one another by gap junctions. The conductivity of the latter is very sensitive to changes in pH on extracellular K^+ and Ca^{2+} and can therefore be modulated under various physiological and pathological conditions (Huang et al., 2005). Furthermore, the volume of the extracellular space may change under various physiological and pathological conditions, which will also be reflected in changes of tissue conductivity.

From the biophysics we may state that there is no accumulation of charge anywhere in the medium, in that currents flowing in or out of the neuronal membranes at the active synaptic sites are compensated by currents flowing in the opposite direction elsewhere along the neuronal membrane. This is described in more precise terms in the next section. Consequently, in the case of an EPSP, in addition to the active sink at the level of the synapse, distributed passive sources occur along the soma-dendritic membrane. The opposite occurs in the case of an IPSP: in addition to the active source at the level of the synapse, distributed passive sinks are formed along the soma-dendritic membrane.

Therefore we may state that synaptic activity at a given site of the soma-dendritic membrane of a neuron causes a sink–source configuration in the extracellular medium around the neurons. In the context of the present discussion, the most important point to take into consideration is the *geometry* of the neuronal sources of electrical activity that gave rise to the scalp EEG or MEG signal. The neurons that give the main contribution to the MEG or the EEG are those that form "open fields" according to the classic description of Lorente de Nó (1947); i.e., the pyramidal neurons of the cortex, since the latter are arranged in palisades with the apical dendrites aligned perpendicularly to the cortical surface (Figure 1–2). This means that longitudinal intracellular currents flow along dendrites or axons, and thus generate magnetic fields around them—just as happens in a wire, according to the well known right-hand rule of electromagnetism (see also FAQ, Q1).

Pyramidal neurons of the cortex, with their long apical dendrites, generate coherent magnetic fields when activated with a certain degree of synchrony. We may say that these neurons behave as "current dipoles," the activity of which can be detected by sensors placed at a small distance from the skull. Later in this chapter we will consider this issue further in quantitative terms, based on recent computational model studies.

In order to make the next step toward an understanding of how MEG signals recorded outside the skull are generated, we also have to take into consideration the folding of the cortex. The fact that the cortex is folded, forming gyri and sulci, implies that some populations of neurons have apical

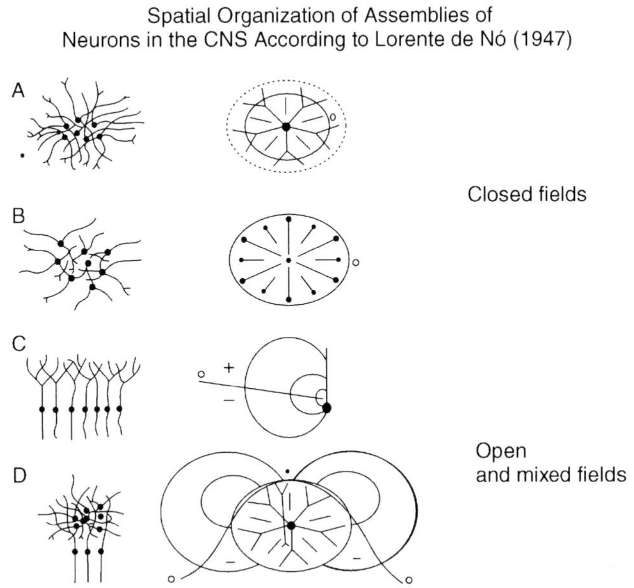

Spatial Organization of Assemblies of
Neurons in the CNS According to Lorente de Nó (1947)

Figure 1–2. Examples of closed (A, B), open (C) and open–closed (D) fields according to Lorente de Nó. The isopotential lines resulting from the activation of the neuronal population are shown on the right side. (Adapted from Niedermeyer & Lopes da Silva, 2005).

dendrites that are perpendicular to the overlying skull, i.e., those that are at the top of a gyrus; whereas others are parallel to the skull, i.e., those that are on the wall of a sulcus. The point to note in this respect is that the orientation of the neurons with respect to the skull influences the resulting MEG signal recorded outside the skull. In fact the MEG "sees" only those magnetic fields that have a component perpendicular to the skull. These magnetic fields are generated by neuronal currents that have a component oriented tangentially to the skull. In contrast, those currents that are oriented radially to the skull do not generate a magnetic field outside the head (Figure 1–3).

A Few Basic Notions of Biophysics

EEG and MEG signals vary in time, but this variation is relatively slow; hence, induction effects can be neglected. This means that Maxwell equations need not be applied, and the behavior of the electric and magnetic fields can be described by the classic Ohm's, Ampère's and Coulomb's laws. For a rigorous treatment of the biophysics of the generation of electric and magnetic fields in the brain[1] one has just to assume that the neural generator, for example a synaptic ionic current, is represented by the impressed current density $\bar{J}_i$ such

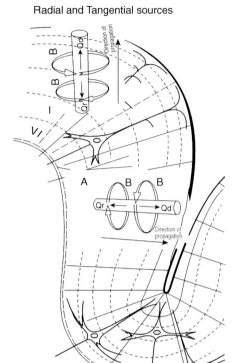

Radial and Tangential sources

Figure 1–3. Schematic drawing of a piece of cortex showing the crown of a gyrus and a sulcus. Two cylinders are drawn to indicate the relation between the direction of the intracellular current and the resulting magnetic fields around the apical dendrite. Sources at the top of a gyrus cause radial fields that are not detectable by MEG. Sources in the fissures cause tangential fields that can be detected at the MEG.

that the total current density field $\overline{J}_t$ consists of $\vec{J}_i$ and a passive part (secondary current) that obeys Ohm's law:

$$\overline{J}_t = \vec{J}_i + \sigma \vec{E} \qquad (1\text{–}1)$$

where σ is the medium conductivity and $\vec{E}$ is the electric field.

Considering that the div $\overline{J}_t$ must be zero, since there is no accumulation of charge anywhere in the medium, we may note that

$$\text{div } \vec{J}_i = -\sigma \text{ div } \vec{E} \qquad (1\text{–}2)$$

assuming that the medium conductivity σ is everywhere constant for simplicity. The relation between $\bar{E}$ and the electric potential V, that is a scalar variable, is given by:

$$\bar{E} = -\operatorname{grad} V \tag{1-3}$$

Accordingly, we may write that the electric potential at a given point $\bar{r}_0$ that results from an impressed current $\bar{J}_i$ at a point $\bar{r}$ is given by the following integral expression:

$$V\left(\bar{r}_0\right) = \left(-1/4\pi\sigma\right)\int div\,\bar{J}_i\left(1/R\right)d^3r \tag{1-4}$$

where R represents the distance between the measuring point $\bar{r}_0$ and the source location $\bar{r}$.

With respect to the magnetic field $\bar{H}\left(\bar{r}\right)$ we should note that it is related to the magnetic flux density field, or induction field, $\bar{B}\left(\bar{r}\right)$ by the following expression:

$$\bar{B}\left(\bar{r}\right) = \mu\bar{H}\left(\bar{r}\right) \tag{1-5}$$

where μ is the magnetic permeability.

According to the equations for electromagnetism we should note that the angular momentum or the curl of a vector field is the amount of "rotation" of the vector, which is denoted by the symbol ∇ (read *del*), such that we may write the following relation between the magnetic field $\bar{H}$ and the current $\bar{J}_t$:

$$\nabla \times \bar{H} = \bar{J}_t \tag{1-6}$$

and since magnetic monopoles don't exist we may write:

$$div\,\bar{B} = 0 \tag{1-7}$$

and

$$\nabla \times \bar{B} = \mu(\bar{J}_i + \sigma\bar{E}) \tag{1-8}$$

where μ is the magnetic permeability.

Here we should note that the passive current field $\sigma\bar{E}$ is conservative; i.e., it can be derived from the scalar potential V as follows:

$$\nabla \times \bar{E}\left(\bar{r}\right) = 0 \tag{1-9}$$

Mathematically, expression (1–7) is equivalent to the statement that $\bar{B}$ can be derived from the vector potential $\bar{A}$ as follows:

$$\bar{B} - \nabla \times \bar{A} \tag{1-10}$$

Combining expressions (1–8), (1–9) and (1–10), we finally arrive at the expression relating the magnetic vector potential $\overline{A}$ to the impressed current $\overline{J}_i$:

$$\overline{A} = \frac{\mu}{4\pi} \int \frac{\overline{J_i}(\overline{r})}{R} \mathrm{d}^3 \mathbf{l} \tag{1–11}$$

assuming an infinite medium with μ and σ constant, as has been proven theoretically by Plonsey (1969; 1982).

In this way we may conclude that this biophysical analysis allows to draw the conclusion that while the electrical potential V depends (expression 1–4) on the divergence of the impressed current (div $\overline{J_i}$), the magnetic vector depends on the impressed current itself $\overline{J_i}$ (expression 1–11).

We should note that 'div $\overline{J_i}$' denotes the current source density (CSD) because the divergence of the impressed current density at a certain site on the membrane of a cell, is the net current that flows per-unit-volume out of the medium into the cell.

It must be emphasized that the expressions introduced here are based on the assumption that the medium is homogenous and infinite. Of course this does not apply to the brain. Indeed, at the microscopic level of one neuron, the influence of inhomogeneous media with different conductivities cannot be neglected, for both electric and magnetic fields. Nevertheless, at the macroscopic level, at which commonly EEG and MEG recordings are made, the brain may be considered a homogeneous medium, in a first approximation, surrounded by layers with different conductivities. In later section we briefly consider this issue of the influence of inhomogeneities.

Figure 1–4 shows schematically the magnetic and electric fields caused by a current dipole in a head approximated as a spherical conductor. Both fields

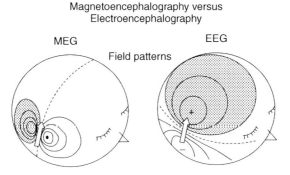

Figure 1–4. Field pattern of MEG, on the left, and EEG, on the right, caused by a current dipole model source in a concentric 4-layer spherical model of a head. The shaded areas indicate the magnetic flux out of the head (MEG) and the positive potential (EEG).
(Adapted from Hari, in Niedermeyer & Lopes da Silva, 2005).

are dipolar but are rotated by 90° with respect to each other. The isocontour lines are tighter in the case of the MEG compared with the EEG. This is mainly due to the influence of the inhomogeneities that smear out the electric potential much more than the magnetic field.

The Contribution of Neuronal Models: In Vitro and Computational Models

Early studies using *in vitro* preparations allowed the simultaneous measurement of both the electric and magnetic fields generated by neuronal activity. A calculation of the magnetic field around an axon was performed by Swinney and Wikswo (1980) using a preparation whereby an isolated axon was kept in a bath with saline, *in vitro*, and was stimulated electrically. They found that the magnetic field resulted from the intracellular current flowing inside the axon in the axial direction, whereas the contribution of the transmembrane current was negligible, and that of the return passive-current flows in the medium was very small. Relative to the intracellular current, the former was estimated to be only 10^{-11} and the latter 10^{-2}. Plonsey (1982) similarly calculated a value of 10^{-7} for the ratio between the secondary current sources and the primary current.

Some computational modeling studies have analyzed the relationship between the activity of neuronal sources and the resulting magnetic fields. An original approach was followed by van Rotterdam (1987), who developed an algorithm to calculate electric and magnetic fields generated by populations of neurons with various geometrical arrangements. This was implemented by sampling the tissue volume using a 3-dimensional lattice, where the sampling distance corresponds to the uncertainty in the measurements. The electric and magnetic fields are calculated for each node as the output of a linear feedback system, using the impressed currents originating at some level along the soma-dendritic membranes as the input. By way of a feedback loop, the reflection phenomena at the boundaries between media of different conductivity are taken into account. However, with this model only very simplified neuronal sources were analyzed; for example, a population of pyramidal cells arranged regularly so that they can be simulated by a half-circular layer of impressed current vectors.

More realistic models have been proposed by Yoshio Okada and colleagues. These authors adapted the detailed compartmental models of Traub and collaborators (1994; 1991) and applied them to a section of a hippocampal slice kept in an *in vitro* bath, while measuring simultaneously the intracellular electric potentials of CA3 pyramidal cells, the extracellular field potentials, and the magnetic fields, using four detection coils connected to superconducting quantum interference devices (SQUIDs). The coils were placed 2 mm above the slice, and were arranged as shown in Figure 1–5. The slice was electrically stimulated with different configurations of stimulating electrodes, in

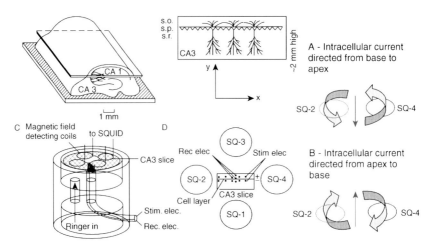

Figure 1–5. Longitudinal hippocampal slice preparation and experimental arrangement (C, D) for electrical stimulation and recording field potentials and magnetic fields. Above: two anatomical fields of the *Cornus Ammonis* (CA1 and CA3) are shown, along with a slice of CA3 where pyramidal cells are schematically indicated with 3 layers: s.o., *stratum oriens*; s.p., *stratum pyramidale*; s.r., *stratum radiale*. C: measurement set-up: The slice is placed in a bath, and stimulating and recording electrodes are placed from below; magnetic fields are recorded using 4 coils connected to SQUIDs (SQs) placed 2 mm above the slice, as shown in more detail in D. A and B: The orientation of the magnetic fields caused by an intracellular current flowing from the soma/basal dendrites to the apex (A) and in the opposite direction (B) are schematically illustrated.
(Adapted from Murakami et al. 2002).

order to elicit different kinds of evoked activities. Measured electric and magnetic activities, *in vitro*, were compared with the theoretical results of the computer model (Figure 1–6). In essence the model consisted of 100 excitatory pyramidal and 20 inhibitory neurons. Each cell was simulated as a set of 19 compartments (8 compartments for the basal dendrites, 1 for the soma, and 10 for the apical dendrites). In addition, different types of synaptic inputs were simulated (glutamatergic and GABAergic) and 6 types of active ion-gated conductances. According to Murakami et al. (2006), the intracellular current of a given compartment k is the vector quantity $\overline{Q}_k(t) = IL\overline{dr}$, where I is the current along the longitudinal axis of the neuron, L is the length of a compartment and $\overline{dr}$ is the unit direction vector for the compartment. In the model, the component of the magnetic field normal to the slice surface was computed at the center of the detection coils. The spatial distribution of the evoked magnetic field generated by the pyramidal neurons above the slice was dipolar, and it appeared to be dominated by the longitudinal current in each neuron: this corresponds to the impressed current $\overline{J}_i$ of equation 1–11.

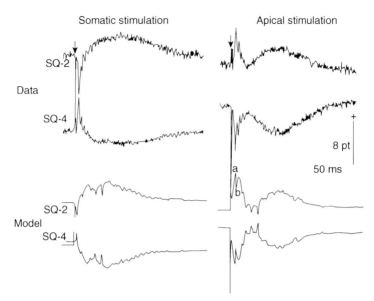
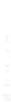

Figure 1–6. Magnetic fields recorded from the CA3 hippocampal slice as indicated in Figure 1–5, and results obtained with a computer model of a population of pyramidal cells. The magnetic fields recorded from SQ2 and SQ4 are shown for two conditions: on the left, after stimulation at the level of the soma; on the right, after stimulation at the level of the apical dendrites. Positivity (deflection upwards) indicates magnetic field directed out of the bath. Note the general similarity of the waveforms of the experimental and the theoretical results. Note also the difference in polarity between early and late components.
(Adapted from Murakami et al. 2002).

The simulations showed, among other effects, that the magnetic field corresponding to the evoked initial spike was directed into the slice at SQ-2 and out of the slice at SQ-4 (Figure 1–5), which indicates that the intracellular current is directed from the basal to the apical dendrites of the pyramidal neurons. The slow wave that follows the spike shows the opposite polarity, indicating that it is generated by an intracellular current in the reversed direction (Figure 1–6). This model allows one to analyze different patterns of dendritic branching, and how the distribution of the density of ion channels along the soma-dendritic membrane may be reflected in the magnetic fields. Interestingly, this experimental and modeling study showed that sodium spikes can be detected magnetically and electrically in this preparation. Murakami et al. (2002) suggest even that sodium spikes would be also detectable in EEG and MEG recorded from the scalp, "if the geometry of the distribution of neurons is favorable". However, this condition is most likely not sufficient, because a high degree of synchrony is also necessary for spikes of this kind to be recordable at the scalp.

Subsequently, Murakami et al. (2003) investigated, along the same lines, the relative contribution of different ionic conductances to the MEG and EEG signals. Surprisingly, they showed that the relatively slow conductances g_{Ca} and $g_{K(Ca)}$ generate intracellular currents that are one order of magnitude larger than the currents associated with g_{Na} and $g_{K(DR)}$. Furthermore, the contribution of the former currents was also stronger than that of synaptic currents; but this may depend on the fact that in this model, synaptic activity was only generated in one compartment along the soma-dendritic membrane, which is not a very realistic scenario.

More recently, Murakami et al. (2006) applied the same kind of approach to a more complex brain structure, the neocortex. This study is particularly relevant because it may yield some results that may help to interpret EEG and MEG recordings from the scalp. These authors constructed a computer model, based on that proposed by Mainen and Sejnowski (1996), of the four main types of cortical neurons taking into account their realistic shapes. Each neuron is described as a three-dimensional compartmental model, where each compartment has its typical geometric dimensions, passive electrical properties (membrane capacitance and resistance, intracellular resistance), and five voltage-dependent ionic conductances. The quantitative values of these variables were taken from the literature. For example, the maximal sodium conductance g_{Na} was assumed to be 40 pS μm^{-2} based on the measurements of Stuart and Sakman (1994), but several values were used in a trial-and-error way to reproduce experimental results. Neuronal activity was obtained by stimulating each neuron with an intracellular current injected at the soma. As in the hippocampal model, the intracellular current is the vector quantity $\overline{Q}_k(t) = IL\overline{dr}$.

The magnitude of this quantity is the current dipole moment, and is represented by Q. The population Q for a group of pyramidal neurons was calculated by computing the sum of the dot product[2] of each current dipole, and the unit vector orthogonal to the cortical surface. The same was done for the stellate cells, with a modification due to the fact that these neurons are differently oriented. Taking the cortical population as a whole, the primary current (that corresponds to $\overline{J}_i$ in the notation used previously) is equivalent to the population Q, and the secondary currents (corresponding to the passive current given by $\sigma \vec{E}$ in equation 1–1) can be computed from Q given the properties of the volume conductor. In this model, the magnetic flux density field $\overline{B}$ is assumed to be generated by the tangential component of Q, with respect to the inner skull surface, and the electric field is due to both the tangential and radial components. This implies that $\overline{B}$ is mainly caused by neuronal activity in sulci, since Q is directed perpendicularly to the pial surface, whereas both radial and tangential components contribute to the electric field. This investigation led to another result of practical interest, namely it gave some direct indications about how to interpret the magnitude of the magnetic fields recorded in man. According to the model, the overall magnitude of Q for the activity of pyramidal neurons of layers V and II/III is on the order of 0.29 – 0.90 pAm. Apparently this value deviates appreciably from that estimated previously for a cell by Hämäläinen et al. (1993), which was just 0.02pAm. That larger value, however, is of the same order of magnitude as values estimated for hippocampal pyramidal neurons (0.2 pAm per cell in CA1 and 0.17 pAm per cell in CA3; see Kyuhou and Okada, 1993 and Okada et al., 1997). Murakami et al. (2006) point out that assuming a Q of 0.2 pAm per cortical pyramidal neuron, a population of 50,000 synchronously active cells would generate a field with a magnitude of 10nAm, which corresponds precisely to the value measurable from the human cortex according to Hämäläinen et al. (1993). Assuming that a cortical minicolumn with a diameter of 40μm contains 100 cells (Mountcastle, 1997), the cortical surface that would correspond to 50.000 cells should form a patch of about 0.63 mm^2 in area. If this cortical patch had a circular form, its diameter would be about 0.9 mm (for more details see FAQ, Q5).

In order to translate a cortical surface to a number of cortical cells, in which the synchronous activity is responsible for the signal measured, one must have a good estimate of the density of pyramidal cells in the cortex. These kinds of estimates, however, are rather imprecise, and those based on the quantitative computational models described above are to be preferred.

We have already discussed the possibility of spikes contributing to the magnetic field measured at a distance. This computer model offers more insight into this issue. According to the calculations performed in the model, a sodium spike corresponds to a Q with the magnitude of 1pAm. Therefore, to reach the measurable value of 10nAm, it would be sufficient that 10,000 neurons generate such spikes synchronously. Although this is not impossible, as these authors note, it is unlikely to occur outside situations of forced synchronization, since there is considerable jitter in the ongoing cortical neuronal activity (de Munck et al., 1992). This model study revealed, in addition, two particularly interesting and unexpected results: first, the activity of basal dendrites may contribute significantly to the MEG and EEG signals; second, the magnitude of Q was unexpectedly large for a spiny cell, since it was estimated to be 0.27pAm, whereas it was only 0.06 for an aspiny cell. Nevertheless, we cannot conclude that spiny cells will make an important contribution to MEG signals, since the dendrites of these neurons are not oriented parallel to each other (as are those of pyramidal neurons) but have quite variable orientations.

The Transfer of Magnetic Signals from the Brain to the Skull

We have assumed until now that the electric and magnetic fields are generated in a homogeneous, isotropic and infinite medium. However, this is not what happens in the brain. At the macroscopic level we have to distinguish different layers with different electric properties in the medium: white and gray matter, meninges and cerebrospinal fluid, skull, and scalp. Also, at the microscopic level the organization of the tissue is far from homogeneous. The extracellular space appears to be constituted by a complex mesh that has been called by Nicholson (1980) the "extracellular jungle." Furthermore, extracellular shifts of ionic concentrations, the role of glial cells and gap junctions, all must be taken into account. Nonetheless, to model the electric and magnetic phenomena as measured from the scalp, a macroscopic description is, in general, adequate. It is not within the scope of this chapter to deal with the mathematics of how electric and magnetic fields are influenced by the boundaries between media with different conductivities. We will consider only whether, and if so, how, the magnetic phenomena are affected by the existence of layers with different conductivities.

It is sometimes argued that these layers affect the EEG but not the MEG signal; in other words, that these inhomogeneous media would be transparent to MEG signals. This is, however, not entirely accurate. In general, the magnetic induction field $\overline{B}$ only depends on the rotation of the current field, as shown above, and that the passive current field $\sigma\overline{E}$, being conservative, has no influence on the vector magnetic potential $\overline{A}$. In a volume conductor with varying conductivity, however, the passive current field can also have rotational components at the boundaries of media with different conductivities. A rigorous mathematical treatment of this matter is given by van Rotterdam (1987).

Frequently Asked Questions

Q 1. What does it mean, at the cellular level, that in MEG the current usually flows away from the cortical surface?

In the cortex, the main neuronal population that contributes to the magnetic field is formed by the pyramidal cells. Let us compare this situation with the example shown in Figure 1–5 for a hippocampal slice. Here we see that the magnetic field of the initial spike peak was directed *into* the slice at SQ-2 and *out of* the slice at SQ-4. The flow of the intracellular current, which resulted from stimulation at the level of the soma, was from the hippocampal slice surface (s.o.), i.e., the basal side of the pyramidal neurons, to the deep layers (s.r.), i.e., their apical side. This follows from the "right-hand rule" for the induced magnetic field. The latter states that magnetic field lines around a long wire that carries an electric current form concentric circles around the wire; the direction of the magnetic field is perpendicular to the wire and is in the direction the fingers of the right hand would curl if one wrapped them around the wire with the thumb in the direction of the current. In this example, the slow wave that follows the spike shows the opposite polarity, indicating that it is generated by an intracellular current in the reversed direction, from the apical to the basal side. In the case of the neocortex, the situation differs from that of the hippocampus in its geometry, since the cortical pyramidal cells, contrary to those of the hippocampus, have apical dendrites oriented toward the cortical surface, and the soma and basal dendrites are in deeper layers. A positive current would flow from the pial surface to deep layers, as the consequence of an excitatory synaptic stimulation at the level of the apical dendrites. This is not, however, the only possible interpretation, as will be discussed further in the next question.

Q 2. On the basis of the direction of fields in MEG, or the polarity of scalp potentials in EEG, can one say something about whether we record excitatory or inhibitory PSPs?

In general, this question cannot be answered in a simple way. Different configurations of EPSPs and IPSPs can give rise to magnetic fields with the same direction, or to electric potentials with the same polarity at the cortical surface. The reason is that an EPSP arising in the apical dendrites, or an IPSP arising in the soma or basal dendrites, may result in an intracellular current with the same orientation. In the former case there is an intracellular current carried by positive ions from the apex to the base of a pyramidal cell; in the latter, there is an intracellular current carried by negative ions from the base to the apex, which is equivalent to a positive current in the opposite direction. In both cases one would have a sink at the apex and a source at the base. Thus, in order to be able to give an unambiguous reply to this question one would need to have additional information about the *site* along the pyramidal cell where the current is initiated.

Q 3. Can we state as a rule that the direction of current flow is from the cortical surface to the depth of the cortex?

In general, we cannot. As described in the answer to Q 2. above, one can have situations where the direction of the intracellular currents reverses. For example, in the case of the experimental studies in hippocampal slices (Murakami et al., 2002) we may observe, in a response to electrical stimulation of pyramidal cells, an initial component of the magnetic field due to a current directed from the basal to the apical sites, followed by a second component due to reversed currents (Figure 1–6). It is likely that the same process may occur in the neocortex. For example, the MEG evoked responses, elicited by stimulation of the tibial nerve in man, show, as a function of time, a rotation of the magnetic field patterns (Hari et al., 1996). This rotation may depend on changes of the cortical areas being activated, but also on changes in the direction of intracellular currents of the pyramidal cells in one particular cortical area that is engaged in these responses. It should be noted, however, that the major part of the electric currents that cause a field that is measurable at a distance flows perpendicular to the cortical surface.

Q 4. How many neurons, synchronously active, are necessary to generate a recordable signal in the human MEG?

A precise answer to this quantitative question cannot be given. Nonetheless, recent model studies suggest the likely order of magnitude. Murakami and

Okada (2006) computed that the current dipole of cortical pyramidal cell is in the order of 0.2 pAm/cell. Considering that, according to Hämäläinen et al. (1993), the weakest measurable cortical signals are on the order of 10nAm, we may assume that such magnetic fields can be produced by about 50,000 cells synchronously active.

Q 5. How large is the cortical area within which neurons must be synchronously active to produce a measurable MEG signal at the scalp?

To answer this, we must take into consideration the estimates of the quantitative distribution of neurons in the cortex. First, it is important to understand some classic concepts about cortical organization. The cortex is organized according to the columnar principle as proposed by Mountcastle in the 1970s (see review, Mountcastle, 1997), which means that the basic unit of the mature neocortex is the *minicolumn*: "a narrow chain of neurons extending vertically across the cellular layers II/VI, perpendicular to the pial surface," having a cross-section with a diameter of about 50µm. A minicolumn in primates contains about 80 to 100 neurons, although this number may vary between areas; in the striate cortex the cell density appears to be 2.5 times larger. Many minicolumns are bound together by short-range horizontal connections, sharing "static and physiological dynamic properties" and thus forming what has been denominated *cortical columns* or *cortical modules* (Mountcastle, 1997). These columns, in the somatic sensory cortex, contain about 80 minicolumns and are roughly hexagonal with a width of about 300–400µm (Favorov & Diamond, 1990). Of course, these numbers are just estimates. Nonetheless, based on these estimates we can attempt to give a rough answer to the question formulated here. Assuming that a column with a diameter of 40µm contains 100 cells, the cortical surface that would correspond to 50,000 cells should form a patch with about 0.63 mm^2 in area. If this cortical patch had a circular form, then its diameter would be about 0.9 mm. It should be noted that this columnar cortical organization is encountered throughout the sensory and motor cortex, albeit with some peculiarities depending on cortical area and sensory/motor modality as reviewed by Buxhoeveden and Casanova (2002). Interestingly, these authors note that from a functional perspective, cortical columns may exist in different dynamic states. They coined the term "physiological macrocolumn" to indicate a set of cortical columns that cooperate in a given functional state or process. These physiological macrocolumns must be considered as dynamic ensembles consisting of a number of columns that may vary as a function of time. In the context of the present question, it is important to note that neurons in separate columns can present oscillatory synchronous activities, mediated by tangential and recurrent connections between different columns (Freiwald et al., 1995; Gray et al., 1989).

Q 6. Can action potentials make a significant contribution to MEG signals?

The most common answer to this question is that the contribution of action potentials is minimal compared to that of synaptically meditated activity and other slow waves. There are two reasons for this. First, the influence of action potentials on recordings at a distance attenuates much more strongly than postsynaptic potentials. Second, the probability that action potentials of different cells synchronize precisely is rather low, since action potentials are very short and there is always a considerable jitter between the discharges of different cells. Nevertheless, Murakami and Okada (2006) in their computer study showed that sodium spikes may have dipolar moments considerably stronger than previously thought. Assuming that the dipolar moment of a spike of a cell is about 1pAm, 10,000 perfectly synchronized neurons could produce a field on the order of 10nAm, which corresponds to the strength of a measurable cortical generator. This would, however, imply that these action potentials should be perfectly synchronized—which may be the case during epileptiform spike discharges, but is not likely to occur under normal conditions. Nevertheless, synchronized population action potentials may contribute to very-high-frequency MEG signals on the order of 600 Hz (Curio et al., 1994 and Hashimoto et al., 1996). Ikeda et al. (2002) detected such MEG signals outside the pig brain, elicited by peripheral electrical stimulation; these authors showed that the high-frequency oscillations consisted of a presynaptic component generated by the specific thalamocortical axonal terminals in layer IV, and another postsynaptic component due to activation of cortical neurons.

Q 7. Is it possible to record, outside the head, MEG signals generated by deep subcortical sources?

In considering this question as applied to human MEG recording, we should note that not all types of magnetic sensors have the same sensitivity to distant sources. In descending order of sensitivity to the depth of sources, magnetometers are most sensitive, followed by first-order axial gradiometers, second-order gradiometers and, finally, planar gradiometers (Figure 1–7). Planar gradiometers have maximum sensitivity to sources directly under them, i.e., superficial cortical sources (Hämäläinen, 1995), which makes them less sensitive to artifacts and distant disturbances.

Experimental evidence supporting a direct answer to this question has been provided by Hashimoto et al. (1996), who recorded, in pigs, somatosensory evoked magnetic fields (SEFs) that were generated by neuronal populations at the level of the thalamus. It should be noted that the latter were elicited by electrical stimulation of peripheral structures, causing a high degree of synchronous neuronal activity. This indicates that deep-lying structures in the brain can generate sufficiently strong MEG signals to be detectable at a distance from the brain surface, at least in the pig head.

In addition, studies using MEG arrays with partial head coverage in humans have suggested the presence of generators of the P3 component of auditory evoked responses in deep-lying source areas, including the hippocampus (Okada et al., 1983), and thalamus (Rogers et al., 1991). However, in these studies the evidence is indirect, since the localization of the sources

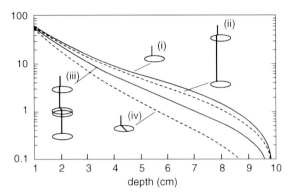

Figure 1–7. Strength (vertical axis) of a magnetic field (arbitrary units) as function of the depth (horizontal axis) for different types of magnetic sensors: (i) magnetometer; (ii) first-order axial gradiometer; (iii) second-order axial gradiometer; (iv) planar figure-of-eight gradiometer. (Adapted from Hari, in Niedermeyer & Lopes da Silva, 2005).

was estimated using approximate source models, in order to obtain estimates of solutions to the non-unique electromagnetic inverse problem. It should be added that Ioannides et al. (1995) identified generators for the same kind of evoked responses in amygdala and hippocampus, which were made plausible when the results obtained in normal subjects using magnetic field tomography were compared with those obtained from a patient who had undergone lobectomy, which removed these structures. Furthermore, Tesche and Karhu (2000) estimated hippocampal oscillatory activities based on surface MEG, using an elaborate signal analysis algorithm. Finally, it should be noted that if adequate prior knowledge exists of the location of the electrical sources, then spatial filtering techniques like beam formers or signal space projection can enable us to reconstruct temporal changes of electrical activities at these deep-lying source locations.

Q 8. Is it possible to record DC MEG or EEG? And if so, what would be the physiological meaning?

There are a number of physical limitations (electrode impedances, electrode polarization, skin/electrolyte junction) that do not allow recording of EEG signals down to 0 Hz, which would correspond to real DC, or "direct current." With MEG, environmental low-frequency noise also imposes limitations, with similar consequences. The aim, however, is not to record down to a real DC level of 0 Hz but to extend the effective frequency band to very low frequencies in the order of 0.1 Hz. (For a discussion of misconceptions of what "DC" means in electroencephalography see Niedermeyer's footnote in Speckmann and Elger, 2005). The recording of ultraslow MEG/EEG signals can be achieved using appropriate techniques, for example as discussed for

EEG by Vanhatalo et al. (2005) and for MEG by Burghoff et al. (2004). Phenomena such as the Contingent Negative Variation (CNV) first described by Walter et al. (1964), and the Bereitschaftspotential (readiness potential) first described by Kornhuber and Deecke (1965), are typical examples of very slow shifts of electric potential or of magnetic fields that can be recorded using appropriate recording and analysis techniques. During slow-wave sleep, EEG ultraslow frequency components of around 0.5 Hz have been recorded (Achermann and Borbely, 1997; Amzica and Steriade, 1997; Massimini and Amzica, 2001; Mölle et al., 2002) and the same is the case with MEG (Simon et al., 2000). These components correspond to the ultraslow oscillations found in cat neocortex during sleep, or anaesthesia, recorded intracellularly from cortical neurons in layers II to VI. These oscillations consist of prolonged depolarizing and hyperpolarizing components, and have been analyzed in detail by Steriade and collaborators (2006). The study of ultraslow oscillations in MEG and EEG is an active area of research, in conditions ranging from studies of peri-infarct depolarisations in stroke patients, and cortical spreading depression in migraine patients (Leistner et al., 2006), to recordings of preterm neonates (Vanhatalo et al., 2005). The underlying neurophysiological mechanisms of ultraslow shifts of cortical activity are well known in respect to the changes in neuronal membrane potentials caused by increases of CO_2 tension and hypoxia in cerebral tissue (Speckmann and Elger, 2005), and basic mechanisms of spreading depression in neurons and glial cells have been put in evidence (Kager et al., 2002; Somjen, 2001).

General Conclusions

In this overview we have briefly covered some of the basic concepts of neurophysiology and biophysics that are important in understanding how magnetic and electric fields are generated in the brain, and give rise to measurable signals at the scalp. A number of recent experimental and modeling studies have provided new insights in this respect. The approach outlined here is that of quantitative neurophysiology, in which the forward problem of MEG/EEG is modeled. We currently have a comprehensive set of methodologies that allow estimation of MEG/EEG signals measured at a distance, namely at the level of the scalp, given a number of sources of electrical/magnetic activity at the cellular level. In this context, the combination of neurophysiology and computational models appears to be essential. The forward problem, however, becomes more complex when we take into consideration the 3-dimensional geometry of neuronal sources within the cortex and its convoluted structure. For instance, when we state that to reach a MEG signal with the magnitude of 10nAm it is necessary that 50,000 pyramidal neurons are synchronously active (since each cortical pyramidal neuron has a Q of 0.2 pAm), the forward problem is not completely solved. In fact, the estimate will be different depending on (i) how these 50,000 neurons are distributed within the cortex, (ii) how the cortex is oriented in relation to the pial surface, and on (iii) the degree of synchrony. Such data are not readily available for most phenomena of interest, and investigations at the level of the neocortex, combining basic neurophysiology with computer models of the forward problem with simultaneous MEG/EEG recordings and structural/functional (fMRI) data, are therefore necessary for a fuller understanding. Ongoing work using these methodologies remains an active esearch area.

Acknowledgments

I thank Bob van Dijk and Stiliyan Kalitzin for their comments and suggestions on the first draft of this paper.

Notes

1 For a more extensive mathematical treatment of this subject the reader may consult Lopes da Silva, & van Rotterdam (2005) and Plonsey (1969).

2 The dot product can be defined for two vectors $\overline{X}$ and $\overline{Y}$ by

$$\overline{X} \cdot \overline{Y} = |X| \cdot |Y| \cos \theta$$

where θ is the angle between the vectors and $|\overline{X}|$ is the norm. It follows immediately that $\overline{X} \cdot \overline{Y} = 0$ if is $\overline{X}$ perpendicular to $\overline{Y}$. The dot product therefore has the geometric interpretation as the length of the projection of $\overline{X}$ onto the unit vector $\overline{Y}$ when the two vectors are placed so that their tails coincide.

References

Achermann, P., & Borbely, A. A. (1997). Low-frequency (< 1 Hz) oscillations in the human sleep electroencephalogram. *Neuroscience, 81,* 213–222.

Amzica, F., & Steriade, M. (1997). The K-complex: its slow (<1-Hz) rhythmicity and relation to delta waves. *Neurology, 49,* 952–959.

Burghoff, M., Sander, T. H., Schnabel, A., Drung, D., Trahms, L., & Curio, G., et al. (2004). DC-Magnetoencephalography: direct measurements in a magnetically extremely-well-shielded room. *Appl Phys Lett, 85,* 6278–6280.

Buxhoeveden, D. P., & Casanova, M. F. (2002). The minicolumn hypothesis in neuroscience. *Brain, 125,* 935–951.

Cohen, D. (1968). Magnetoencephalography: evidence of magnetic fields produced by alpha-rhythm currents. *Science, 161,* 784–786.

Curio, G., Mackert, B. M., Burghoff, M., Koetitz, R., Abraham-Fuchs, K., & Harer, W. (1994). Localization of evoked neuromagnetic 600 Hz activity in the cerebral somatosensory system. *Electroencephalogr Clin Neurophysiol, 91,* 483–487.

de Munck, J., Vijn, P., & Lopes da Silva, F. (1992). A random dipole model for spontaneous brain activity. *IEEE Trans Biomed Eng, 39,* 791–804.

Favorov, O. V., & Diamond, M. E. (1990). Demonstration of discrete place-defined columns—segregates—in the cat SI. *J Comp Neurol, 298,* 97–112.

Freiwald, W. A., Kreiter, A. K., & Singer, W. (1995). Stimulus dependent intercolumnar synchronization of single unit responses in cat area 17. *Neuroreport, 6,* 2348–2352.

Gray, C. M., Konig, P., Engel, A. K., & Singer, W. (1989). Oscillatory responses in cat visual cortex exhibit inter-columnar synchronization which reflects global stimulus properties. *Nature, 338,* 334–337.

Hämäläinen, M. S. (1995). Functional localization based on measurements with a whole-head magnetometer system. *Brain Topogr, 7,* 283–289.

Hämäläinen, M. S., Hari, R., Ilmoniemi, R. J., Knuutila, J., & Lounasmaa, O. (1993). Magnetoencephalography-theory, instrumentation, and applications to noninvasive studies of the working human brain. *Reviews of Modern Physics, 65,* 413–497.

Hari, R. (2005). Magnetoencephalography in clinical neurophysiological assessment of human cortical functions. In: E. Niedermeyer & F. H. Lopes da Silva (Eds.) *Electroencephalography, basic principles, clinical applications and related fields.* (5th Ed., pp. 1165–1198). Philadelphia: Lippincott Williams & Wilkins.

Hari, R., Nagamine, T., Nishitani, N., Mikuni, N., Sato, T., Tarkiainen, A., et al. (1996). Time-varying activation of different cytoarchitectonic areas of the human SI cortex after tibial nerve stimulation. *Neuroimage, 4,* 111–118.

Hashimoto, I., Mashiko, T., & Imada, T. (1996). High-frequency magnetic signals in the human somatosensory cortex. *Electroencephalogr Clin Neurophysiol Suppl, 47,* 67–80.

Huang, T. Y., Cherkas, P. S., Rosenthal, D. W., & Hanani, M. (2005). Dye coupling among satellite glial cells in mammalian dorsal root ganglia. *Brain Res, 1036,* 42–49.

Ikeda, H., Leyba, L., Bartolo, A., Wang, Y., & Okada, Y. C. (2002). Synchronized spikes of thalamocortical axonal terminals and cortical neurons are detectable outside the pig brain with MEG. *J Neurophysiol, 87,* 626–630.

Ioannides, A. A., Liu, M. J., Liu, L. C., Bamidis, P. D., Hellstrand, E., & Stephan, K. M. (1995). Magnetic field tomography of cortical and deep processes: examples of "real-time mapping" of averaged and single trial MEG signals. *Int J Psychophysiol, 20,* 161–175.

Kager, H., Wadman, W. J., & Somjen, G. G. (2002). Conditions for the triggering of spreading depression studied with computer simulations. *J Neurophysiol, 88,* 2700–2712.

Kornhuber, H. H., & Deecke, L. (1965). Changes in the brain potential in voluntary movements and passive movements in man: readiness potential and reafferent potentials. *Pflugers Arch Gesamte Physiol Menschen Tiere, 284,* 1–17.

Kyuhou, S., & Okada, Y. C. (1993). Detection of magnetic evoked fields associated with synchronous population activities in the transverse CA1 slice of the guinea pig. *J Neurophysiol, 70,* 2665–2668.

Leistner, S., Wuebbeler, G., Trahms, L., Curio, G., & Mackert, B. M. (2006). Tonic neuronal activation during simple and complex finger movements analyzed by DC-magnetoencephalography. *Neurosci Lett, 394,* 42–47.

Lopes da Silva, F. H., & van Rotterdam, A. (2005). Biophysical aspects of EEG and Magnetoencephalographic generation. In: E. Niedermeyer & F. H. Lopes da Silva (Eds.). *Electroencephalography, basic principles, clinical applications and related fields.* (5th Ed., pp. 1165–1198). Philadelphia: Lippincott Williams & Wilkins.

Lorente de Nó, R. (1947). Action potential of the motoneurons in the hypoglossus nucleus. *J Cell Comp Physiol, 29,* 207–287.

Mainen, Z. F., & Sejnowski, T. J. (1996). Influence of dendritic structure on firing pattern in model neocortical neurons. *Nature, 382,* 363–366.

Massimini, M., & Amzica, F. (2001). Extracellular calcium fluctuations and intracellular potentials in the cortex during the slow sleep oscillation. *J Neurophysiol 85,* 1346–1350.

Mölle, M., Marshall, L., Gais, S., & Born, J. (2002). Grouping of spindle activity during slow oscillations in human non-rapid eye movement sleep. *J Neurosci, 22,* 10941–10947.

Mountcastle, V. B. (1997). The columnar organization of the neocortex. *Brain, 120*(4), 701–722.

Murakami, S., Hirose, A., & Okada, Y. C. (2003). Contribution of ionic currents to magnetoencephalography (MEG) and electroencephalography (EEG) signals generated by guinea-pig CA3 slices. *J Physiol, 553,* 975–985.

Murakami, S., & Okada, Y. (2006). Contributions of principal neocortical neurons to magnetoencephalography and electroencephalography signals. *J Physiol, 575,* 925–936.

Murakami, S., Zhang, T., Hirose, A., & Okada, Y. C. (2002). Physiological origins of evoked magnetic fields and extracellular field potentials produced by guinea-pig CA3 hippocampal slices. *J Physiol, 544,* 237–251.

Nicholson, C. (1980) Dynamics of the brain cell microenvironment. *Neurosci Res Program Bull, 18,* 175–322.

Okada, Y. C., Kaufman, L., & Williamson, S. J. (1983). The hippocampal formation as a source of the slow endogenous potentials. *Electroencephalogr Clin Neurophysiol, 55,* 417–426.

Okada, Y. C., Wu, J., & Kyuhou, S. (1997). Genesis of MEG signals in a mammalian CNS structure. *Electroencephalogr Clin Neurophysiol, 103,* 474–485.

Plonsey, R. (1969). *Bioelectrical phenomena.* New York: McGraw Hill.

Plonsey, R. (1982). The nature of sources of bioelectric and biomagnetic fields. *Biophys J, 39,* 309–312.

Rogers, R. L., Baumann, S. B., Papanicolaou, A. C., Bourbon, T. W., Alagarsamy, S., & Eisenberg, H. M. (1991). Localization of the P3 sources using magnetoencephalography and magnetic resonance imaging. *Electroencephalogr Clin Neurophysiol, 79,* 308–321.

Salmelin, R., Hari, R., Lounasmaa, O. V., & Sams, M. (1994). Dynamics of brain activation during picture naming. *Nature, 368,* 463–465.

Simon, N. R., Manshanden, I., & Lopes da Silva, F. H. (2000). A MEG study of sleep. *Brain Res, 860,* 64–76.

Somjen, G. G. (2001). Mechanisms of spreading depression and hypoxic spreading depression-like depolarization. *Physiol Rev, 81,* 1065–1096.

Speckmann, E. J., & Elger, C. E. (2005). Introduction to the neurophysiological basis of EEG and DC potentials. In: E. Niedermeyer and F. H. Lopes da Silva (Eds.). *Electroencephalography, basic principles, clinical applications and related fields.* (5th Ed., pp. 17–29). Philadelphia: Lippincott Williams & Wilkins.

Steriade, M. (2006). Grouping of brain rhythms in corticothalamic systems. *Neuroscience, 137,* 1087–1106.

Stuart, G. J., & Sakmann, B. (1994). Active propagation of somatic action potentials into neocortical pyramidal cell dendrites. *Nature, 367,* 69–72.

Swinney, K. R., & Wikswo, J. P. Jr. (1980). A calculation of the magnetic field of a nerve action potential. *Biophys J, 32,* 719–731.

Tesche, C. D., & Karhu, J. (2000). Theta oscillations index human hippocampal activation during a working memory task. *Proc Natl Acad Sci U S A, 97*, 919–924.

Traub, R. D., Jefferys, J. G., Miles, R., Whittington, M. A., & Toth, K. (1994). A branching dendritic model of a rodent CA3 pyramidal neurone. *J Physiol, 481*(1), 79–95.

Traub, R. D. and Miles, R. (1991) *Neuronal networks of the hippocampus.* New York: Cambridge University Press.

Van 't Ent, D., Manshanden, I., Ossenblok, P., Velis, D. N., de Munck, J. C., Verbunt, J. P., & Lopes da Silva, F. H. (2003). Spike cluster analysis in neocortical localization related epilepsy yields clinically significant equivalent source localization results in magnetoencephalogram (MEG). *Clin Neurophysiol, 114*, 1948–1962.

van Rotterdam, A. (1987). Electric and magnetic fields of the brain computed by way of a discrete systems analytical approach: theory and validation. *Biol Cybern 57*, 301–311.

Vanhatalo, S., Voipio, J., & Kaila, K. (2005) Full-band EEG (fbEEG): a new standard for clinical electroencephalography. *Clin EEG Neurosci, 36*, 311–317.

Walter, W. G., Cooper, R., Aldridge, V. J., McCallum, W. C., & Winter, A. L. (1964). Contingent Negative Variation: an Electric Sign of Sensorimotor Association and Expectancy in the Human Brain. *Nature, 203*, 380–384.

2

Instrumentation and Data Preprocessing

Lauri Parkkonen

- Feasible detection of the weak MEG signals is currently possible only with superconducting SQUID sensors
- Ambient magnetic fields are several orders of magnitude stronger than MEG. Therefore, magnetic shielding and interference suppression systems are mandatory
- MEG results are often visualized on anatomical MRIs, which requires bringing the two modalities in the same coordinate system
- Pre-processing techniques such as averaging and filtering in time and space are required to boost the low signal-to-noise ratio of MEG

Introduction

This chapter reviews the methods and technology required for magnetoencephalographic (MEG) measurements.

The magnetic fields due to neural activity are extremely weak, thus the task of measuring them is challenging both in terms of required sensitivity, and also in the ability to suppress interference several orders of magnitude stronger than the signals of interest. Therefore, an appropriate combination of multiple techniques, both physical and computational, is required to make MEG measurements feasible.

Prior to analysis, MEG data often undergoes several preprocessing steps. These include noise reduction, artifact detection and removal, filtering, and averaging.

The physics and mathematics in this chapter are kept relatively simple to serve readers with various backgrounds. New concepts are described verbally rather than by equations. The mathematically inclined reader may refer to the cited text-books and reviews for a more thorough mathematical treatment of the subtopics.

Instrumentation

Review of Relevant Electromagnetic Concepts

- **Electric current** is the flow of charge carriers. The strength of the current I is measured in Amperes (A).
- All currents generate a **magnetic field** around them. A magnetic field is a vector field; it has a direction at each point in space. The field vector can be expressed as components, e.g., as the field strength to the x, y and z-directions of the 3-dimensional space. Two distinct quantities are referred to as magnetic fields: the magnetizing field or auxiliary magnetic field **H** (measured in Amperes/meter), and the magnetic flux density or magnetic induction **B** (measured in Teslas), commonly called the magnetic field.
- **Magnetic flux** is the net magnetic field through a given surface (taking into account only the field component perpendicular to the surface). Magnetic flux ϕ is a scalar quantity and its unit is Weber (Wb).
- **Spatial derivative** of the magnetic field is the rate of change of the field along a certain direction. It is measured as Teslas per meter (T/m). If all spatial derivatives are zero, the field is said to be homogeneous. Field derivative is a tensor quantity; there are 9 first-order derivatives (3 field components × 3 directions of the derivatives) at each point in space. For example, the derivative of the z-component along the x-direction at location **r** is denoted as $\partial B_z(\mathbf{r})/\partial x$.
- A time-varying magnetic flux induces an electromotive force (a voltage) in the circuit. Similarly, a circuit moving in a magnetic field experiences an electromotive force.
- Magnetic **permeability** indicates the extent to which a material magnetizes when subjected to an external magnetic field. Permeability μ is the ratio of the internal and applied fields. Permeability of vacuum relates the magnetization **M** and the magnetizing field **H** to the magnetic field: $\mathbf{B} = \mu_0 (\mathbf{H} + \mathbf{M})$.
- **Ferromagnetic** materials remain magnetic after being exposed to a magnetic field ("permanent magnets"). They usually have a high permeability.

- **Paramagnetic** materials amplify applied fields (permeability larger than unity); however, they do not retain the magnetization.
- **Diamagnets** also react to applied fields, but by weakening them.

MEG Signal Strength

To motivate the development and use of the relatively complex and costly MEG instrumentation, let us compare the strength of the MEG signals to some ambient magnetic fields. As shown in Figure 2–1, magnetic fields due to brain activity are 8–9 orders of magnitude (about one billion times) smaller than the Earth's static magnetic field, which orients the compass needle. Even the magnetic noise, (mostly generated by various electric devices and moving magnetic objects) encountered in a typical laboratory environment is often more than a thousand times stronger than any magnetic signal due to the activity of neurons in the brain.

Sensors

Superconductivity

In order to understand the physical principles behind the sensors employed in all modern MEG systems, we should familiarize ourselves with a remarkable property exhibited by certain materials: when cooled down to a sufficiently low

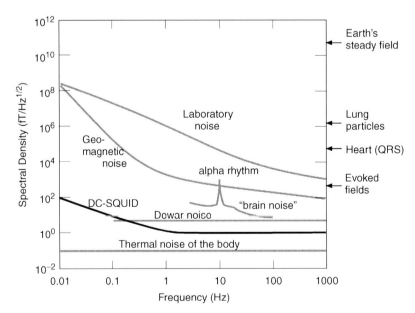

Figure 2–1. Magnetic field strengths of various sources.
Adapted from Hämäläinen et al., (1993).

temperature, these materials lose electrical resistance completely, i.e., they become *superconductors*. An electric current flows in these materials without "friction" and when arranged to circulate in a loop, the current does so infinitely, provided that the low temperature is maintained. This perpetual current, like any electric current, generates a magnetic field. The converse is also true with superconductors: an applied static magnetic field gives rise to a continuous *shielding current* on the surface of a superconductor, which in turn generates a magnetic field exactly cancelling the impinging external field, thus preventing the external field from entering the superconducting material. Superconductors are thus perfect *diamagnets*; external magnetic fields cannot penetrate them, except to a very shallow *penetration depth* of typically less than 100 nm.

The characteristic transition temperature, or *critical temperature T_c*, at which the material switches from the normal to the superconducting state, depends on the material and is typically below 20 Kelvin ($-253°C$). A typical material utilized in MEG sensors is niobium with $T_c = 9.2$ K. Other common superconductors are lead ($T_c = 7.2$ K) and mercury ($T_c = 4.2$ K). The most commonly employed coolant to achieve these very low temperatures is liquid helium, whose boiling point is 4.2 K or $-269°C$.

The required extraordinarily low temperatures and associated thermal isolation have effectively prevented the wide-spread use of superconductors, despite their exploitable properties. Therefore, the discovery of compounds — consisting primarily of copper and oxygen — with much higher T_c's in the 1980's evoked great interest. These high-temperature, or high-T_c, superconductors have critical temperatures up to 134 K, or $-139°C$, and thus allow inexpensive liquid nitrogen (boiling point 77 K) to be used as the coolant. Unfortunately, the high-T_c materials are in crystalline form, and are therefore difficult to manufacture reliably as wires or films to be used in MEG sensors. In addition, until now the noise levels attained with high-T_c sensors are too high for practical MEG work.

The transition between the normal and superconducting states is not only governed by the temperature. Superconductors also have a characteristic *critical field B_c* (typically ranging between 1 mT and 100 T) and a *critical current I_c*; exceeding either of these limits reverts the material to the normal state, even if the temperature is kept well below the critical value. Thus, superconductors do not withstand arbitrarily large magnetic fields, nor electric currents, passing through them. These three quantities (T_c, B_c and I_c) have a complex interdependence; e.g., the critical field diminishes when the temperature of the material rises and approaches the critical value.

The BCS theory by Bardeen, Cooper and Schrieffer (1957) explains the transition to the superconducting state as pairing of the electrons, which are normally responsible for electrical conduction as invidivals, but in a superconductor as *Cooper pairs*, governed by a common macroscopic wavefunction.[1]

The wavefunction describing the electron pairs in a superconducting ring has to be continuous around the ring. It can be shown that this condition leads to the quantization of the magnetic flux threading the ring; the flux can only assume a value equal to an integral number of a *flux quantum* Φ_0 = 2.07 Weber. The applied field gives rise to a shielding current I_s (inducing a flux $\Phi = LI_s$ where L is the inductance of the ring) that maintains a constant flux $n \cdot \Phi_0$ through the ring. If the shielding current exceeds the critical current I_c, a flux quantum may "slip" into the ring, elevating the flux to $(n + 1) \cdot \Phi_0$ and lowering the shielding current accordingly. With this in mind, it is possible to understand many of the qualitative characteristics of the SQUID sensors employed in MEG systems.

SQUID

The weakness of the cerebral magnetic fields necessitates a very sensitive magnetic field detector. The sensors that measure magnetic fields in devices such as a video tape recorder or an electronic compass are far from being sensitive enough for MEG. The only sensor that provides sufficient sensitivity for practical MEG work is the SQUID, or Superconducting Quantum Interference Device. To fully understand the internal workings of a SQUID requires an elaborate quantum mechanical treatment beyond the scope of this book. However, equipped with the phenomenological descriptions of superconductivity given in the previous section, we can elucidate the operating principles of a SQUID.

Let us consider a superconducting ring placed in a magnetic field. As described in the previous section, the field induces a shielding current around the ring, and this current depends on the applied field. Thus, the shielding current would provide an indirect measure of the applied magnetic field. However, that current cannot be readily measured, since a conventional current measurement would destroy the continuous superconducting loop and the flux quantization would disappear. If the ring is broken by a very thin layer of an electrical insulator, the electron pairs may still tunnel through the insulator even if there is no electric field driving them to do so; this phenomenon was theoretically predicted by Brian D. Josephson (1962), later awarded the Nobel Prize in physics. These *Josephson junctions*, or *weak links*, allow for an interference of the wavefunctions describing the electron pairs, and this interference gives rise to a measurable physical quantity, namely a dynamic, flux-dependent resistance across the SQUID. If we feed a constant bias current I_B through the SQUID, changes in the applied magnetic flux will alter the average voltage measured over the SQUID; see Figure 2–2.

The dynamic resistance depends on the applied flux in a nonlinear way; changing the flux threading the ring exactly by an integral number of flux quanta does not alter the resistance, although any other change does. This periodic relationship is also manifested in the *characteristic curve*, that is, the voltage-vs-flux function of a SQUID; changing the flux by one flux quantum does not change the SQUID output; see Figure 2–3b. Thus, with a SQUID one cannot measure the absolute flux and, hence, not the absolute magnetic field, but only its variation in time.

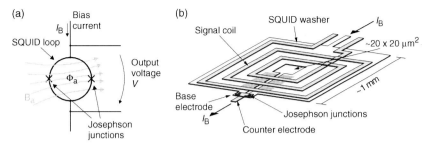

Figure 2–2. A dc-SQUID with two Josepson junctions. **(a)** A schematic illustration of the SQUID loop in the magnetic field B_a which causes magnetic flux Φ_a in the SQUID loop. **(b)** A modern thin film dc-SQUID and the signal coil on top of the SQUID loop.
Adapted from Hämäläinen et al., (1993).

The first SQUIDs were designed and made by James Zimmerman (1970) in the late 1960s. At that time, most SQUIDs comprised only a single Josephson junction because fabricating a properly working junction took a great deal of care and effort. This kind of SQUID is read via an inductive coupling to an external circuit operating at radio frequencies. Hence, these single-junction SQUIDs are called rf-SQUIDs. Later, when manufacturing processes developed in the semiconductor industry allowed a relatively cheap "mass production" of Josephson junctions, the two-junction dc-SQUID became more popular, as it outperforms the rf-SQUID in many respects—most importantly, by having a lower noise level and by allowing much simpler electronics and minimal crosstalk between channels. All these factors are indispensable for MEG, and thus all modern MEG systems are equipped solely with dc-SQUIDs.

Negative feedback

The periodic response of the SQUID to the variation of the applied flux, as shown in Figure 2–3, prevents us from using the SQUID output directly as a measure of the magnetic signal of interest; changes larger than half a flux quantum would lead to ambiguous results. Therefore, in MEG systems, the SQUIDs are operated in a *flux-locked loop* by providing them a feedback signal that cancels the effect of the signal we are measuring. In other words, the output of the SQUID is held constant by artificially generating an additional magnetic flux that "undoes" the effect of the actual flux to be measured. It is easy to see that this additional artificial signal, or feedback signal, depends directly on the signal to be measured; it only has the opposite sign and hence the term *negative feedback*.

By using negative feedback, the SQUID is locked to a certain *operating point* as illustrated in Figure 2–4b; changes in the measured signal only

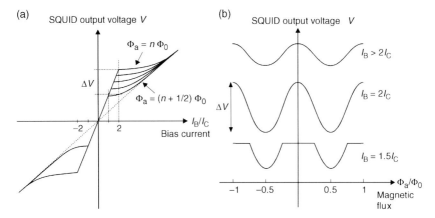

Figure 2–3. Characteristic curves of a dc-SQUID. **(a)** SQUID output voltage as a function of the bias current I_B fed through the SQUID, and **(b)** as a function of the applied flux Φ_a. The maximum change in the output voltage ΔV for different flux values is the *modulation depth* of the SQUID. It depends on the bias current and peaks when $I_B = 2 \cdot I_c$. The extremities of the curve family in **(a)** correspond to flux values that are an integral number of quanta, or just in between (*n* is an integer).

deviate the SQUID output slightly from the operating point until the *feedback controller* reacts and adjusts the negative feedback signal accordingly to again perfectly cancel the measured signal. Thus, the signal that the MEG system outputs and stores into a computer is not the SQUID output as such, but the inverted negative feedback signal, which linearly tracks the true measured signal, even if it undergoes variations larger than a flux quantum.

Sensor Coils

To optimize the sensitivity, SQUIDs are made rather small, typically less than 1 mm in outer diameter. Due to the small surface area, SQUIDs have rather poor coupling to the magnetic field. In MEG applications, SQUIDs cannot be used as they are; the coupling must be enhanced with *flux transformers* that "squeeze" more magnetic flux into the SQUID loop by collecting it from a much larger area. This is not a drawback, since the use of flux transformers allows us to measure different components of the magnetic field without changing the SQUID geometry.

Like SQUIDs, the flux transformers are made of superconducting material. They comprise a *pick-up coil* closest to the brain, an optional, more distant *compensation coil*, and a *signal coil* on top of the SQUID loop (Figure 2–4a,c). These coils are typically connected in series so that the net shielding current induced by the magnetic fields at the pick-up and compensation coils circulates through the signal coil, and thus generates a magnetic

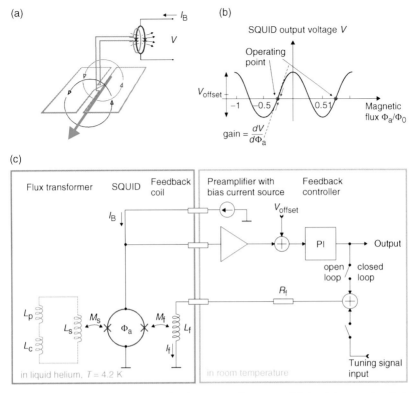

Figure 2–4. (a) The principle of a flux transformer, which picks up the field due to a neural current (green arrow) and couples it to a SQUID (blue ring). **(b)** Illustration of the operating points at which the SQUIDs locks when used in a flux-locked loop, and **(c)** a simplified block diagram of the sensor electronics (utilizing direct readout) of one MEG channel.

field and flux to the SQUID loop. Because of superconductivity, flux transformers work also at DC, whereas normal transformers do not, since a static magnetic field does not induce currents in normal, stationary conductors.

The simplest configuration is a *magnetometer*: a single pick-up coil and no compensation coil (Figure 2–5a). This setup measures the magnetic field component along the direction perpendicular to the surface of the pick-up coil, usually denoted as B_z. While being very sensitive to nearby sources, such as neural currents in the brain, a magnetometer is sensitive also to sources far away. To decrease the sensitivity to distant sources, one may add a compensation coil that measures mostly the interfering signal; this configuration is a *gradiometer* (see Figure 2–5b,c), which measures a spatial gradient of a magnetic field component rather than the field component itself. The underlying idea is that the far-away interference sources manifest themselves as homogeneous magnetic fields, i.e., the field is about the same at close-by spatial locations.

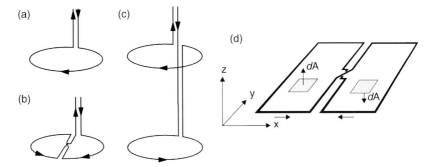

Figure 2–5. Flux transformer geometries: **(a)** magnetometer, **(b)** planar gradiometer, **(c)** axial gradiometer. **(d)** Integrating the flux that threads a planar gradiometer measuring dB_z/dx; see the text for details.

Thus, the interference field at the pick-up coil and compensation coil is about the same. When those coils are wound in opposite directions, the interference fields produce no net shielding current, and thus do not couple to the SQUID, making the sensor blind to sources distant enough to be seen as homogeneous fields.

The two coils of a gradiometer can be arranged in several ways to sensitize the sensor for different spatial derivatives of the field. Perhaps the most intuitive configuration is shown in Figure 2–5c, where the coils are along the same radial axis, but the pick-up coil is typically 5 cm closer to the head. This is called an *axial gradiometer* and it measures the change of the radial field component along the radius.

Another option is to place the coils side-by-side in the same plane to form a *planar gradiometer* (Figure 2–5b). Both of these arrangements are insensitive to homogeneous fields but their responses to nearby sources are very different; the signal from an axial gradiometer peaks for sources around the rim of the sensor while planar gradiometers give the maximum signal for sources right beneath them. Formally, these spatial sensitivity patterns can be described with the concept of *lead field*. It is a fictitious vector field whose value at a spatial location gives the direction of the current that yields the maximal output at that location, and the gain with which the source current affects the output of the sensor. Thus, each sensor type, or pick-up coil geometry, has a specific lead field, some of which are illustrated in Figure 2–6. Knowing the lead field $\mathbf{L}_i$ of the i'th sensor, the output of that sensor, b_i, can be expressed mathematically as

$$b_i = \int_G \mathbf{L}_i(\mathbf{r})\, \mathbf{j}_p\, dG. \tag{2–1}$$

where the integration is carried out throughout the volume G where currents can flow, and $\mathbf{r}$ points to the center of the integration element dG.

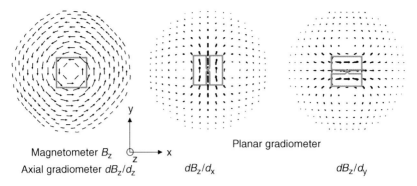

Figure 2–6. Lead fields of a magnetometer/axial gradiometer, and two orthogonal planar gradiometers with the field components they measure. The lead fields of magnetometers and axial gradiometers are not shown separately, as they are very similar. The directions x and y are in the plane of the paper as shown by the coordinate axis, while the z direction points towards the reader. When the sensors are arranged into a roughly spherical array, the approximate radial direction r in the sphere is often used instead of z.

The lead field can be estimated by virtually scanning the volume G with a set of three orthogonal unit-strength test current dipoles. At each spatial location, the signals elicited by the x, y and z-directed dipoles are the corresponding components of the lead field vector at that location. Assuming that we can calculate the total magnetic field $\mathbf{B}(\mathbf{r})$ at location $\mathbf{r}$ due to a current dipole in a conducting volume, the output of the i'th channel is

$$b_i = \int_A \mathbf{B}(\mathbf{r}) \cdot d\mathbf{A} \approx \sum_{k=1}^{N} w_k \mathbf{B}(\mathbf{r}_k) \cdot \mathbf{n}_k \qquad (2\text{–}2)$$

where the integral is calculated over the surface A of the pick-up and compensation coils, taking the winding direction of the coil into account, and with $\mathbf{r}$ pointing to the center of the surface patch dA (see Figure 2–5d); the approximation by N points involves the unit normal vectors $\mathbf{n}_k$ and surface areas w_k associated with each point k.

Lead fields have practical relevance also when interpreting MEG data visually. Figure 2–7 shows auditory evoked responses measured with an array comprising only magnetometer sensors, and with a similar array of planar gradiometers. In this experiment, there was significant activity only in the left and right auditory cortices at about 100 ms after the presentation of a short tone. For the source in either auditory cortex, there is a group of magnetometers showing a positive deflection (field coming out of the head), another group with a negative deflection (field going into the head). The magnetometers right above the underlying source current do not show any signal. The situation is quite the opposite for the planar gradiometers shown in the same

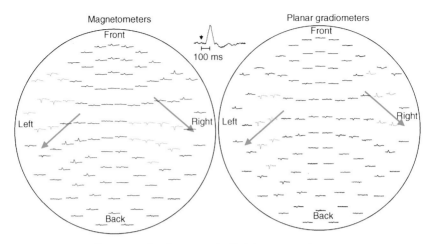

Figure 2–7. Auditory evoked magnetic fields as seen by a magnetometer and a planar gradiometer sensor array (only one direction of the planar gradiometers is shown). The largest deflections are highlighted, and the source currents in the brain are shown schematically by the green arrows. Magnetometer signals exhibit two maxima with opposite signs, somewhat off the active brain region, while the planar gradiometer signals show a single peak on top of the source.

Figure; they peak just on top of the neural current. Thus, knowing the sensitivity pattern of the sensors is essential for the correct interpretation of the data. Proper source modeling algorithms, to be discussed in the subsequent chapters, take the different lead fields automatically into account, so that the source currents can be localized correctly. Nevertheless, for the human observer who wants to get a rough idea of the source locations, or needs to disentangle the contributions of different neural sources at the sensor level, understanding the sensitivity pattern is essential.

Sensor Arrays

The first MEG measurements with SQUIDs (Cohen, 1972) were done with a single-channel instrument. While this is sufficient for the mere detection of the signal, a proper mapping requires multiple measurements at distinct spatial locations. Such mapping can be done even with a single-channel system by repeating the measurement multiple times with the measurement probe at different locations. This is not only cumbersome and time-consuming, but also prevents studying, e.g., induced synchronization between two brain areas. During the 1980s several MEG systems with the number of channels ranging up to 37, covering approximately one lobe of the brain at a time, were developed. In 1992, the first whole-head MEG system, comprising 122 planar

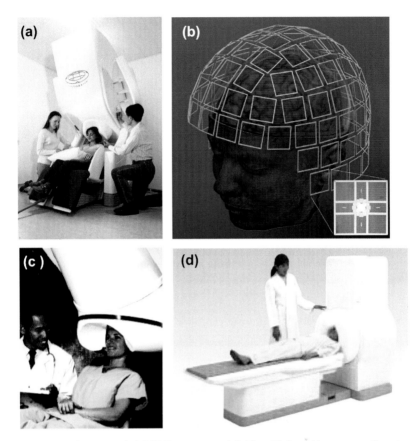

Figure 2–8. Commercial MEG systems. **(a)** The Elekta Neuromag®system (Elekta Oy, Helsinki, Finland) features 306 channels on 102 planar sensor elements **(b)**, each comprising a magnetometer measuring B_z and two orthogonal planar gradiometers measuring dB_z/dx and dB_z/dy. **(c)** The Magnes®3600 WH system (4-D Neuroimaging, San Diego, CA, USA) incorporates 248 magnetometers (B_z) or axial gradiometers (dB_z/dz) depending on the configuration. **(d)** MEGvision (Yokogawa Electric Corp., Tokyo, Japan) comprises 160 axial gradiometer channels.

gradiometer channels, was introduced (Ahonen et al., 1993b) and since then, the MEG market has been dominated by whole-head systems.

Several factors and trade-offs are to be considered in the design of the sensor array. For example, larger pick-up coils yield higher signal-to-noise ratios (considering only the intrinsic system noise), but the larger the loops the fewer of them fit on the head surface. In addition, the distance from the most superficial neural sources sets a limit on the highest spatial frequencies present at the pick-up coils, thus, packing the sensors more densely increases the spatial resolving power of the array only up to a limit. Instead of increasing the density of sensors that measure one particular field component, one can measure multiple independent components of the field at each sensor location to increase the total information captured by the array (Ahonen et al., 1993a).

The optimal size of the pick-up coil depends also on the noise level of the SQUID: lower SQUID noise allows a reduction in the size of the pick-up coil without an adverse effect on the signal-to-noise ratio for a given source. Strictly speaking, this is true only if we assume the instrument to be the sole source of noise in the measurement. In practice, the "brain noise," i.e., the brain activity not of interest, dominates among the noise sources, which complicates the pick-up loop optimization further.

The coverage of the sensor array is another difficult optimization task. A sensor helmet as extended as possible would be optimal in capturing the neuromagnetic fields; however, practical limitations exist—for example, the MEG device should not severely limit the visual field of the subject. The overall size of the array should also be optimized to fit a high percentage of the population while minimizing the average distance from the sensors to the scalp.

Dewar and Cryogenics

The distance between the sensor coils and the head surface should be minimized to maximize the neuromagnetic field at the pick-up coils. Further, the coils must be superconducting, i.e., their temperature should remain below the critical value while the head surface is at body temperature. Maintaining this high temperature difference (about 300 K or °C) across a relatively small distance of 2–3 cm without excessive use of the coolant requires elaborate thermal isolation. A special container called *Dewar*, after the inventor James Dewar, comprises two concentric vessels with a vacuum jacket and radiation shields in between. The vacuum prevents heat conduction from the outside to the inside vessel, and the shields block thermal radiation. The sensors reside in the inner vessel[2] immersed in the coolant (liquid helium, $T = 4.2$ K). An MEG Dewar has to be strictly nonmagnetic not to distort the fields being measured.[3] The Dewars are usually built of glass-fibre composites which are magnetically transparent. Unfortunately, helium atoms slowly diffuse to the vacuum through the glass-fibre wall of the inner vessel. Therefore, the outer surface of the inner vessel is usually covered with a medium that absorbs the helium atoms.

Despite the extreme thermal isolation, there is still heat leakage, albeit small, into the inner vessel, causing the liquid helium to slowly evaporate. The gaseous helium exits the Dewar along an *exhaust line* which guides the gas out of the system and the magnetically shielded room. The helium gas is either collected into pressurized containers for reliquification, or just let out into the open air outside of the building. The feasibility of re-collection depends on the local price of liquid helium, and is seldom profitable for just one MEG system alone.

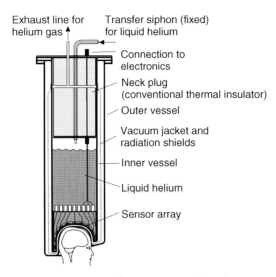

Figure 2–9. Schematic cross section of a Dewar employed in an MEG system.

A typical whole-head MEG system boils 10–20 liters of liquid helium per day. The helium reservoir of the Dewar is usually 70–90 liters, thus a refill is required 1–3 times a week to keep the system operational. Liquid helium is transferred from a storage Dewar by means of a vacuum-isolated *siphon*. The storage Dewar is pressurized by gaseous helium to "push" the liquid along the siphon into the MEG Dewar. Some liquid evaporates when cooling the siphon from room temperature down to 4.2 K. Typically, up to 10 liters of liquid per transfer should be budgeted for such losses.

Care should be taken to do the refills in time. If all liquid helium has evaporated and the temperature of the inner vessel thus starts to increase, the helium atoms trapped in the absorbant are released in the vacuum due to their increased thermal energy, and they start contributing to the heat conduction from the outer to the inner vessel. In such an event, the Dewar usually cannot be cooled down simply by transferring liquid helium; instead, the vacuum jacket has to be re-evacuated first.

Gantry

The mechanical system supporting the Dewar is called the *gantry*. It often allows adjusting the elevation and angle of the Dewar to accomodate subjects of different heights and in different measurement positions, such as seated or supine. Alternatively, the height adjustment can be addressed by moving the seat up/down. The gantry should be very rigid, since even minute movements of the sensors in the remanent field inside the shielded room gives rise to artifacts.

Electronics

The output signal of a SQUID sensor has to be processed extensively before it is possible, or feasible, to store it. The following paragraphs illustrate the required steps, implemented in hardware and software of a MEG system. A more detailed treatment of this topic is available, e.g., in Clarke and Braginski (2004).

A SQUID is a challenging signal source due to its low output impedance; the output voltage is so low that the voltage noise levels of even the best amplifiers available today clearly exceed that of the SQUID. Thus, additional measures are required to prevent the preamplifier from contributing more noise than the SQUID itself does. To this end, the output impedance of the SQUID should be stepped up to better match the input impedance of the amplifier. Such matching can be achieved by two techniques: (i) using a transformer between the SQUID and amplifier, and (ii) feeding back the amplifier output to the SQUID via the feedback coil, which effectively increases the SQUID output impedance. The transformer of the first option—as any transformer— works only when the SQUID outputs an ac signal, which generally is not the case. However, by adding a periodic magnetic flux component $\pm\Phi_0$ to the total flux applied to the SQUID, the output is guaranteed to be alternating. This approach is known *as flux modulation.* The modulation frequency is typically 100–200 kHz. The real input signal is recovered by demodulating the amplified output.

The feedback scheme (the second option) does not require a transformer nor flux modulation and is thus called *direct readout* (Seppä et al., 1991; Clarke and Braginski, 2004). The proper amount of feedback depends on the gains of the amplifier and SQUID; in practice, the feedback has to be adjustable to attain optimal noise performance. The direct readout is simpler to implement than flux modulation and it is less prone to electronics-based cross-talk between channels; however, occasional tuning might be required for best performance.

After amplification (and possible demodulation), the SQUID signal is conveyed to the feedback controller, which adjusts the negative feedback to the SQUID (see above discussion) to optimally null the changes at the SQUID output. As explained earlier, this negative feedback loop effectively linearizes the flux-to-voltage response of the SQUID. The signal to be processed further is the feedback, not the SQUID output. The feedback controller can be implemented either in the hardware, using analog electronics ("analog flux-locked loop"), or in the software, employing analog-to-digital and digital-to-analog converters and a digital signal processor or comparable digital circuitry ("digital flux-locked loop").

Modern MEG devices often include the option to measure EEG in addition to MEG. The EEG electronics include preamplifiers with rather stringent requirements for the noise level, as the electric signals on the scalp are typically on the order of a few microvolts only. For the safety of the subject, the electric ground of the preamplifier should be floating so that no excessive currents can pass through the EEG electrodes and amplifiers, should any electric system connected to the subject break and supply dangerously high voltages. The preamplifier ground is, therefore, often referred to as the *isolated ground*, or iso-ground. The required galvanic isolation is provided either by a special isolation unit, or by converting the EEG signal to a digital form already in the preamplifier and using an optic fiber to convey the samples to subsequent processing stages.

In addition to the MEG and EEG signal processing, complete MEG systems also feature electronics for driving the head-position tracking coils and the artificial sources in a phantom, and for monitoring the level of liquid helium in the MEG Dewar.

Data Acquisition

With the advent of digital SQUID electronics, the boundary between the electronics and data acquisition became fuzzy; traditionally, the acquisition system sampled and stored the amplified and filtered analog signals from the electronics, whereas nowadays the conversion to the digital domain happens much earlier on the signal path, and many of the acquisition system tasks are handled by the main electronics. The theoretical background remains the same: sampling theory and relevant performance criteria are reviewed briefly in the following paragraphs.

Frequency Range and Dynamics of MEG Signals

The bulk of the MEG activity occurs in the conventional *Berger bands*, defined by Hans Berger in 1920s after his first EEG measurements (Berger, 1929). MEG responses typically contain frequencies up to about 100 Hz with a gradual fall-off towards higher frequencies as shown in Figure 2–10. More recently, the higher frequency bands, up to 700 Hz, have also received attention following the discovery of certain fast oscillatory responses measured directly on the cortex, and also noninvasively by EEG and MEG. The 600-Hz burst response to electric nerve stimulation (Curio, 2000; Hashimoto, 2000; Okada et al., 2005) contains probably the highest-frequency oscillatory components so far detected by MEG. Responses from peripheral nerves, generated by compound action potentials and not much studied by magnetic measurements, extend above 1 kHz in frequency content. Generally, for MEG and EEG, as for most physical systems, it appears that the higher the frequency, the weaker the signal. The 600-Hz response, for example, is hidden in the noise due to the background brain activity and instrumentation, and can be recovered only by averaging hundreds of responses to a specific stimulus type.

The ratio of the maximum to the minimum signal amplitude, or the *dynamic range*, is rather low in the MEG signals that really originate in the brain; however, the residuals of the environmental interference, as well as the artifactual signals from the subject, may exceed the brain signals by orders of magnitude.

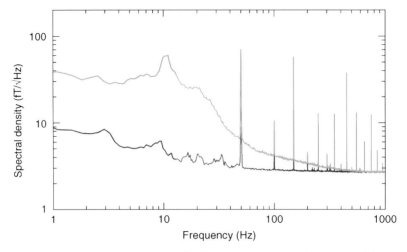

Figure 2–10. Average spectrum of all magnetometer channels without a subject (blue) and with a resting subject (green).

The dynamic range D is often expressed in decibels as

$$D[\mathrm{dB}] = 20\,\mathrm{dB} \cdot \log_{10} \frac{B_{\mathrm{max}}}{B_{\mathrm{min}}} \qquad (2\text{--}3)$$

where B_{max} and B_{min} are the maximum and minimum magnetic signal amplitudes, respectively, usually given as rms (root-mean-square) values.

The brain-signal dynamic range as seen by MEG is difficult to quantify, since the largest brain responses are typically associated with neurological pathologies. The MEG sensors pick up both brain and interference signal, and this combination may span a dynamic range of several tens of decibels. Although the residual interference is usually not of interest, the MEG system has to be able to represent such signals, since the post-measurement noise compensation methods rely on a faithful picture of not only the brain signals but of the interference as well.

Temporal Sampling and Amplitude Quantization

Most physical quantities, including magnetic field and its derivatives, are represented by a temporally continuous signal, that is, the signal has a value at every point in time. If there is a limit to the rate at which the signal can vary, all available information is retained by considering the amplitude of the continuous signal only at certain intervals. Indeed, it can be shown that it is sufficient to sample the continuous signal at a rate that is twice the frequency of any component of the signal, and yet to perfectly reconstruct the original signal from the discrete samples. This important result is known as the *sampling theorem*. It should be stressed here that all signal components, whether of interest or noise, must be below half the sampling rate; as a result of the sampling process, those signals that are above will fold along the frequency axis to appear as lower frequencies. This undesirable phenomenon, called *aliasing*, can be avoided by low-pass filtering the signal before sampling to ensure that there is no signal above half the sampling rate, or the *Nyqvist frequency*. This low-pass filtering just prior to sampling to avoid aliasing is often referred to as *anti-alias filtering*. Figure 2–11 illustrates sampling of continuous signals.

Given the MEG signal frequencies and the Nyqvist condition described above, the sampling rates range between 300 Hz and 4 kHz. It is often desirable to temporally oversample the signal of interest to avoid the non-idealities of the anti-alias filters such as phase distortion and the finite fall-off rate, and also to allow for an easier reconstruction of the original signal by linearly interpolating the values between the samples instead of using the optimal, but computationally expensive, sinc interpolation.

Converting a signal from the analog to digital domain involves the discretization of the signal amplitude as well. This process is often referred to as *quantization*, since the graded analog amplitude values are represented with a finite number of amplitude bins. The height of each amplitude bin, or the quantization step size, determines how faithfully the amplitude of the original signal can be represented in the digital domain. A smaller step size allows more precise reconstruction of the signal, but also requires more bits and thus more storage space to encode the steps. Assuming a certain step size, the signal dynamics determines how many such steps are required in the quantization.

Practically all quantizers utilized in MEG/EEG data acquisition systems are linear and memoryless, i.e., the quantization step size does not depend on the signal amplitude (see Figure 2–12) nor does the output depend on its previous values. Analyzing the dynamics of such a quantizer is straightforward if we assume that the signal amplitude has a uniform probability distribution when considering the amplitudes that would fall within a single quantization step. Let L be the number of steps of size Δ and $q(t)$ the quantization error, i.e., the difference between the original and quantized signals. This error can be considered as an uncorrelated noise source even though $q(t)$ is a deterministic function of the input signal. The variance of the quantization error

$$\sigma_q^2 = \int_{-\infty}^{\infty} q^2 p_q(q)\, dq \qquad (2\text{–}4)$$

where $p_q(q)$ is the probability distribution of the error term, which can be assumed to be uniform provided that the input signal does not exceed the normal range of the quantizer; the probability density function is thus

$$p_q(q) = \begin{cases} 1/\Delta & |q| < \Delta/2, \\ 0 & \text{otherwise.} \end{cases} \qquad (2\text{–}5)$$

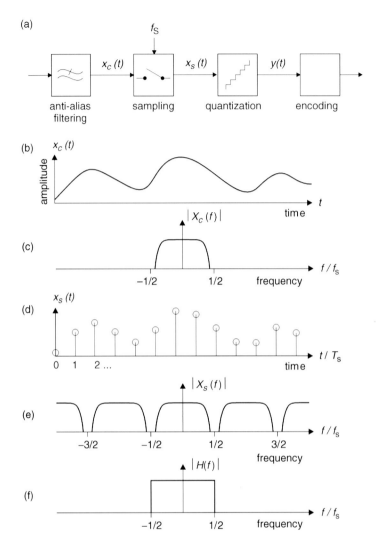

Figure 2–11. (a) Conversion of a timevarying analog signal to its digital counterpart. **(b)** The temporal waveform and **(c)** the spectrum of the band-limited continuous signal. **(d)** The sampled temporal waveform and **(e)** its spectrum, which shows also the aliased images. The original spectrum, and hence the original temporal waveform, can be recovered from the samples by **(f)** a reconstruction filter which suppresses the aliased images. Functions in lower and upper case refer to the time and frequency domain representations, respectively. f_s denotes the sampling frequency, and $T_s = 1/f_s$ is the corresponding sampling period, i.e., the time interval between two consecutive samples.

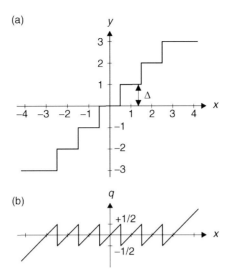

Figure 2–12. Amplitude quantization. **(a)** The transfer characteristics of a uniform quantizer with $L = 7$ amplitude steps, input x and output y. **(b)** The corresponding quantization error q as a function of the input amplitude x.

Substituting this into Equation (2–4), the variance $\sigma_q^2 = \Delta^2/12$.

The signal-to-noise ratio of a quantizer is typically expressed in decibels

$$\text{SNR}[\text{dB}] = 10\,\text{dB} \cdot \log_{10} \frac{\sigma_x^2}{\sigma_q^2} \qquad (2\text{–}6)$$

where σ_x^2 is the variance of the input signal. For an input signal with a uniform distribution

$$p_x(x) = \begin{cases} 1/(L\Delta) & |x| \le L\Delta/2, \\ 0 & \text{otherwise} \end{cases} \qquad (2\text{–}7)$$

the SNR is $\sigma_x^2 = L^2\Delta^2/12$. Substituting the variances into Equation (2–6) yields

$$\text{SNR} = 20\,\text{dB} \cdot \log_{10} L = 20\,\text{dB} \cdot \log_{10} 2^N \approx 6.02\,\text{dB/bit} \cdot N \qquad (2\text{-}8)$$

where N is the number of bits required to encode L quantization steps. Thus, to accomodate a dynamic range of 60 dB, we need 60 dB/6.02 dB/bit $\approx$ 10 bits for each sample. Modern MEG systems employ 16–32 bits per sample to allow for dynamic ranges in excess of 96 dB.

Until now, we have considered temporal sampling and amplitude quantization as separate processes; however, high temporal sampling rate can be traded for a larger dynamic range provided that there is some uncorrelated noise on top of the signal. This perhaps counterintuitive effect is best explained with an example; consider a slowly varying signal with an amplitude 1.7 at some point in time. When this signal is fed to a quantizer whose step size $\Delta = 1$, the quantizer output will be 2 since the value 1.7 falls into the bin [1.5, 2.5] centered around 2. On the other hand, if broadband noise (whose variance is larger than the step size) is added to the input signal, and this signal is sampled at a rate which is several times higher than what is required by the sampling theorem, the quantizer output is 2 for most of the samples, 1 almost as often, and may, less frequently, also assume other values if the noise variance is large. The average of multiple such samples approaches 1.7 without a limit when the number of samples tends to infinity. Thus, temporal *oversampling* is able to extend the dynamic range at the small-signal end. When the sampling rate is dropped, i.e., the signal is *downsampled*, additional accuracy is gained; it can be shown that downsampling by a factor F yields

$$N_{ds} = \log_2 \sqrt{F} \qquad (2\text{-}9)$$

bits in the small-signal end, provided that the original signal contains enough wideband noise.

Averaging trials (see previous section) has the very same effect; the average signal can show brain responses whose amplitude is smaller than the quantization step size of the raw signal, provided that the implementation of the averager is such that it preserves the emerging "sub-bits." In other words: if the quantization step is much smaller than the system noise amplitude in the frequency band of interest, the step size does not limit the smallest discernible brain response, since averaging is required anyway to recover the response amid noise.

Acquired Signals

The number of MEG channels in todays whole-head systems ranges from 100 to 300. The data acquisition system samples all these channels in parallel.

The MEG systems do not only acquire MEG data; many MEG devices feature a built-in EEG system to be used for simultaneous MEG/EEG measurements. The EEG systems have channels for scalp EEG, and some also for intracranial EEG, for monitoring muscular (electromyogram or EMG) and cardiac (electrocardiogram or ECG) activity, as well as eye movements and blinks (electrooculogram or EOG). The amplitudes of these electric signals range from the sub-microvolt-level scalp EEG to the millivolt peak amplitudes of ECG. To optimally acquire all these signals, the EEG systems typically have an adjustable gain, or sensitivity, separately for each input channel. The EEG systems operated with MEG typically have 32–128 channels.

The timing of the stimuli given to the subject, and the subject's behavioral button-press responses, are usually recorded by special *trigger channels*.

MEG systems typically include 8–32 independent trigger lines, or bits, which are encoded on one or more trigger channels.

MEG experiments may also involve recording additional signals from the subject such as the gaze direction (provided by an eye tracker), position of fingers or limbs, or speech. These can be acquired using the auxiliary analog inputs provided by most MEG systems.

All the above input signals are usually sampled synchronously at the same sampling rate and stored into a single data file. Common sampling rate usually implies equivalent low-pass or anti-alias filtering of all signal; however, the trigger signals are sampled without filtering. Since filtering involves a delay, the trigger signals must be shifted accordingly in time, or the trigger event timing has to be compensated mathematically off-line to ensure perfect synchronization of all acquired signals.

Acquisition Modes

Raw MEG/EEG signals can be recorded either continuously or as epochs. In the continuous mode, trigger signals are recorded together with MEG/EEG— but triggers do not affect the timing of the recording itself. In the *epoch mode*, the trigger events control the extraction of predefined windows of raw data, and these windows are stored consecutively in the file. The epoch mode yields smaller files, since the uninteresting periods between the events are not stored. However, the discontinuities at the epoch boundaries may give rise to problems when processing the recording.

For evoked response studies, many MEG systems can accumulate the average response in the course of the measurement and provide the operator with a display of the average during data collection. This capability is referred to as *on-line averaging*, and it is useful as a quality assurance method during the measurement, even if an off-line average calculated from the continuous or epoch mode recording would serve as the primary output data.

Figure 2–13 illustrates the three data collection modes described above.

Interference Suppression

As discussed earlier in this chapter, MEG signals are several orders of magnitude weaker than the ambient magnetic noise due to sources like powerlines, electric appliances, and traffic. Detecting MEG signals in a magnetically silent environment is already challenging, and doing it in normal surroundings is even more so. Sufficient suppression of environmental magnetic interference involves a combination of multiple methods. The mostly widely applied techniques are briefly reviewed in this section.

Maqnetically Shielded Rooms

The traditional, and still the most important, means to protect MEG against environmental interference is to employ a passive *magnetically shielded room*.

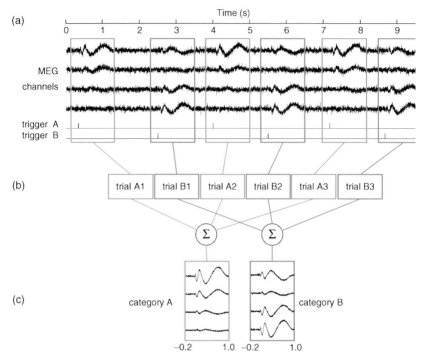

Figure 2–13. Data collection modes provided by MEG systems. The raw MEG/EEG signals can be stored either **(a)** continuously, **(b)** in short windows about a trigger event (epoch mode), or **(c)** as on-line averages. Often the continuous or epoch mode and on-line averaging can be engaged simultaneously. Here, the simulated experiment involves two different stimuli whose onsets are marked by triggers A and B, and accordingly, two sets of average responses are computed.

The shielding properties of such a room at low frequencies are attributable to the high-permeability *mu-metal* (an alloy consisting mostly of nickel and iron) which provides the impinging magnetic field with a low-reluctance path along the walls of the room, thus reducing the field strength within the room. At higher frequencies the shielding relies on the eddy currents flowing in a high-conductivity material, usually aluminium. To allow both shielding methods to work efficiently, the walls are typically made of a combination of mu-metal and aluminium plates (Kelhä et al., 1982).

Practical shielded rooms employ multiple such shells, or layers, to increase the shielding factor, particularly at low frequencies. This effect is evident in Figure 2–14, which illustrates typical shielding factors attained with different constructions of the walls. Most shielded rooms comprise either 2 or 3 shells. Recently, single-shell light-weight shielded rooms, supported by active compensation systems, have been successfully employed with MEG (De Tiège et al., 2008).

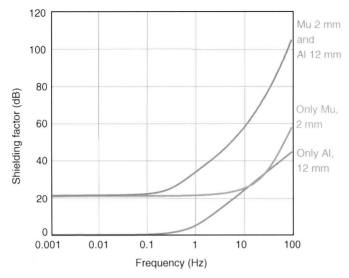

Figure 2–14. Estimated shielding factors as a function of frequency obtained with different shielded room wall structures. Note that mu-metal is exclusively responsible for the shielding at low frequencies whereas aluminum provides good shielding at higher frequencies.
Figure courtesy of Dr. Juha Simola.

The inside dimensions of a shielded room are typically $4 \times 3 \times 2.5$ meters (*length × width × height*). Accounting for the thick walls and the space needed around the room, a standard two-layer room requires at least $15m^2$ of floor space, excluding the space for the electronics, stimulators, patient preparation and operator's area, which all have to be in the immediate vicinity of the shielded room.

Multi-shell rooms are bulky; a two-shell construction weighs typically about 10 tons and three-shell about 15 tons. Therefore, such rooms are usually located in the basement and even then the building floor may require additional reinforcement to support the room. These requirements can be relaxed considerably for the single-shell construction.

Mechanical vibrations of the building (due to traffic, for example) may be transmitted to the room structure and may thus appear as artefactual signals. To prevent such conduction, the shielded room foundations can be isolated from the rest of the building by having the room to rest on its own concrete slab.

Mu-metal is costly; its main ingredient, nickel, is expensive, and so is the complex manufacturing process of high-quality mu-metal sheets. Thus, a shielded room with several tons of mu-metal presents a considerable share of the investment to a new MEG laboratory.

Active Noise Compensation Systems

Passive magnetic shields can be enhanced by active systems that measure the interference field and generate a compensating field to cancel the interference at the location of the MEG system. The typical active compensation system comprises a flux-gate sensor, driver electronics, and pairs of Helmholtz coils outside of the room to supply the cancellation fields. Such a setup can provide 10–30 dB of additional shielding if the interference sources are far away (tens of meters or more), so that their fields are approximately homogeneous at the location of the room. Unfortunately, nearby sources may turn problematic, since proper compensation would require the spatial derivatives of the field to be taken into account. Tuning the setup against a particular nearby source may still give satisfactory results.

Noise Cancellation within MEG Devices

Despite all the effort of suppressing ambient magnetic fields, some residual interference is typically still present within the shielded room. Thus, further noise reduction techniques have to be applied within the MEG systems themselves.

Gradiometrization. As discussed earlier in this chapter, employing gradiometers instead of magnetometers is a straightforward method to protect the MEG sensors from far-away interference sources; a gradiometer's response to a source falls off much faster with distance than that of a magnetometer. A carefully manufactured (well-balanced) gradiometer can attenuate homogeneous fields by as much as 60 dB (factor 1,000). On the other hand, fields from the most distant brain regions are picked up better by magnetometers than gradiometers.

Reference sensor array. Interference can also be measured explicitly and then subtracted from the signals. *Reference sensors* located some tens of centimeters away from the MEG helmet do not measure brain signals, but capture mainly the interference. By optimally coupling the output of the reference-sensor array to the MEG channels proper, the interfering signal can be removed. This arrangement works well with homogeneous interference field; however, the presence of gradients may degrade the performance, as the interference at the helmet must be extrapolated from the measurements at the reference sensors. For this purpose, the reference sensor arrays usually include both magnetometers and gradiometers. The reference-sensor approach can also be considered as a higher-order gradiometrization (Vrba & Robinson, 2001).

The optimal couplings ("weights") from the reference sensors to the MEG sensors can be determined either by direct calculation, if the geometry is known to a high precision, or adaptively from real measurements of external interference by the same array.

When performing correlation or coherence analysis of MEG data, it should be noted that the couplings to the reference sensors may introduce spurious correlations between the MEG channels, if not explicitly addressed.

Signal-space projection. Interference can also be suppressed without a reference-sensor array by exploiting the fact that external interference and brain sources evoke different spatial patterns on the sensor helmet. The benefit of this reference-free approach is that no extrapolation is required, since the interference is measured at the very location it should be suppressed. To understand this approach, the concept of signal space comes in handy; each channel spans one dimension of that virtual space. Thus, the output of an n-channel sensor array at any time instant can be expressed as a vector, or a point, in the n-dimensional signal space. The spatial pattern is equal to the direction of the corresponding vector in the signal space, while the overall strength of the signal defines the length of that vector, or distance from the origin. If the interference subspace is known, the measurement data can be projected onto a hyperplane orthogonal to that subspace, thus completely removing the contribution of the unwanted subspace; the method is called *signal-space projection* (SSP) (Uusitalo and Ilmoniemi, 1997; Parkkonen et al., 1999). An analogous situation arises when taking a 2D picture of a 3D object (a 3-channel "measurement") at such an angle that, say, the depth of the object (the "interference direction") is completely hidden.

Projected data are rank-deficient, i.e., after projecting out an m-dimensional subspace from an n-channel measurement, there are only $n - m$ linearly independent signals, or equivalently, degrees of freedom. Since m is usually only 3–8 and $n > 100$, the mere loss of degrees of freedom is not a problem as such, but to correctly interpret the spatial aspect of projected data, the SSP operator should be taken into account. For example, SSP may introduce slight changes in the signal topography. In source modeling, the projection operator has to be applied also to the result of the forward computation (see Chapter 5) to ensure unbiased estimation.

The interference subspace is usually determined by principal component analysis (PCA) of a short measurement without a subject. Selecting 3–5 components associated with the highest eigenvalues for the subspace typically reduces the variance of the interference down to acceptable levels. Such subspaces appear very stable over time, even months or years, provided that the magnetic environment does not change drastically.

Signal-space separation. Instead of determining the interference subspace statistically, the known physical properties of magnetic fields — expressed in Maxwell's famous equations — can be exploited to mathematically construct the subspace where all signals due to sources external to the sensor helmet must reside. Similarly, another subspace can be spanned for all signals whose sources are inside the sensor helmet. These two subspaces are linearly independent thus providing a unique way of separating the measured data to contributions from outside and inside of the sensor helmet. Interference suppression can now be performed simply by dropping out the outside contribution. This recent method is called *signal-space separation* (SSS) (Taulu et al., 2004, Taulu & Kajola, 2005).

The SSS subspaces are derived from series of spherical harmonic functions. In the SSS framwork, the data are first expressed as two multipole expansions, one for the inside and the other for the outside contribution, in the spherical harmonic spaces. Subsequently, the sensor-level data are reconstructed using only the inside expansion. Both series are truncated to stay within the limits imposed by the number of channels in the system; the inside expansion typically corresponds to about 100 degrees of freedom.

The SSS method is data-independent and time-invariant, however, it does require precise information on the geometry of the sensor array; with 0.1 percent calibration accuracy, the shielding provided by SSS is roughly 40 dB.

Co-registration

The MEG source estimate, i.e., the estimated spatial distribution of the neural (primary) currents given the MEG measurements, is usually visualized superimposed on the anatomical MR-image of the subject. In addition, the estimate can be mapped into a normalized space, such as Talairach, the Montreal Neurological Institute (MNI) standard brain, or other atlas brains; see, e.g., Fischl et al. (1999); Mazziotta et al. (2001); Van Essen (2005); Toga et al. (2006). On the other hand, the MEG measurements are taken at locations known only with respect to the MEG device itself, instead of the anatomy of the subject. For subjects with smaller heads, the MEG helmet typically allows for head movements as large as a few centimeters; not knowing the head position within the sensor array would lead to drastic errors when superposing the MEG sources onto an individual anatomical MRI. Therefore, MEG devices include a subsystem to determine the position of the head with respect to the MEG sensors.

Since MEG — unlike MRI — cannot directly measure the position of the head, small coils generating magnetic fields at known locations on the scalp of the subject are employed in the *head position measurement*. When the coils are energized, the MEG sensor array can be used to localize the coils, just like it is used to localize neural currents in the brain. If we could place the coils at anatomical locations that are accurately identifiable on anatomical MRIs, this step would be sufficient to provide us with a coordinate transformation between the *MEG device coordinate system* and the *MRI device coordinate system*. Unfortunately, such anatomical locations are either not covered by the MEG sensor array (nasion and the tip of the nose) or they are inconvenient as coil locations (preauricular points). This necessitates the definition and use of a *head coordinate system*, which is based on landmarks identifiable accurately both in the MRIs and on the real head. By measuring the coil locations in the head coordinate system with a 3D digitizer, and combining that information with the locations of the coils in the MEG device coordinate system, we are able to bridge the gap between the MEG and MRI device coordinate systems and thus to translate MEG results onto the MRI space.

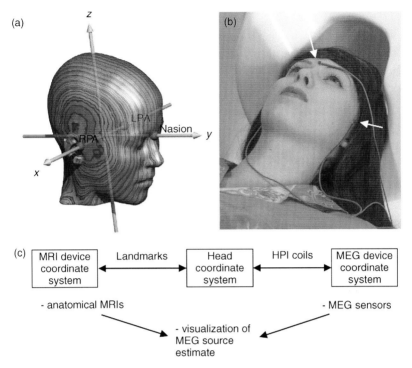

Figure 2–15. **(a)** One definition of an orthonormal right-handed head coordinate system; x-axis passes through both left (LPA) and right (RPA) preauricular points and points to the right, y-axis intersects x-axis at a right angle and passes through nasion, and z-axis is normal to the xy-plane and points upwards (the Elekta-Neuromag convention; other MEG vendors have different systems, albeit based on the same landmarks). **(b)** Three head-position indicator coils attached to the head of the subject. Note that the coils do not correspond to the landmarks, and thus the coil locations must be digitized prior to the head position measurement in the MEG system. **(c)** The relevant coordinate systems and the ways to move between them.
3D rendering courtesy of Dr. Mika Seppä

Within the MEG system, the head position is determined by feeding small currents through the 3–5 indicator coils either sequentially or simultaneously at different frequencies, measuring the elicited magnetic fields and then estimating the coil locations. This procedure is usually carried out in the beginning of each recording block, during which the position of the head is assumed to be stable.

With some subject groups, most notably children, the assumption of a stable head position (within a few millimeters) for longer than some seconds is not necessarily valid. Continuous head position tracking should be used in these cases.

Safety

MEG is inherently very safe; it measures magnetic fields that are always present outside of the head, and does not employ high magnetic fields, as does (f)MRI, or radioactive tracers, as does PET. The only safety concern is liquid helium, utilized as a coolant for the superconducting parts of the MEG system. Helium is nontoxic and nonflammable but may replace oxygen when present in the air in large quantities. Helium gas is lighter than air, so it concentrates at the ceiling level. Liquid helium may also cause severe frostbites because of its very low temperature.

During normal operation, the helium gas evaporating inside the MEG Dewar is fed outside through an exhaust line. Should this line be blocked, the pressure inside the Dewar starts to rise gradually. To prevent the system from eventually exploding, the Dewars are fitted with safety valves that let out the excess gas by releasing it to the air inside the shielded room. Therefore, the shielded room must have proper ventilation, arranged in such a way that the air outlet is near the ceiling.

A sudden loss of the vacuum isolation of the MEG Dewar leads to a rapid boil-off of liquid helium. Since one liter of liquid helium expands to about 750 liters of gas at room temperature and normal atmospheric pressure, many of the MEG Dewars are equipped with a high-capacity safety exhaust line to provide a low backpressure path to the outside air.

Stimulators

Most MEG measurements involve stimulation of the subject by, e.g., sounds, touch, images, video clips, or their combinations. Delivering stimuli without interferring with the MEG signals is often challenging, as many conventional devices that could be used for generating the required sensory input also produce unwanted magnetic signals that are picked up by the MEG. In addition, stimulus delivery should be temporally precise; sloppy timing yields smeared responses, particularly in the primary sensory areas. The following sections describe the principles of MEG compatibility and highlight the most commonly employed stimulation setups for MEG. Developing, selecting and applying stimulators is a large undertaking; this section is merely an brief introduction.

Electromagnetic Compatibility

An MEG recording may suffer from interference of several kinds: magnetic materials, electric currents and radio-frequency signals can all disturb the MEG recordings. The next paragraphs address these issues in more detail.

Magnetic material that moves within the shielded room naturally interferes with the recording. The level of such interference depends on the distance to the MEG sensors, on the amplitude of the movement, and on the magnetization of that moving object. Even though, in theory, perfectly stable yet magnetic objects would not interfere, it is often exceedingly difficult to immobilize them so that no interference would be seen. Particularly the devices in contact with the subject do always move due to breathing and pulsation, not to mention normal muscular movements. Even if magnetic objects are only on the floor of the shielded room, the minute vibrations or bending of the floor may be sufficient to generate observable interference. Thus, to be on the safe side, devices within the shielded room should be made of nonmagnetic materials. In practice, few materials are strictly nonmagnetic. Testing for sufficiently low magnetism is fortunately straightforward with the MEG system itself: the material to be tested is periodically moved back and forth with an amplitude of a couple of centimeters, and slowly brought from a distance toward the MEG sensor helmet while someone else is watching the MEG traces for periodic deflections that clearly exceed the background fluctuations. Commonly used nonmagnetic materials include aluminum, brass, copper, silver, gold, high-quality stainless steel, rubber, glass, wood, and many plastics. Even these should be tested with the above procedure since some samples may contain magnetic impurities, and certain coloring agents are magnetic. When constructing or using electronic devices, it should be noted that the commonly used gold-plated electrical connector pins typically include a layer of nickel, which is strongly magnetic.

Currents in electric devices generate magnetic fields around them, just like the very weak currents in neurons. The strength of the field due to a current is directly proportional to the strength of the current and to the surface area of the current loop. Therefore, to minimize the interference, the currents must be kept as low as possible and the current loops as small as possible. Accurate analysis of the current path may be elaborate, but observing the following guidelines should yield satisfactory results: (i) circuits should be powered with a single cable where the feed and return wires are carefully twisted around each other for the entire length of the cable to ensure that the net surface area of the loop is close to zero; (ii) circuits and devices should be grounded only at a single point, and the ground connections should form a star-like structure, thus preventing the formation of accidental "ground loops," which can be large and thus give rise to significant stray field; (iii) the current path and consumption should be as constant as possible, so that if a measurable field is generated it is only a DC field that can easily be compensated for; and (iv) the signal input/output connection should carry only a very low current (a balanced differential line is optimal) to avoid loops formed by the power-feed and signal-output wires.

As mentioned earlier, external radio-frequency (RF) signals may interfere with the operation of a SQUID. RF signals decrease the modulation depth, increase the white noise level, and may introduce a DC shift in the output signal. Many modern stimulators include digital circuitry that operates at relatively high frequencies, and unfortunately these devices often emit spurious RF noise. The regulatory directives that govern the level of these emissions are not strict enough for MEG compatibility, and thus a fully compliant device may still be unusable with MEG. Even if the generator of RF signals, e.g., a cell phone, is outside of the shielded room, directly or indirectly (capacitively or inductively) coupled wires may act as antennas and carry the unwanted interference into the room. Therefore, all cables entering the shielded room should be properly low-pass-filtered at the feedthrough to remove any RF contamination. Omitting feedthrough filtering may result in a setup that works most of the time if the environment is relatively RF-free, but exhibits spurious artifacts when RF sources happen to be in the vicinity.

Timing

MEG is a time-sensitive method; it allows tracking the neural responses down to millisecond timescales. The latencies of the early responses from, e.g., primary sensory regions, are rather constant across healthy individuals—however, such measures are of diagnostic value only if the stimulus timing is known with adequate precision, typically within a millisecond. Trigger-to-stimulus timing can be broken into two components: a constant delay between a trigger signal and the actual physical delivery of the stimulus, and a random, or at least uncontrollable, variation of that delay about the average value, also known as jitter. A constant delay can be readily compensated for, and generally does not compromise the quality of the MEG data in any way, whereas jitter destroys the fine details and reduces the amplitude of the response; see Figure 2–16. Note that this stimulus vs. trigger jitter should not be confused with the sometimes desirable random variation of the interstimulus intervals.

The timing errors are most often attributable to the stimulus generator, nowadays often a PC running special software. The PCs with standard operating systems are not hard realtime devices, and thus there is no way to guarantee that the stimulus and the corresponding trigger pulse are both sent out at any precise moment in time. With fMRI, the requirements for timing accuracy are not so demanding; a system targeted for fMRI might not be accurate enough for MEG and EEG. Usually the only way to verify the timing — and to record the trigger-to-stimulus delay — is to measure it with an additional device that generates a trigger pulse when a sound (recorded by a microphone) or an image (captured by a photodetector on the screen) is received.

Auditory

The quality of an auditory stimulation system is characterized by its frequency response, distortion level, channel separation (crosstalk), dynamic range, accuracy of loudness control, and maximum distortion-free sound pressure level. The experiment at hand sets the standard: a moderate-quality system serves well in studies concerning, e.g., the processing of semantics of spoken language, while a high-fidelity system is needed for studying the auditory system *per se*.

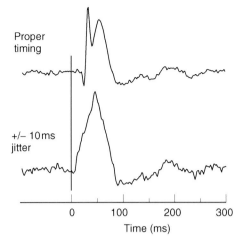

Figure 2–16. Demonstration of the stimulus-to-trigger timing accuracy; the evoked response to electric median nerve stimulation with precise timing (upper curve) and with uniformly distributed timing jitter upto ±10 ms (lower curve). The jitter abolishes the fast components of the response.

Normal loudspeaker—comprising a permanent magnet, a voice coil and a cone—cannot be operated within the shielded room without interferring with the MEG recording. Therefore, a common setup is to have the loud-speakers outside of the room and convey the sound to the ears of the subject via plastic tubes. With large-diameter tubes, their proper matching to the driver elements, and an equalization unit, it is possible to achieve relatively high sound quality. The downside of this approach is the clumsiness of the tubes and the necessity to wear earpieces.

Electrostatic loudspeaker elements, if not located in the very vicinity of the sensors, do not interfere with MEG, as the drive currents are rather low and no magnets are involved. A properly directed electrostatic element, mounted on the wall of the shielded room, provides a good-quality binaural auditory stimulus. The lack of monaural or stereo stimulation and attenuation of background noise limits the applicability of this setup. On the other hand, many studies utilize only binaural stimulation, and the shorter setup time and increased comfort due to the subject not having to wear earpieces should not be overlooked.

Insert earphones (e.g. "EAR-Tone" by Etymotic Research Inc., IL, USA) are commonly utilized with MEG. They comprise a small driver unit, thin plastic (often silicon) tubing and an earplug. The frequency response of the insert earphones is typically limited to 4–5 kHz, but they allow stimulating the ears independently and are relatively convenient to use. The driver unit may emit magnetic interference at the stimulus frequency; thus, particularly with stimuli that contain low-frequency components, one should ensure that the units are sufficiently far from MEG sensors to avoid artifactual responses.

It is often desirable to present the stimuli at a certain level with respect to the hearing threshold, say at 60 dB-SL[4], to reduce the response variability due to differences in stimulation. Since hearing thresholds vary across people, and the seating of the earpiece affects the conduction of the sound wave to the ear (Saunders & Morgan, 2003), the threshold should preferably be measured with the same stimulation setup and in the same session as the actual MEG data.

Visual

The MEG environment is challenging also for presenting high-quality visual stimuli interference-free. The de facto standard is a setup where a video projector, located outside of the shielded room, beams through an opening in the wall to a semitransparent back-projection screen in front of the subject. With the projector at an appropriate location, direct projection to the screen usually works for seated subjects, whereas mirrors might be required for the supine position of the subject.

The whole setup should be considered for parameters such as luminance, contrast, geometric fidelity and the available range of visual angles. The projector determines most of the other parameters: resolution, temporal synchronization (delay + jitter, if any), response time and its symmetry, linearity, the depth and temporal simultaneity of color reproduction. Again, the required fidelity of the image or video reproduction depends on the experiment: a high-quality system is required for studying certain aspects of the early visual cortices while a moderate system may suffice for other purposes. One should be aware that the projector types on the market behave quite differently in many important respects: LCD (Liquid Crystal Display) projectors may exhibit asymmetric black/white/black transition times and colors may not be drawn simultaneously, which, although not usually perceived, can alter responses from the visual system. DLP (Digital Light Processing, arrays of micro-mirrors whose angle can be controlled electronically) projectors often have better contrast and symmetric transition times. The more expensive models feature separate DLP units for the main colors, thus allowing them to be drawn simultaneously.

The light bulbs in the projectors wear out, and the luminance drops accordingly (in some cases by as much as 50%). For experiments where the absolute illumination matters, it is thus important to regularly measure the luminance on the projection screen.

Most, if not all, video projectors keep at least one full image frame in an internal buffer before showing it, which corresponds to a constant delay (the duration of one frame is 16.7 ms at the 60-Hz refresh rate). Projectors draw the frames usually at few fixed rates, typically only at 50 or 60 frames per second. When driving a projector at a higher rate, it may adapt by simply dropping out a frame every now and then. This coarse downsampling gives rise to jittering on top of the constant delay. This jitter cannot be compensated for, except by triggering each trial by measuring the stimulus onset directly on the screen with a photodetector. Note that this elaborate arrangement is not required to remove the effect of a constant delay, yet it is always worthwhile to verify with a photodetector that a new setup (including the stimulation software, graphics hardware and driver, video projector and the employed resolution and refresh rate) works flawlessly.

Somatosensory

The human somatosensory system can be stimulated peripherally and noninvasively by touching the skin mechanically, by heating and cooling, and by applying brief electric pulses to directly activate a nerve.

Tactile stimuli are usually delivered by feeding pressurized air either directly to skin or to a small container with an elastic membrane in contact with the skin. Such pneumatic devices come with multiple channels to stimulate, e.g., fingertips independently. Due to the dispersion of the pressure wave, these stimuli have significant rise and fall times (on the order of 20 ms). A bundle of optic fibers shaped in the form of a brush can also be used as a tactile stimulator; the light reflected from the skin when tapping it with the brush is utilized to obtain accurate timing information (Jousmäki et al., 2007).

The skin can be heated locally by a laser beam, which provides a way for controlled pain stimulation. Such stimulation yields a sensation of mild pricking pain.

Sensory nerves can also be stimulated directly; electric pulses applied via cutaneous electrodes trigger action potentials in the nerve fiber. The applied pulses are very brief, typically 100–200 μs. Stimulators can operate either by keeping the current or the voltage constant. Since the constant current drive is less affected by changes in the electrode impedance, it is more widely used. When stimulating the median nerve at the wrist, the current at the motor threshold is typically 5–10 mA.

Since nerve stimulators are electrically connected to the subject, they have to include an isolation system to protect the subject in case of a potentially lethal failure in any electric system that could be in contact with the subject. This isolation can be achieved either optically or by a transformer. Optical isolation is always MEG-compatible but the transformer isolation, in some devices, employs RF pulses that severely contaminate the MEG signals. Irrespective of the isolation type, the stimulator should be kept outside of the shielded room and only the electrode leads should enter the room. Unfortunately, normal feedthrough filtering is difficult to arrange to comply with the regulations on the protective isolation. Therefore, an RF-shielded enclosure with a direct feed-in to the shielded room is the preferred location for such a stimulator.

Other Modalities

Auditory, visual and somatosensory stimulation covers almost all MEG experiments. Yet, there is room for studies concerning the olfactory, gustatory and proprioceptive systems, for example. Commercial stimulators for these modalities are scarce, and even more so when considering only MEG-compatible devices. Thus, these stimulators are often developed in the MEG laboratories.

Recording Behavioral Responses

In many experiments, in addition to MEG data, behavioral responses are of interest. Certain paradigms, e.g., recording motor-evoked fields or responses related to speech production, rely on behavioral responses for timing the averaging of MEG data.

Normal response buttons can be used with MEG, provided that they are nonmagnetic and that their operation is silent to avoid confounding auditory responses due to the button presses. Optical switches, in which a light beam is interrupted by the finger press, are well-suited for this task. The light source and detector, connected to the switch by optic fibers, can be placed outside of the shielded room. Nonmagnetic electric switches can also be employed, provided that the associated cabling is appropriately filtered for no RF leakage.

The onset of speech can be recorded with a microphone and preamplifier whose output is either directly fed to an auxiliary analog input available in most MEG systems, or to a trigger input, after thresholding it to a binary signal ("speech on" vs. "speech off").

Preprocessing

Signal-to Noise Ratio and Averaging

The MEG signal amplitude is affected by several factors: the extend of the activated area, the level of neuronal synchrony, the anatomical location and orientation of the source, and cancellation effects due to opposing coincident nearby activations. Signal amplitude may also change due to medication and pathologies. Therefore, MEG response amplitudes span a wide range, from few femtotesla to a picotesla.

Noise from several sources hampers MEG. Brain activity not of interest ("brain noise"), biological noise from sources other than the brain, instrumentation and ambient magnetic interference, all contribute to the noise seen in MEG recordings. The relative strengths of these sources depend on the frequency: in rough terms, at the lowest frequencies (below 1 Hz) the ambient and biological noise are usually most prominent; the mid-frequency band (1–100 Hz) is dominated by brain noise (except at the line frequency of 50/60 Hz), and at higher frequencies most of the noise originates in the MEG instrument itself.

Single evoked responses often have a poor signal-to-noise ratio (SNR), on the order of one. To improve the SNR to allow, e.g., accurate detection and localization of the underlying sources, multiple responses can be averaged. Averaging reduces the noise as $1/\sqrt{N}$, where N is the number of averaged trials, provided that the noise in the data is temporally uncorrelated from trial to trial. Figure 2–17 illustrates the improvement in SNR due to averaging. Since the response amplitude often decreases with frequent presentations of the same stimulus, and biological noise may increase with a prolonged mea-surement (frequent eye blinks, muscle artifacts due to neck tension etc.), the SNR improvement in practice is somewhat worse than predicted by the formula above. See Chapter 4 for more information.

Averaging can also be done in the spatial domain: signals at neighboring channels can be added together, often after squaring to avoid cancellation due to field sign changes, to gain in SNR by trading off spatial resolution. This approach is well-suited when accurate localization is not the main point in the analysis.

Filtering

Signal-to-noise ratio of MEG data can be improved also by limiting the window of frequencies so that only the band where the response's energy lies is retained. This operation is *filtering*, also referred to as *time-domain* or *temporal* filtering in order not to confuse it with *spatial filtering*.

To understand how filtering may reduce the noise level, a simple example comes in handy: If the noise spectrum can be assumed white,[5] the RMS (root-mean-square) amplitude of noise $n = B_n \sqrt{\Delta f}$ where B_n is the spectral density of noise and Δf is the bandwidth. For example, if the white noise level $B_n = 5\text{fT}/\text{cm}/\sqrt{\text{Hz}}$ and the pass-band is 0–100 Hz thus $\Delta f = 100$ Hz, the observed noise amplitude $n = 50$ fT/cm$_{RMS}$. If we know that the responses of interest are confined to 0–25 Hz and we filter the data accordingly, the noise

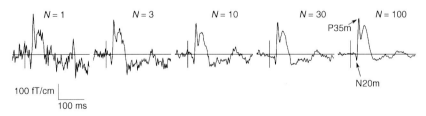

100 fT/cm

100 ms

Figure 2–17. Averaging somatosensory evoked fields. Single planar gradio-meter channel above the S1 hand region shown. *N* refers to the number of trials averaged. The responses are elicited by electric stimulation of the median nerve at the wrist of a healthy adult. Note that the earli-est responses (N20m and P35m) are apparent already in the single trial response, and that their amplitudes decrease slightly when more trials are presented.

amplitude drops to 25 fT/cm$_{RMS}$, i.e., to one half. Here, the gain in SNR achieved by filtering is equivalent to prolonging the experiment fourfold.

Some responses have lower- and higher-frequency components which can be separated by filtering. The somatosensory response of the previous example (Figure 2–17), if measured with a wide enough pass band, comprises the traditional low-frequency responses and a high-frequency burst-like response around 600 Hz, which react to experimental manipulations differently and likely reflect partially different neural events (Curio, 2000; Hashimoto, 2000; Okada et al., 2005). Figure 2–18 shows such an average response and its low- and high-frequency components.

Low-pass filters limit the frequency band at its upper end, i.e., attenuate all frequencies above their *corner frequency*, usually denoted as the frequency at which the filter drops the signal amplitude by 3 dB (to 71 percent), assuming unity gain at DC. Similarly, *high-pass filters* remove the frequency components below their corner frequency. These two types can be combined into a *bandpass filter*. Conversely, a contiguous range of frequencies can be removed by a *band-stop filter*, and when this range is very narrow the filter is often called a *notch filter* as it has a "notch" in the frequency response. Regularly-spaced notch filters form a *comb filter*, which is useful in removing a signal with a harmonic structure, e.g., the line frequency with the fundamental at 50/60-Hz and its harmonics (100/120 Hz, 150/180 Hz, etc.).

No filter has an infinitely steep transition from the pass-band to the stop-band but filters rather exhibit a certain roll-off rate, often expressed as dB per octave (doubling of the frequency). This value is influenced mostly by the *order* of the filter; the attenuation of a 2nd-order low-pass filter typically

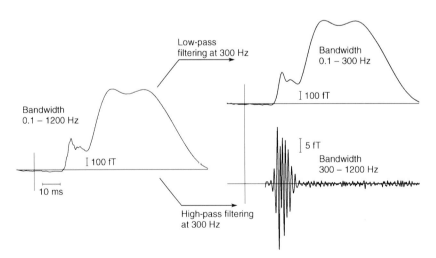

Figure 2–18. Separating the low- and high-frequency components of somatosensory evoked responses to electric median nerve stimulation.

increases 12 dB/octave, whereas that of an otherwise similar but 6th-order filter increases 36 dB/octave.

The above simple characterization does not describe any filter fully: in addition to the *amplitude response*, the filter has a *phase response* that indicates how the filter changes the phase of the signal as a function of frequency. Here, filter design becomes relevant: a *Bessel* filter has a maximally linear phase response but less attenuation, whereas a *Chebyshev* filter is optimized for maximum attenuation but trades off the linear phase response. A *Butterworth* is a good compromise of the two. All these filters can be implemented either as analog electronic circuits, or digitally on a signal processor or computer. In the digital domain, these "analog" filters are often referred to as *infinite impulse response*, or IIR, filters as their output would (in theory) last infinitely long for a delta spike at the input. Both the analog and digital versions are *causal*, that is, the output of the filter depends only on the past input.

In addition to the above filters, digital systems allow implementing filters that would be very cumbersome to build in the analog world. *Finite impulse response* filters have guaranteed zero output in a certain time after applying a delta impulse at the input. FIR filters feature linear phase response and they are inherently stable; both very desirable properties. A close relative is *a frequency-domain filter*, also referred to as an FFT (fast Fourier transform) filter, which realizes the filter function by transforming the input signal to the frequency domain, shaping the complex-valued spectra by the desired filter response, and then performing an inverse Fourier transform to provide the filtered time-domain signal. FFT filters process a short segment of the signal at a time, and the frequency-shaping is bounded by the length of the window; for high-pass filters the segment has to be long enough to capture the corner frequency.

FIR and FFT filters can be *acausal*: the output depends not only on the previous input but also on the future input. This somewhat counterintuitive concept simply means that the filter keeps the input signal in memory for a certain duration, and uses the prior and subsequent values to compute the filtered output value, which enables desirable features such as a linear phase response. Unfortunately, there is a price to pay: acausal high-pass filters can generate artifacts. For example, when high-pass-filtering an evoked response at a corner frequency which is higher than the lowest frequency component of the response itself, a fake response may emerge before the actual one, as the filter removes frequency components that are required to confine the response in time.

Suppressing Residual Interference

Despite the suppression systems outlined previously, unwanted signals may still remain in the measured MEG data, either due to their high amplitude (the attenuation provided by suppression methods is always limited) or due to their spatial distribution being generally indistinguishable from that of brain activity. If this residual interference occupies the same frequency range as the brain responses of interest, the simple time-domain filtering cannot be used to remove the interference. However, exploiting the statistical and spatial properties of the interference can still provide a way to clean the data.

Independent component analysis (ICA) is a blind source separation method that seeks for directions in the signal space that are maximally independent in the statistical sense, and expresses the data along these directions; see, e.g., Hyvärinen and Oja (2000) for a thorough description of ICA and its implementations. Since artifactual signals are most often independent of brain activity, ICA suits the task very well (Vigário et al., 2000): however, ICA relies on the user to classify the obtained independent components to reflect either artifacts or brain activity.

If there is *a priori* information about the artifact, the suppression method can take advantage of it. Knowing the precise timing (or determining it from the data if possible) of spatially similar, repeating events—e.g., the magnetic artefact due to a heartbeat—allows us to average several such events for a better signal-to-noise ratio of the artifact itself, and thus obtain its spatial pattern on the sensor array. Once the pattern is known, it can be removed from the data by signal-space projection (see earlier discussion). If the pattern is not stable but undergoes a stereotypical sequence, principal component analysis (PCA) can be employed to extract a small set of patterns from the "artifact average" to be removed from the data.

Within the signal-space separation framework, many artifactual signals can be detected as temporal correlations between the inside and outside spaces. If high correlations are found, the corresponding interference can be removed by projection (Taulu and Simola, 2006); this method is known as temporal signal-space separation, or tSSS.

Notes

1 Wavefunction in quantum mechanics gives the probability of finding the particle at a certain location in space.

2 In some MEG systems the sensor coils are located in the vacuum space and they are thermally linked to the inner vessel.

3 An experimental MEG system by Volegov and colleagues (2004) employs a superconducting magnetic shield inside the Dewar to provide high attenuation towards external interference fields, and to act as a "magnetic mirror" which turns magnetometers into axial gradiometers.

4 Sensation level: decibels with respect to the individually-determined hearing threshold.

5 In a white signal, the spectral density is the same at all frequencies, i.e., the spectrum is "flat." The term is analoguous to white light, which contains all visible wavelengths.

References

Ahonen, A. I., Hämäläinen, M. S., Ilmoniemi, R. J., Kajola, M. J., Knuutila, J. E., Simola, J. T., et al. (1993a). Sampling theory for neuromagnetic detector arrays. *IEEE Trans Biomed Eng, 40*(9), 859–869.

Ahonen, A. I., Hämäläinen, M. S., Kajola, M. J., Knuutila, J. E., Laine, P. P., Lounasmaa, O. V., et al. (1993b). 122-Channel SQUID Instrument for Investigating the Magnetic Signals from the Human Brain. *Physica Scripta T49*, 198–205.

Bardeen, J., Cooper, L. N., & Schrieffer, J. R. (1957). Theory of Superconductivity. *Phys Rev, 108*, 1175–1204.

Berger, H. (1929). Uber das Elektroenkephalogramm des Menschen. *Archiv für Psychiatrie und Nervenkrankheiten, 87*, 527–570.

Clarke, J. & Braginski, A. I. (2004). *The SQUID Handbook: Fundamentals and Technology of SQUIDs and SQUID Systems*, (1st ed.) Berlin: Wiley-VCH.

Cohen, D. (1972). Magnetoencephalography: Detection of the Brain's Electrical Activity with a Superconducting Magnetometer. *Science, 175*, 664–666.

Curio, G. (2000). Linking 600-Hz "spikelike" EEG/MEG wavelets ("sigma-bursts") to cellular substrates: concepts and caveats. *J Clin Neurophysiol, 17*(4), 377–396.

De Tiège, X., Op de Beeck, M., Funke, M., Legros, B., Parkkonen, L., Goldman, S., et al. (2008). Recording epileptic activity with MEG in a light-weight magnetic shield. *Epilepsy Res, 82*(2-3), 227–231.

Fischl, B., Sereno, M. I., Tootell, R. B., & Dale, A. M. (1999). High-resolution intersubject averaging and a coordinate system for the cortical surface. *Hum Brain Mapp, 8*(4), 272–284.

Hashimoto, I. (2000). High-frequency oscillations of somatosensory evoked potentials and fields. *J Clin Neurophysiol, 17*(3), 309–320.

Hyvärinen, A. & Oja, E. (2000). Independent component analysis: algorithms and applications. *Neural Netw, 13*(4-5), 411–430.

Hämäläinen, M., Hari, R., Ilmoniemi, R. J., Knuutila, J. & Lounasmaa, O. V. (1993). Magnetoencephalography: theory, instrumentation, and applications to noninvasive studies of the working human brain. *Rev Mod Phys, 65*, 413–497.

Josephson, B. D. (1962). Possible New Effects in Superconductive Tunnelling. *Phys Lett, 1*(7), 251–253.

Jousmäki, V., Nishitani, N., & Hari, R. (2007). A brush stimulator for functional brain imaging. *Clin Neurophysiol, 118*(12), 2620–2624.

Kelhä, V. O., Pukki, J. M., Peltonen, R. S., Penttinen, A.J., Ilmoniemi, R. J., & Heino, J. J. (1982). Design, Construction, and Performance of a Large-Volume Magnetic Shield. *IEEE Trans Magn, MAG-18*(1), 260–270.

Mazziotta, J., Toga, A., Evans, A., Fox, P., Lancaster, J., Zilles, K., et al. (2001). A probabilistic atlas and reference system for the human brain: International Consortium for Brain Mapping (ICBM). *Philos Trans R Soc Lond B Biol Sci, 356*(1412), 1293–1322.

Okada, Y., Ikeda, I., Zhang, T., & Wang, Y. (2005). High-frequency signals (> 400 Hz): a new window in electrophysiological analysis of the somatosensory system. *Clin EEG Neurosci, 36*(4), 285–292.

Parkkonen, L., Simola, J. T, Tuoriniemi, J. T., & Ahonen, A. I. (1999). An Interference Suppression System for Multichannel Magnetic Field Detector Arrays. In: *Proc. 11th Intl. Conf. on Biomagnetism*, pp. 13–16. Sendai, Japan: Tohoku University Press.

Saunders, G. H., & Morgan, D. E. (2003). Impact on hearing aid targets of measuring thresholds in dB HL versus dB SPL. *Int J Audiol*, *42*(6), 319–326.

Seppä, H., Ahonen, A., Knuutila, J., Simola, J., & Vilkman, V. (1991). DC-SQUID Electronics Based on Adaptive Positive Feedback: Experiments. *IEEE Trans Magn*, *27*(2), 2488–2490.

Taulu, S., Kajola, M., & Simola, J. (2004). Suppression of interference and artifacts by the Signal Space Separation Method. *Brain Topogr*, *16*(4), 269-275.

Taulu, S., & Kajola, M. (2005). Presentation of electromagnetic multichannel data: The signal space separation method. *J Appl Phys*, *97*(12), 124905–124910.

Taulu, S., & Simola, J. (2006). Spatiotemporal signal space separation method for rejecting nearby interference in MEG measurements. *Phys Med Biol*, *51*(7), 1759–1768.

Toga, A.W., Thompson, P. M., Mori, S., Amunts, K., & Zilles, K. (2006). Towards multimodal atlases of the human brain. *Nat Rev Neurosci 7*(12), 952–966.

Uusitalo, M., & Ilmoniemi, R. (1997). Signal-space projection method for separating MEG or EEG into components. *Med Biol Eng Comput 35*(2), 135–140.

Van Essen, D. C. (2005). A Population-Average, Landmark- and Surface-based (PALS) atlas of human cerebral cortex. *Neuroimage*, *28*(3), 635–662.

Vigário, R., Särelä, J., Jousmäki V., Hämäläinen, M., & Oja, E. (2000). Independent component approach to the analysis of EEG and MEG recordings. *IEEE Trans Biomed Eng 47*(5), 589–593.

Volegov, P., Matlachov, A., Mosher, J., Espy, M. A., & Kraus, R. H. (2004). Noisefree magnetoencephalography recordings of brain function. *Phys Med Biol*, *49*(10), 2117–2128.

Vrba, J., & Robinson, S. E. (2001). Signal processing in magnetoencephalography. *Methods*, *25*(2), 249–271.

Zimmerman, J.E., Thiene, P., & Harding, J. T. (1970). Design and Operation of Stable rf-Biased Superconducting Point-Contact Quantum Devices and a Note on the Properties of Perfectly Clean Metal Contacts. *J Appl Phys*, *41*(4), 1572–1580.

3

Measurements

Lauri Parkkonen and Riitta Salmelin

- A careful measurement and a good experimental design are the keys to good-quality data
- Interfering signals may arise from the subject, environment, or the measurement setup; the sources should be identified and removed if possible
- Results of MEG measurements replicate accurately even within single subjects

Introduction

Running successful MEG measurements requires not only understanding the principles of MEG but also mastering various practical points which impact the quality of the acquired data. Investing time and effort in the MEG recordings most often pays off; nothing facilitates data analysis more than a well-planned experiment and good-quality data.

This chapter addresses the practical issues encountered when conducting MEG measurements.

Quality Assurance

The MEG environment and the system may change over time. New interference sources (magnetic or radio frequency), flux traps in the MEG sensors, incorrect or suboptimal settings of the MEG system or stimulators etc. may all reduce the amount of useful information in the MEG recordings. Equipment may also malfunction. In the worst case, such degradations could hamper the detection and localization of neural sources.

Quality assurance measures are thus recommended. A typical procedure comprises (i) noise measurements without a subject — "empty room measurements" — to spot changes in the magnetic environment or MEG sensors, (ii) verification of the localization accuracy with the help of a phantom head that includes current sources, and (iii) checking the proper operation of the stimulus delivery system. Quality assurance checks can be done on a daily or weekly basis depending on the usage of the system and the risk factors involved.

Monitoring the data quality should eventually save time by allowing the experimenter to concentrate on the particulars of the experiment instead of the system and setup. Sometimes it may be difficult to tell whether data are compromised because of interference from the subject or from the environment or the system itself; having a recent "fingerprint" of the signals without the contribution from a subject helps to resolve these cases. Similarly, an apparently incorrect source localization cannot necessarily be traced to any particular device or procedural step if regular checks are not performed.

In addition to periodic quality assurance measurements, it is good practice, prior to each MEG experiment and before bringing in the subject, to reserve ample time to check that all the hardware and software components are fully functional. A test run of the MEG data acquisition also provides an opportunity to record "empty room" data (2–3 min) for reference. If multiple groups share the MEG system, it is particularly important to check that the stimulation devices and the possible software scripts, as well as response buttons or microphones, if needed, are connected as required by the experiment and function as expected.

Careful pre-tests improve the data quality as the subject's time and attention can be focussed on the experiment instead of debugging the measurement setup.

Subject Preparation

Before starting the actual MEG recording and even prior to guiding the subject into the magnetically shielded room, several preparatory steps are necessary. A typical procedure is outlined below.

1. **Consent**. The subject receives a clear explanation of the experimental procedures and reads and signs the consent form.

2. **Demagnetization**. All objects that contain metal (earrings, hairpins, neck-laces, piercings on the head, wrist watch, underwire bra, belt, etc.) should be removed. Clothing can include magnetic buttons, rivets and zippers so it is best to change to known non-magnetic clothes. Shoes are frequently magnetic and should be removed. Make-up and hair dyes can contain magnetic metal particles. Magnetization of, e.g., dental work can be reduced by a demagnetizer; refer to the instructions of the demagnetizer for correct operation, incorrect use may even increase the magnetization. Note that a demagnetizer exerts substantial force on ferromagnetic objects; if there is any possibility that such objects are within the body, a demagnetizer should not be applied.

3. **Test for magnetization**. With new subjects and patients, it is worthwhile to do a quick test before proceeding with the preparations. This test is con-ducted simply by having the subject to sit in the MEG system while the experimenter checks the raw signals for possible contamination; cf. "Artifacts" section below. The body can be magnetic due to, e.g., dental work, metal particles from previous surgery, and implants. Iterate demagnetization and testing if necessary.

4. **EEG**. If scalp EEG is to be measured, the EEG cap is applied and the elec-trode impedances verified to be low enough, typically less than 10 kilo-ohms (the limit depends on the amplifier). If the cap does not include the reference electrode, a separate single electrode should be applied as the reference. An elec-trode for the isolated ground of the EEG amplifier should be attached as well.

Single scalp electrodes are often placed according to the international 10–20 system, which was originally designed for just 21 electrodes (Jasper, 1958) but now has modern derivatives supporting denser electrode arrays (Oostenveld & Praamstra, 2001). In these systems, the on-scalp distances between the preauricular points and nasion and inion are divided into predefined sec-tions, which form a grid for the electrodes. EEG text books (see, e.g., Niedermeyer & Lopes da Silva, (2004) describe the standards on placing the electrodes.

Whole-scalp EEG is usually measured with an EEG cap instead of single electrodes. Detailed instructions on how to apply the cap are provided by the vendor.

5. **EOG**. Electrodes are applied for monitoring eye movements and blinks. A pair of electrodes attached diagonally (below the left eye and above the right eye, or vice versa) allow catching both eye movements and blinks for auto-matic rejection of contaminated trials. Applying two pairs, one horizontally and another one vertically, enables more sensitive monitoring of eye move-ments. The impedance of EOG electrodes is not as critical as that of scalp EEG electrodes but should still be below 100 kilo-ohms.

6. **EMG/ECG**. If required, electrode pairs for monitoring muscular (skeletal and cardiac) activity are attached. The EMG electrodes should be placed roughly at the ends of the muscle for maximum signal, palpation and muscle contraction aid in positioning the electrodes. Again, impedances should be verified.

7. **Coils.** Head position indicator coils are attached on the scalp. Using three coils is the absolute minimum, but for improved accuracy and desirable redundancy at least four coils should be employed, if that option is supported by the MEG system. With four or more coils the system is able to cope with situations where one coil detaches or moves prior to the MEG measurement. The locations should be chosen such that the coils can be firmly attached to the scalp, not to the hair, and that they are all covered by the MEG sensor array once the subject is seated in the system. At the same time, they should be as far apart as possible to ensure most stable and accurate co-registration. When using four coils, two of them are typically placed behind the earlobes as high up as possible, and the other two wide apart on the forehead, again as high up as possible so that they can be properly covered by the MEG sensor array.

There are various ways to attach the coils: they can be embedded in the EEG cap, attached to the scalp with tape, or even glued to the skin with collodium. Note that the coils are electrically isolated, and they should not be in an electrical contact with the scalp.

8. **Digitization.** The locations of the indicator coils must be known with respect to the anatomy for co-registration, e.g., with MRI, and the locations of the scalp EEG electrodes for EEG source modelling. This information is obtained by a digitizer device that records the coordinates of a stylus in the 3D space. The digitization procedure begins by identifying the anatomical landmarks that span the head coordinate system (see Chapter 2). After that, the locations of the head position indicator coils and EEG electrodes can be digitized, and both expressed in the head coordinate frame. If no scalp EEG electrodes are digitized, the head shape should be digitized to allow for a more accurate and verifiable co-registration with anatomical MRIs. Some tens of scalp points taken along contours from the tip of the nose to the back of the head, and from one ear to the other, already help in obtaining a better match with the MRIs. Some systems support a continuous digitization mode which allows quickly collecting thousands of points on the head surface.

These steps may take just a few minutes, or even up to an hour if a high-density EEG cap is applied.

Measurement

After the preparation steps described above, the subject can be guided in to the shielded room. The actual measurement is typically preceded by the following steps.

1. **Seating.** Head position indicator coils and EEG electrode wires and cap cables should be connected to the MEG/EEG system. Stimulator devices (e.g., auditory or somatosensory), if used, should be connected to the subject and tested.

The subject should also try out the response buttons and microphones, if they are needed in the experiment.

The setup should be made as comfortable as possible for the subject; if the position is not comfortable, being immobile even for a short time easily becomes painful, which distracts the subject. Tense neck muscles add wideband noise to the MEG, and thus deteriorate the quality of the recording.

Unlike in fMRI, in MEG subjects may see the movement of, e.g., the hand when using response keys. Looking at such a movement evokes visual responses that do not vanish in the averaging, as they are synchronized to the trials. Such additional responses may unnecessarily complicate the data analysis. Similarly, response buttons emitting an audible click may give rise to time-locked auditory responses, and movements that are mechanically transmitted to other limbs may lead to additional somatosensory responses. Thus, care should be taken to prevent or mask unwanted sensory input.

When recording children, or certain kinds of patients, it may be advisable to have an assistant in the shielded room with the subject. The above demagnetization guidelines apply also to the assistant. During data collection, the assistant should remain immobile and as far from the MEG sensor helmet as possible.

2. **Instructions**. The subject is reminded of the task and given specific instructions. In most MEG experiments, the subject should also be asked not to move during the recording, to avoid eye movements, and — depending on the experiment — to try to blink only during certain periods of the stimulus sequence. In addition, the subject should be told how and when to communicate with the experimenter.

3. **Checking for artifacts**. After the door of the shielded room has been closed and the data acquisition system started, the MEG traces should be examined visually for any artifacts. Movement-related and biological artifacts are the most common; refer to the following section to identify artifacts. Requesting the subject to take a couple of deep breaths helps in verifying that there is no magnetic material on the subject's person; see the next section.

4. **Checking the EEG signals**. Scalp EEG signals should be inspected visually. Excessive noise or line frequency interference are likely signatures of bad electrode contacts. With high-density electrode caps, it is often unavoidable that some channels lose proper contact to the skin; aiming to have every single EEG cap electrode working may not be the most productive approach. On the other hand, the reference and isoground electrodes must be fully functional, as losing them spoils the whole EEG recording.

The operation of the EOG channels can be verified by asking the subject to blink a few times, move the gaze to left and right, followed by up and down movements, while the experimenter is watching the EOG traces: blinks and vertical movements should evoke clear signals, in excess of 200 microvolts, in the vertical EOG channel whereas horizontal movement is mainly visible in the horizontal EOG channel. A single diagonal EOG channel picks up all these movements but with a lower signal-to-noise ratio than separate horizontal and vertical channels.

Contracting the muscle monitored by EMG should give rise to bursting high-frequency activity. In studies of cortico-muscular coherence where the subject has to maintain a steady contraction, it is a good idea to give feedback of the proper level of contraction (clear bursting on the EMG channel) at this stage.

5. **Head position measurement**. The position of the subject's head with respect to the MEG sensor is determined by briefly energizing the head position indicator coils. Depending on the MEG system, the coils are activated either sequentially or simultaneously at distinct frequencies. The signals emitted by these coils are captured by the MEG sensors. Based on these signals, the coil locations are estimated in the MEG device coordinate system (see above). With the help of the information from the digitization, the transformation between the head and MEG device coordinate systems is calculated.

Just prior to the head position measurement, the subject should be asked to take a comfortable position and remain as immobile as possible until the end of the measurement block. If continuous head position tracking is enabled, small movements are acceptable, however, the subject should still avoid large head movements, as the associated motor activity and sensory input may have an effect on the data.

When measuring a subject for the first time in MEG, it may be advisable to perform a short test run prior to the actual measurement and re-adjust the position when the subject is more relaxed.

6. **Data collection**. After a successful head position measurement, MEG data collection can be started. The experimenter should monitor the raw MEG data throughout the experiment; simple visual inspection allows judging whether the noise level is acceptable. All deviations should be detected as early as possible in order to avoid recording useless data.

In addition, on-line averaging should be employed and the accumulating average monitored. Even when the data are to be re-averaged off-line, the online average reliably shows the response amplitude. This direct measure of signal-to-noise ratio allows the researcher to decide when to stop data collection, instead of always acquiring a fixed number of trials. It also helps in detecting unwanted trial-locked responses due to, e.g., movement.

7. **Breaks between blocks**. Subjects can typically concentrate on a task no more than 10 to 15 minutes continuously. Therefore, longer experiments are often split in multiple blocks (see Chapter 4). Between the blocks, the subject can rest and relax, blink and move the eyes freely. Head movement between the blocks may also be allowed, if the blocks are analyzed separately or if the researcher is prepared to apply specific post-processing and analysis methods to the data. In any case, it is advisable to measure the head position at the beginning of each block.

If continuous head position tracking is not available or applied, the within-block stability can be verified by performing an additional head position measurement at the end of each block; if it differs substantially from the measurement at the beginning of the block, the experimenter should consider discarding and re-measuring that block; however, experiments that rely on the novelty of stimuli may not allow such repeats.

8. **Finishing the recording**. Once a sufficient amount of data is collected and the measurement finished, the subject can be guided out of the shielded room, and EEG caps, electrodes and head position indicator coils carefully detached. EEG caps and electrodes should be cleaned soon after the experiment to remove any residual electrode paste before it dries.

Besides the actual measurement, time should be budgeted for the checks listed above, which typically add up to 10 minutes to the recording time.

Artifacts

MEG signals can, unfortunately, be hampered by unwanted signals from several sources. Contaminating interference can be a result of strong ambient magnetic fields or by sources — biological or artifactual — in the subject. The ambient sources include interference from power lines and electromotors (at 50 or 60 Hz and harmonics) and from large moving magnetic objects such as cars, elevators, and even hospital beds. The signals from moving objects are characterized by temporal scales similar to the movement; the frequency content is predominantly below 1 Hz. Reduction of this type of interference is discussed in Chapter 2.

The experimenter is more often confronted by interference from the subject rather than from the environment. Common biological sources disturbing MEG include the cardiac muscle, skeletal muscles, and the eyeballs. Each of these sources has a distinct temporal waveform; see Figure 3–1. Cardiac artifact reflects either the pulsation or the magnetic counterpart of the QRS complex of the electrocardiogram (Jousmäki and Hari, 1996). It is characterized by relatively brief pulses occuring at the heart rate, and it appears more prominently on magnetometers than gradiometers. Other muscles, when they contract, emit continuous or bursting high-frequency noise, which is naturally stronger the closer the muscle is to the sensor array. Both head and eye movements are associated with shifts of the steady (DC) magnetic field level seen by the MEG sensors; eye movements and blinks are manifested as sub-second deflections on the frontal channels, whereas large head movements evoke such changes on most channels.

Artifacts may also arise from nonbiological sources in or on the subject. Dental work, fillings and braces, often give rise to large-amplitude magnetic signals that amplify when the subject is moving the jaw. These signals may be so strong even after demagnetization that the subject has to be excluded from research studies. However, cleaning the data with post-processing methods

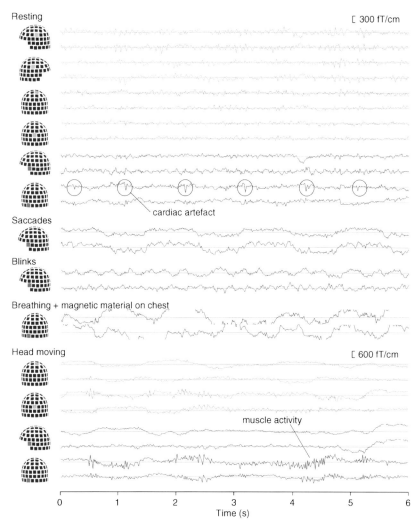

Figure 3–1. Normal vs. artifactual signals on representative MEG channels (planar gradiometer pairs). Top rows show typical raw MEG traces from a resting subject (note the regular cardiac artifact on the lowest sensors), whereas the lower traces display typical biological artifacts and a breathing-induced signal from a magnetic particle on the chest of the subject.

described in Chapter 2 may enable detection and localization of the relatively fast brain signals from, e.g., primary sensory areas and epileptic foci.

If the subject has magnetic particles on the body, particularly on the chest, breathing evokes slow periodic magnetic signals seen on several channels, more strongly on magnetometers than gradiometers. If in doubt, a suspect respiration-related source can easily be verified by asking the subject to first hold the breath, and then to take a couple of deep breaths while the experimenter is monitoring the MEG signals: if the slow variation first disappears and then increases, the source is likely related to the small movements associated with breathing. To trace the source further, the subject can be asked to move one limb at a time. Most often the magnetic material is in the clothing.

Replicability of MEG Results

The reliability of MEG responses can be verified by repeating the experiment and comparing the results. Physiological factors such as vigilance are beyond the scope of this text, but purely technical aspects may also contribute to differences between measurements. They pertain mostly to co-registration of the MEG and MRI coordinate systems; head movements, if not monitored and compensated for, result in displacement of the source on the MRI anatomy.

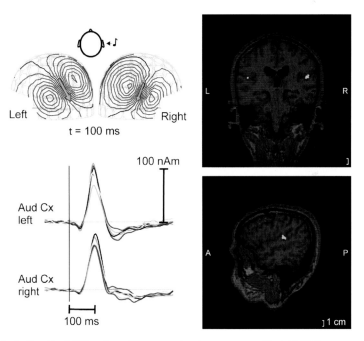

Figure 3–2. Replicability of auditory evoked responses. Eight MEG measurements performed on the same subject over a period of two years all yield consistent responses to stimulation of the right ear with short 1-kHz tone pips. The locations of the N100m sources (modeled as equivalent current dipoles; see Chapter 6) estimated from the responses are shown as blue dots on the structural MRI of the subject. The corresponding source waveforms vary slightly in amplitude, whereas the peak latency remains similar.

When the underlying neural sources are strong and exhibit simple field patterns, so that they are easy to model, co-registration procedures are responsible for most of the localization errors. When the experiments are performed carefully, such sources can repeatedly be localized to a few millimeters.

Differing sensor-level responses from two recordings of the same subject may be simply due to different head positions. This problem can be rectified either by preprocessing the data with movement compensation methods (Uutela et al., 2001; Taulu et al., 2005) to align the signals to a reference head position, or by performing the comparison in the source space instead of sensor space.

The overall replicability of MEG responses is good. Figure 3–2 shows the results of the same auditory experiment performed multiple times on a single subject. The locations of the N100m sources, reflecting a response from the primary auditory cortex, are within a few millimeters of each other, and the source waveforms differ only by amplitude, partly attributable to variations in the stimulus intensity.

References

Jasper, H. H. (1958). The ten-twenty electrode system of the International Federation of Electroencephalography and Clinical Neurophysiology. *Electroencephalogr Clin Neurophysiol, 10*, 371–375.

Jousmäki, V., & Hari, R. (1996). Cardiac artifacts in magnetoencephalogram. *J Clin Neurophysiol 13*(2), 172–176.

Niedermeyer, E., & Lopes da Silva, F. (2004). *Electroencephalography: Basic Principles, Clinical Applications, and Related Fields*(5th ed.). Philadelphia: Lippincott Williams & Wilkins.

Oostenveld, R., & Praamstra, P. (2001). The five percent electrode system for high-resolution EEG and ERP measurements. *Clin Neurophysiol, 112*(4), 713–719.

Taulu, S., & Kajola, M. (2005). Presentation of electromagnetic multichannel data: The signal space separation method. *J Appl Phys 97*(12), 124905–124910.

Uutela, K., Taulu, S., & Hämäläinen, M. (2001). Detecting and correcting for head movements in neuromagnetic measurements. *Neuroimage, 14*(6), 1424–1431.

4

Experimental Design

Riitta Salmelin and Lauri Parkkonen

- Experimental setups that work well for fMRI are often suboptimal for MEG, and vice versa
- Designs used in behavioral studies may serve as good starting points for MEG experiments
- Interstimulus interval, stimulus duration, and number of trials per experimental condition, all influence the neural response

Introduction

In order to design efficient functional neuroimaging experiments, one needs to consider (i) the dynamics of the measured neural variable, and (ii) the rate at which this variable can be sampled. The bulk of the MEG (and EEG) signal reflects synchronous post-synaptic current flow in a large number of neurons. These are very fast processes, in the millisecond range, and the signal can also be sampled at a very high rate, up to several kHz, i.e., in submillisecond range. Accordingly, the response can be tracked with good temporal accuracy in each trial (Figure 4–1). In contrast, fMRI signal reflects changes in the oxygen consumption, which lags the neural activation by 5–10 s and varies slowly, over a period of several seconds. Whole-head fMRI images with a reasonable spatial resolution can usually be collected every 2 seconds, at best,

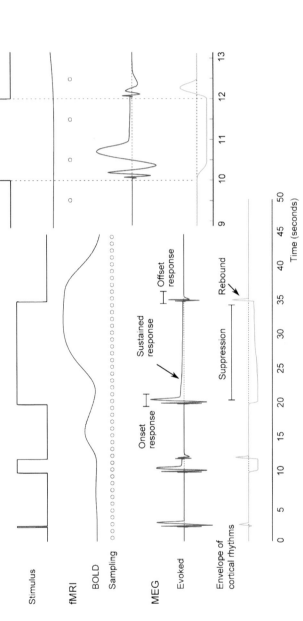

Figure 4–1. Comparison of fMRI BOLD and MEG/EEG signals; schematic responses to stimuli of 200 ms, 2 s and 15 s in duration. A prominent BOLD effect is obtained only with stimulation persisting for several seconds, whereas MEG/EEG evoked responses are primarily elicited by stimulus onsets and offsets, with possibly a relatively weak sustained response. Cortical rhythms seen by MEG/EEG (mainly alpha around 10 Hz and mu with 10- and 20-Hz components) may undergo suppression and rebound modulation, whose time course is more comparable to that of BOLD. Due to the sluggishness of the BOLD signal, it is sufficient to sample it 0.5–2 times per second; here, the dots denote sampling at a rate of 1/second (repetition time TR = 1 s). The MEG/EEG onset responses typically last for less than a second and change orders of magnitude more rapidly than BOLD, thus necessitating sampling rates above 300 Hz.

with the sampling rate limited by the image acquisition process. Because of that, single trials can typically not be sampled with high enough temporal resolution. The shape of the response can be estimated by combining multiple single trials which were sampled at different times with respect to stimulus or task onset (event-related design with jittered stimulus timing). The commonly applied analysis to a block design experiment effectively sums up the fMRI signal over 20-30-s periods when the subject continuously receives similar stimuli, or performs the same task—thus, the result carries no temporal information on the responses.

Thus, a major difference between neurophysiological and hemodynamic neuroimaging methods is that the signatures of neural activity recorded in MEG (and EEG) are fast and they are oversampled in time whereas those detected with fMRI and PET are slow and they are undersampled (see Figure 4–1). This difference affects experimental design to a large extent and, in particular, often renders good fMRI designs suboptimal for MEG and vice versa. In fact, the designs used in behavioral studies, where one collects manual or oral reaction times, tend to be better suited as starting points for MEG/EEG experiments than those typically used in fMRI/PET studies.

Owing to its combined temporal and spatial sensitivity, MEG can identify different processing stages as they unfold. Because of that, negligence in stimulus preparation tends to immediately manifest in the neural signals. For example, differences in the fade-in envelope of sound stimuli may cause much larger effects in the early auditory responses than behaviorally highly relevant differences in the stimulus content, e.g., speech vs. nonspeech sounds. Therefore, the basic physical properties of sensory input need to be controlled carefully (either matched or completely randomized) in order to extract meaningful information about different levels of processing. For this same reason, MEG studies do not readily accommodate an approach frequently applied in fMRI/PET studies in which one assumes that, e.g., when the same type of manual response has been given in two tasks, those tasks can be directly contrasted and the movement effects so removed. MEG data may well reveal that particularly the timing of the neural processes leading to the manual response, and the sensorimotor activation itself, are influenced by the experimental condition. This great advantage (or curse, depending on the situation) of the MEG method has to be kept in mind when designing and piloting new experiments.

Measures of Brain Activity

The choice of experimental parameters is influenced by the type of information one wishes to extract from the brain signals and by the type of analysis one plans to use in that endeavor. Here we briefly review the most common response types relevant for MEG (and EEG) studies.

Evoked Responses

Most MEG studies, so far, have focused on evoked responses, i.e., neural activation that occurs at the same time, phase-locked, with respect to stimulus or task onset (or offset) from trial to trial. Evoked responses are typically detected within about 1 s from the stimulus presentation or execution of the task. Evoked *single-trial responses* may be detectable in favorable conditions; however, most often some tens or hundreds of trials are collected to yield an average evoked response with a good signal-to-noise ratio. The earliest salient responses, i.e., those of shortest latency, are typically transient (short-lasting) and tightly locked to the stimulus, and thus yield sharp responses even when averaged across multiple trials. The longer-latency responses tend to progressively increase in duration and are likely to exhibit more jitter with respect to the stimulus timing; in the average, they appear as sustained responses with slow fade-in and fade-out phases. Figure 4–1a illustrates these dynamics in a schematic way.

Evoked responses can be considered to reflect changes in the sensory input: a long-lasting stimulus gives rise typically only to a transient MEG/EEG evoked response at the onset and offset of the stimulus, whereas the fMRI BOLD response may persist throughout the entire duration of the stimulus, although delayed overall due to the sluggishness of the BOLD signal. Moderately long stimuli may generate sustained components in the evoked response.

Modulation of Cortical Rhythms

Event-related modulation of cortical rhythmic activity—i.e., time-dependent variation of the amplitude of oscillations within a frequency band of interest, often referred to as *stimulus- or task-induced responses*—may reveal effects that occur systematically across trials, but are less strictly time-locked to the stimulus or task timing. It should be noted that such oscillatory signal itself is generally not phase-locked to the stimulus presentation or task, and these components typically vanish in the time-domain averaging commonly employed to recover evoked responses.

Modulation of rhythmic activity often extends over several seconds, thus providing a time frame that is complementary to that accessible with evoked responses. There may be spatial limitations, however, as salient rhythmic activity tends to be concentrated to specific areas in the cortex, in and around the primary sensory and motor areas. Non-averaged data collected during continuous stimulation or task performance (or during rest) lends itself to analysis of spectral power.

Changes in Interareal Synchronization

Measures such as coherence and phase synchronization between brain regions are employed to search for functionally connected networks and to characterize their dynamics. The relevant time courses of these signatures range from transient phase-locking of some tens of milliseconds induced by sensory stimulation, to coherent activity lasting several seconds in a complex cognitive task.

In the following, we will consider the practical influence of various experimental parameters on the collection of evoked, event-related, and non-averaged MEG data.

Timing and Number of Trials

The number of experimental conditions, the number of trials per condition, the stimulus or task duration, the intertrial interval and the total duration of the experiment are all tied together. *The number of trials per experimental condition* needs to be high enough to enable data analysis in single subjects. Ideally, when focusing on stimulus-locked evoked responses, one would aim for about 100 accepted trials per condition which, with a realistic estimate of 15–20% of the trials contaminated by eye blinks or other types of artifact signals (see Chapter 3), requires about 120 trials per condition. In some subjects, auditory responses (N100m) to short tones may be so strong that even responses to single stimuli can be detected among the task-unrelated background noise, and 40–50 trials may be quite sufficient for source analysis. However, the strength of cortical responses varies considerably between individuals. In practice, about 60 artifact-free trials may provide a good enough signal-to-noise ratio. In cognitive tasks, in which each trial may be fairly long and one needs to limit the total duration of the experiment in order to keep the subjects alert and motivated, 60–80 accepted trials (out of a total of 80–120 trials) is often a realistic goal. When the focus is on event-related modulation of cortical rhythms, as few as 40–50 trials may be adequate (although a higher number is preferable), as source analysis is typically performed on data integrated over extended time intervals, or on non-averaged signals. If possible within a reasonable recording time, one may test the reproducibility of the neural responses by presenting twice the minimum required number of stimuli, dividing the trials randomly into two groups, and averaging the responses. This type of approach is most suitable for simple sensory stimuli.

Stimulus duration has a strong effect on the MEG (and EEG) signal. For example, a short tone pip elicits a transient N100m response, which for a longer sound is followed by another, more sustained response. For an auditory, somatosensory or visual stimulus of long duration, separate responses may be detected to both stimulus onset and offset. When the focus is on evoked responses, stimuli of short duration (< 100–200 ms) are a good option, unless there is a specific need to choose otherwise. The phase-locked synchronized response is strongest to the onset of the stimulus, with little added value provided by an extended duration, and shorter stimulus duration helps to limit the full length of the experiment. In the visual domain, the risk for saccades (and problematic artifacts) is significantly reduced by presenting the stimulus for less than 150–200 ms. If one needs to use stimuli or tasks of very long duration, on the order of seconds, it may be worthwhile to consider whether, instead of phase-locked evoked responses, a more suitable approach might be spectrotemporal analysis on averaged event-related data, or on blocks of non-averaged data, and design the experiment accordingly.

The interstimulus interval (ISI) should be long enough to allow the neural responses to return to the base level ('rest') for at least 200 ms in the case of evoked responses, or for 500–1000 ms in the case of event-related modulation of rhythmic activity. Thus, when the focus is solely on evoked responses, stimulus onset asynchrony (SOA) falls typically within 1–3 s, depending on the amount of sustained activity the stimulus or task elicits, and on the speed at which the subject can process the stimuli or perform the task. SOAs up to 5–10 s may be required for comprehensive tracking of event-related modulation of cortical rhythms. The choice between fixed or variable ISI/SOA is at the discretion of the experimenter. MEG analysis does not set any requirements in this regard, owing to the high time resolution. In MEG (or EEG) experiments the effective ISI/SOA within each stimulus or task category often varies considerably because the order of the trials belonging to the different categories is usually randomized. Randomization is recommended, as the vigilance of the subject thus varies, on average, similarly for all experimental conditions and renders them more comparable. Nevertheless, should it be required by the neuroscience question, a blocked design is obviously equally feasible from the MEG point of view. Even in that case, randomized mini-blocks may often be a better option than one extended block of each stimulus/task type. Blocked design is obviously the choice when using continuous tasks or stimuli, and the analysis is performed on non-averaged data. In that case, it may be useful to introduce short rest periods also within blocks (and not just longer periods between blocks) to serve as a baseline condition.

As an example, let us assume that we are interested in how the left and right auditory cortex respond to 1–kHz tones, 50 ms in duration, presented to the left or right ear or to both ears simultaneously. Since the stimuli are short tone pips, cortical activation is concentrated to the first 100–200 ms. Thus, the SOA could, in principle, be as short as 600 ms. However, the auditory cortex responds more strongly with increasing SOA. A reasonable setup might be as follows: 3 conditions (randomized) x 100 stimuli x 2–s SOA = 600 s = 10 min of effective recording time. This is a very short experiment, and one could easily double the number of stimuli, and thus test for reproducibility of the responses. Alternatively, one could enhance the neural responses by choosing a longer SOA, or the SOAs could be randomized, e.g., between 2 and 6 seconds to reduce expectation. However, one also needs to keep in mind that this is an extremely boring experiment for the subject and, therefore, best results are probably obtained by keeping the experiment as short as possible.

As another example, one might evaluate reading comprehension by showing sentences that create a strong expectation for a certain final word, and replacing that word with another one having different types of relationships to the expected word. Let us assume that we have four different types of sentences, and 100 sentences in each category. The sentences have, on average, 7 words. In order to avoid artifacts from eye movements (saccades), the sentences are presented one word at a time, displayed in foveal vision. The neural response to each word contains a strong sustained component that lasts until 600–800 ms after stimulus onset. A reasonable setup would thus be as follows: 4 types of sentences (randomized) x 100 sentences x (7 words x 1-s SOA within each sentence plus an additional 1-s interval between sentences) = 3200 s = 53 min, divided into 5–6 sequences with short breaks in between, thus resulting in about 80–90 min in total recording time. An experiment should not last much longer than this, for the sake of the subject and data quality.

Collecting Behavioral Responses (or Not)

There is plenty of MEG research on the motor system. However, when the focus is on auditory or visual perception, or cognitive processing, the strong neural activations associated with voluntary movements are essentially artifacts that may seriously hinder the analysis of the primary effects of interest. Therefore, if answering the neuroscience question does not necessarily require reaction times to be collected for each stimulus, it is best not to collect them. This is where design of MEG (and EEG) experiments diverges most from that of purely behavioral experiments.

However, the usual counterargument is that one needs behavioral responses in order to keep the subject alert and to verify that s/he performs the task as instructed. One can think of multiple alternative approaches. One possibility is to require a delayed response, prompted by another stimulus that follows the stimulus of interest, which will interfere less with the primary effects, but allows monitoring of behavior. Another possibility is to require a delayed response only to a part of the stimuli, e.g., a yes/no decision prompted by an occasional question mark, and remove this small subset of trials from the source analysis. Equally well, one could define specific targets which the subject needs to respond to immediately, thus providing reaction times to a subset of stimuli; again, these trials would be removed from the source analysis.

If the experimental question requires behavioral responses in all trials, they can obviously be collected. Eye movements are the most problematic as they generate huge artifacts. Finger movements are often preceded by strong readiness fields, thus easily confounding data in the time window of interest. Use of left vs. right hand is complicated, at the neural level, by the fundamentally different activation patterns. This is a problem also when using different fingers of the same hand, to a somewhat lesser degree. In some cases, verbal responses may work better, as the readiness field tends to be markedly weaker than for hand movements, and the activation is bilateral and quite similar for stereotyped responses such as "yes/no."

The excellent time resolution of MEG facilitates a fairly free choice of parameters. What we have presented here are guidelines, rather than rules, for experimental design. They can be adjusted at will, as long as the experimenter is aware of the possible effects for subject performance, neural responses, and data analysis.

5

The Dowser in the Fields: Searching for MEG Sources

Sylvain Baillet

- Finding sources of MEG/EEG traces can either be viewed as a localization or an imaging problem
- Localization refers to decomposing the data into the respective contributions of a limited number of elementary current source models, e.g. point-like equivalent current dipoles
- The imaging approach produces representations of brain currents distributed in space, e.g. on the cortical surface
- The pertinence of either of these approaches is dictated by the neuroscience question that initially motivated the experiment and the acquisition of data
- Both need to be advantageously complemented by adapted methods for statistical exploration and inference that have recently emerged – at the individual and group levels – thereby considerably reducing the incertitude in the confidence awarded to a given source estimate

Introduction

First: A Metaphoric Detour

Leaving the dowser behind right from the beginning of this chapter, there are plenty of other ecological situations where finding sources of some observations is not obvious to begin with. Imagine that you go bow-fishing in clear waters for the first time ever. This is a well-known situation in many books of lessons about things: "How come the bird will catch the fish before I can?". The answer stays almost immutably the same: "That's because the bird knows about light refraction at the surface of water". As unsatisfactory as this answer might sound, we have to admit *at least* that the bird (and humans) can learn from experience that the fish, being underwater, cannot be caught in the same way as the mouse, running on the ground. This countryside metaphor does not take us too far from our problem here. Indeed, the observations the bird makes are series of distorted images from its prey. The fish here is the source of the observations, which the bird implicitly combines with his model of the influence of the source medium on the observation (light refraction), and a collection of *a priori* information on the expected fish behavior in stressful circumstances.

Maybe the bird catches the fish much faster than we would ever do, but he surely does not know he is solving forward and inverse problems with every dinner.

Historical Roundup and Motivations

The estimation problem of sources of electromagnetic traces collected outside the head has certainly mobilized, initially, most of the early clinical electro-physiologists. Since the late 1940s when electroencephalography (EEG) entered the clinical rooms, the medical community had gathered an impressive corpus of empirical knowledge on the localization of the origins of abnormal scalp recordings from patients (Petit-Dutaillis et al., 1952) – which is still the essence of the EEG clinical practice today. EEG and MEG scientists have subsequently greatly benefited from the decisive contributions of biophysicists initially interested in modeling the origins of electrocardiographic (ECG) signals. David B. Geselowitz became a major contributor to the field by formalizing the concept of *equivalent* generator (Geselowitz, 1963) and the dipole theory in ECG (Geselowitz, 1964). The dipole model later entered the EEG literature as an empirical tool to formally describe the topography of scalp potentials, and yielded a means to infer qualitatively the localization of the main sources of surface signals (Kooi et al., 1969). The ECG community kept the lead, however, by studying the influence of inhomogeneities in body tissues on the empirical localization of a dipole model (Arthur & Geselowitz, 1970), making the first comparison between ECG and magnetocardiographic (MCG) recordings (Geselowitz, 1973), and designing a multiple-dipole source model in a spherical approximation of the geometry of body tissues in the vicinity of surface recordings (Miller & Geselowitz, 1974). Being themselves physicists and MCG experimenters, early MEG scientists like B. Neil Cuffin and David Cohen were naturally connected to the most advanced models from cardiographics (Cuffin & Geselowitz, 1977), and initiated a tradition of modeling and methodological innovations for MEG (Hosaka & Cohen, 1976; Cohen & Hosaka, 1976) that also benefited the analysis of EEG sources. Beyond the visual inspection of field topographies at the sensor level, the

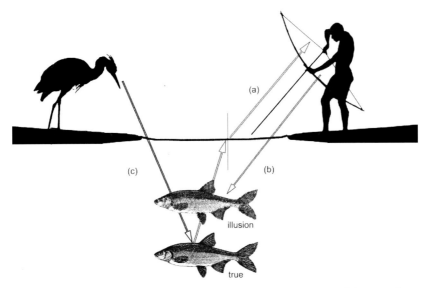

Figure 5–1. A natural metaphor of forward and inverse modeling: refraction of light at the surface of water lets us perceive that the depth of the fish is shallower (illusion) than it is (true). Bird catches prey with forward model learned from experience. The naive bow-fisher does not know about the physics of light refraction at the surface of water, (a) and starts with a wrong forward model ("no light refraction at the water surface") that will lead him to miss his target (b). The heron knows from experience how to catch the prey without explicit knowledge of light refraction (c).

somatosensory cortex then became the playground of computational source estimation challenges and demonstrations in the 1980s. Okada et al., (1984) demonstrated the relative localization power of single dipoles in a spherical head geometry, as an elementary model for the primary cortical projection of fingers and ankle, along the homuncular mediolateral somatotopic organization, originally evidenced by the direct cortical stimulations of Penfield (Penfield & Boldrey, 1937). Finally, MEG source estimation became acknowledged as an *inverse problem* – a concept already well known to physicists, and which addresses a wide range of methodological frameworks and innovations – following the Biomagnetic Inverse Problem Conference in 1985, the proceedings of which (*Biomag*, 1987) contain important contributions that initiated most of the subsequent developments that we shall review, comment, and illustrate with a pragmatic perspective in the next sections of this chapter.

Chapter Overview and Recommended In-depth Reading

This book chapter has no intent to cover an extensive technical review of all methodological tricks relevant to the MEG source-estimation problem.

Indeed, this would cover too wide a spectrum to be compacted in a few pages. Most relevant details to the approaches we will introduce here will be covered – with a focus on applications – in the next chapters of this handbook. Detailed technical reviews are available in journal literature, and are constantly enriched by a productive scientific community. A subjective desert-island selection of useful published review material would include: Hämäläinen et al., (1993) is a classic of MEG at large, and includes detailed descriptions of basic source-estimation approaches; Baillet et al., (2001a) is a detailed review of source estimation and modeling with a signal-processing perspective; Darvas et al., (2004) is complementary reading, as it includes recent developments in statistical appraisal and inference of the estimated source; Hillebrand et al., (2005) reviews the relatively popular spatial-filter approach to the MEG source estimation problem. See also chapters 7 and 8 for updated and technically detailed documentation.

Inverse Problem Theory in a Nutshell

The rapid historical review we have covered in the second section of the introduction above, closes with the statement that MEG (and EEG) source estimation is an inverse problem. Though it is quite acceptable that this indeed might be a problem, it might be less intuitive why this problem is *inverse*.

The Inverse and the Forward (problems)

An inverse problem is something we are all facing in our personal and sometimes professional lives. The bow-fishing metaphor was an attempt to demonstrate this statement. The concept of inverse problem was formalized by physicists in experimental science, where a model is confronted to some observations. Models derive from theories and are supposed to let us make predictions on natural phenomena and, more generally, on the outputs of a system (e.g., the Earth's climate, the stock exchange, or the brain). Hence, a system is a very general concept used in many different situations – from biology to economics. The main motivation here is to formalize how inputs I are transferred to observable outputs O via some transformation $\mathrm{T}()$ – which might include optional feedback loops and additional nuisances – so that:

$$O = \mathrm{T}(I). \tag{5–1}$$

which constitutes a model for the production of O. The *parameters* of the system are quantities that might be changed without fundamentally violating and thereby invalidating the theoretical model. Inputs I and some elements of $\mathrm{T}()$ (such as the refractive index of water n_w in the light refraction problem) are explicit and implicit parameters respectively of the system in (5–1).

The distinction between the implicit and explicit nature of parameters is rather artificial as (5–1) could as well be rewritten:

$$O = \mathrm{T}(I, \theta).\qquad\qquad(5\text{–}2)$$

where θ represents the set of originally implicit parameters in T() (i.e. $\theta = \{n_w\}$ in the context of light refraction). Predicting observations from a theoretical model with a given set of parameters is called solving the **forward** modeling problem.

The reciprocal situation, where observations are used to estimate the values of some parameters of the system, corresponds to the **inverse** modeling problem.

Why MEG Source Estimation is an Inverse Problem

Without further theoretical elaboration, we need to clarify why MEG source estimation – like all other brain imaging techniques – requires us to solve an inverse problem. The system specifically under consideration here concerns the (electro)magnetic activity of the brain. The basic input I is the global electrophysiological activity of neurons. Experimental evidence reports on magnetic fields being measured at the surface of the head in the context of cognitive or clinical neuroscience paradigms. These are the observations O. The theoretical model T at stake here builds on the theory of electrodynamics (Feynman, 1964) which reduces in MEG to the Maxwell equations under quasistatic assumptions (Hämäläinen et al., 1993).

In the context of brain mapping, we are essentially interested in *identifying*, in space and time, the sources of the observed head surface signals – that is, the parameters of I. This identification challenge reduces to the estimation of the free parameters of a source model of mass neural activity detectable at the scalp surface in a specific experimental context, which is an incarnation of an inverse modeling problem as defined previously. Forward modeling in the context of MEG consists in predicting the magnetic fields produced at the sensor level by the source model in question, for any values of parameters in I. Beyond the very choice of a theoretical model to account for mass neural activity, MEG forward modeling considers the parameters in θ as being known and fixed. These include the geometry of the head, conductivity of tissues, sensor locations, etc.

As an illustration, take a single current dipole as a model for the global activity of the brain, at a specific latency of an averaged evoked response O. We might choose to let the dipole location, orientation, and amplitude as the set of free parameters I, to be inferred from the sensor observations. The model T necessitates we specify some parameters θ to solve the forward modeling problem, which consists in predicting how a single current dipole may produce magnetic fields on the sensor array in question. We might, therefore, choose to specify in θ that the head geometry will be approximated as a single

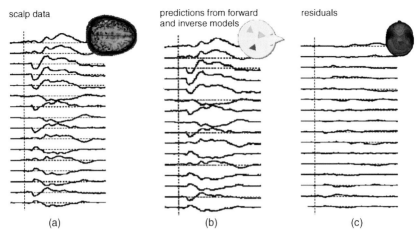

scalp data   predictions from forward and inverse models   residuals

(a)   (b)   (c)

Figure 5–2. Modeling illustrated: unknown brain activity – (a) top view – generates variations of magnetic fields, and electric potentials, at the surface of the scalp. This is illustrated by time series representing measurements at each sensor lead – (a) from bottom to top. Modeling of the sources and of the physics of MEG and EEG is illustrated in (b). As naively represented at the top of (b) forward modeling consists of a simplification of the complex geometry and electromagnetic properties of head tissues. Source models are presented with colored arrows. Their free parameters – e.g. location, orientation and amplitude – are adjusted during the inverse modeling procedure to optimize some quantitative index. This is illustrated here in (c) where the residuals – i.e., the absolute difference between the original data and the measures predicted by a source model – are minimized.

sphere, with its center at some given coordinates. The way the inverse modeling phase will be approached has many branches, as we shall discuss later.

Back to Theory: Important Detours

Before moving forward with the specificity of MEG inverse modeling, we need to discuss a couple of important theoretical considerations.

First, the nature of the parameters to be estimated from the observations depends on the motivation of the experiment. While a physicist might have been motivated in estimating n_w from observations of his favorite goldfish in a water tank, the bird is essentially motivated in identifying the source of the observation, that is, the fish. Both are solving an inverse problem from the same system and observations, but with different objectives.

Likewise, both the naive bow-fisher and the bird are seeking a solution to the same inverse problem (localize the fish), but with different models ($n_w > 1$ for the fish, $n_w = 1$ for the naive fisherman). This thought experiment let us conclude that while two solutions to the forward problem might exactly fit the observations by adjusting the free parameters in the model (here by changing values in I, e.g., the size and the location of the fish), this would lead to multiple – and sometimes radically different—solutions to the inverse problem (a strong bias in fish localization from the naive bow-fisher). Therefore – and this is a general principle – whereas the forward problem has a unique solution in classical physics (as dictated by the causality principle), the inverse problem might accept multiple solutions, which are models that equivalently predict the observations.

In MEG (and EEG), the situation is critical, as it has been demonstrated theoretically by von Helmoltz back in the 19th century that the general inverse problem that consists in finding the sources of electromagnetic fields outside a volume conductor has an infinite number of solutions. This issue is not specific to MEG: geophysicists are also confronted to non-uniqueness of inverse models in trying to determine the distribution of mass inside a planet by measuring the gravity field in the space outside the globe. Therefore, theoretically, an infinite number of source models would equivalently fit MEG and EEG observations, which reduces their predictive power on the system's behavior to null. Fortunately, this question has been addressed with the mathematics of ill-posedness and inverse modeling, which formalize the necessity of bringing additional contextual information to complement a basic theoretical model, as we shall discuss in the next section. This brings us to the second point, where one has to bear in mind that **the inverse problem is a modeling problem**. If we follow the Popperian paradigm that states that a model is valid as long as it is not falsified by failure in predicting new experimental evidence (Popper, 1959), both the bird and naive solutions to the fish problem are valid until the fish needs to be caught, which consists in itself of a new experiment that will eventually invalidate the naive model. Transposed to the MEG world, the fish becomes, e.g., an epileptogenic locus supposedly identified using MEG source modeling and potentially subjected to surgical resection, with terrible consequences if the wrong model was not falsified beforehand.

As we shall now see, these considerations have both philosophical and technical impacts on approaching the general theory and the practice of inverse problems (Tarantola, 2004). An important approach to address this caveat consists in obtaining a measure of the uncertainty on the values of the parameters sought by the inverse model. Situations like the aforementioned, where a large set of values for some of the parameters produce models that equivalently account for the observations, may raise a red flag to both question the quality of the experimental data and, most importantly, falsify the theoretical model.

Therefore, because uncertainty and modeling come in a pair, solutions to the inverse problem should necessarily be complemented or even directly built from probabilistic appraisal or statistical inference. This point will be reviewed below.

Ill-posedness and the Need for A Priori Information

Non-unicity of the solution is one situation where an inverse problem is said to be *ill-posed*. One could think also about the reciprocal situation, where there is no value for the system's parameters to account for the observations. In this case, the data are said to be inconsistent (with the model). The bird is confronted with this situation when seeing an object at the bottom of the water that does not match his representation of what a fish is supposed to look like (e.g., a wrecked car).

Another critical situation, which indeed concerns MEG, is when the model parameters do not depend continuously on data. This means that even tiny changes on the observations (e.g. by adding a small amount of noise) trigger major variations in the estimated values of the parameters. This is critical to any experimental situation, and especially in the biosciences and with MEG in particular, where the data are contaminated by considerable artifacts.

The epistemology and early mathematics of ill-posedness were initiated by Jacques Hadamard (Hadamard, 1902), where he somehow radically stated that problems that are not uniquely solvable are of no interest whatsoever. This statement is obviously unfair to important questions in science such as gravitometry, the backwards heat equation[1], and surely MEG source modeling.

The modern view on the mathematical treatment of ill-posed problems has been initiated in the 1960s by Andrei N. Tikhonov and the introduction of the concept of *regularization*, which spectacularly formalized a *Solution of ill-posed problems* (Tikhonov & Arsenin, 1977). Tikhonov suggested that some mathematical manipulations on the expression of ill-posed problems could make them turn well-posed in the sense that a solution would exist, and be eventually unique.

More recently this approach found a more general and intuitive framework using the theory of probability, which naturally refers to the uncertainty and contextual *a priori* inherent to experimental sciences (see, e.g., Tarantola, 2004).

As of 2008, more than 2000 journal articles referred in the PubMed publication database to the query '(MEG OR EEG) AND source' and about 560 to the more technical query '(MEG OR EEG) AND ("inverse problem" OR "inverse method"'(U.S. National Library of Medicine). This abundant literature may be considered ironically as only a small sample of the infinite number of solutions to the problem, but it is rather a reflection of the many different ways MEG source modeling can be addressed with additional information of various nature.

Such a large amount of reports on the same technical issue has certainly been detrimental to the visibility and credibility of the MEG and EEG brain mapping community within the larger functional brain-mapping audience, where the fMRI inverse problem reduced to the estimation of the BOLD signal – though subject to major detection issues – is well-posed.

Today, it seems that a reasonable degree of maturity has been reached, as all the investigated methods reduce to only a handful of classes of approaches that are now well-identified. Gradually, the methodological research in MEG source modeling is moving from inverse methods to the issue of statistical appraisal and inference, and is joining the concerns shared by other functional brain-imaging communities (Baillet et al., 2001a).

We will now survey this landscape of approaches to the MEG source modeling problem with a pragmatic point of view. Technical details will be usually skipped, to focus on a clearer classification of the methods. More information is delivered in other sections concerning data analysis in this book. In-depth reviews are available in all cited references, and especially those in the early sections of this chapter.

The Many Faces of MEG Inverse Modeling

For purposes of clarity, we will not attempt to formalize in a general way the classes of approaches to the MEG inverse modeling problem. We will rather take the steps from a phenomenological point of view, observing that two main chapels have developed quite separately: the localization and the imaging approaches, respectively. Our purpose here is to note methodological landmarks and focus on differences, similarities, and on the respective assets of the corresponding basic models.

Localization vs. Imaging

We refer to the **localization approach** when the global source model considered in the MEG inverse problem states that the observations are produced by the activity of brain areas, whose locations can be estimated from the data. In this paradigm, each source in the global model accounts for the activity of a brain region which is explicitly separated in space from other active regions in the model.

Imaging approaches have been developed more recently, and were inspired by the plethoric research in image restoration and reconstruction in other domains (early digital imaging, geophysics, and other biomedical imaging techniques). The corresponding global source model does not attempt to estimate location parameters from observations, but rather aims at recovering the distribution of *all* mass neural currents, at a scale compatible with the electrophysiological basis of MEG signals (Chapter 1). The general outcome of this approach is truly a stack of images – hence *imaging* – in the sense that the estimated parameters are restricted to the intensities of distributed elementary models of mass neural activity that spatially sample the brain, just like the pixels of an image sample a region of 2D space. Contrarily to the localization model, there is no sense of source separation in the imaging

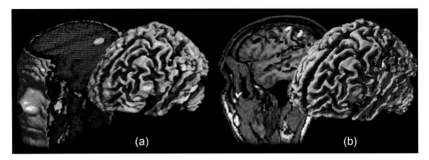

Figure 5–3. Inverse modeling: the localization (a) vs. imaging (b) approaches. Source modeling through localization consists in decomposing the MEG generators in a handful of elementary source contributions; the simplest source model in this situation being the equivalent current dipole (ECD). This is illustrated here from experimental data testing the somatotopic organization of primary cortical representations of hand fingers (Meunier et al., 2001). The parameters of the single ECD have been adjusted on the [20, 40] ms time window following stimulus delivery. The ECD was found to localize along the contralateral central sulcus, as revealed from the 3D rendering obtained after the source location has been registered to the individual anatomy. In the imaging approach, the source model is spatially-distributed using a large number of ECD's. Here, a surface model of MEG generators was constrained to the individual brain surface extracted from T1-weighted MR images. Elemental source amplitudes are interpolated onto the cortex, which yields an image-like distribution of the amplitude and spatial extension of cortical currents.

approach *per se*. Explicit identification of activity issued from distinct brain regions necessitates complementary analysis beyond inverse modeling.

We will now discuss these approaches in the following subsections with a focus on concepts rather than on techniques, which details can be found in the cited references.

The Localization Approach

Empirical Inference on Source Localization

The early attempts for source localization in the context of MEG and EEG started by questioning the elementary source model to be considered, and then by evaluating the number of source parameters that could *reasonably* be estimated from the data.

The seminal achievements of cardiography that we have briefly surveyed earlier exhibited the current dipole as a generic model of massive electrophysiological activity. Indeed, a significant number of publications in the EEG and MEG community have addressed the localization issue by empirical inference on the location of a current dipole susceptible to generating the surface measurements under investigation. This supposed that the electrophysiologist would intuitively solve the MEG forward problem that consists in predicting what is the surface distribution of magnetic fields produced by a dipole, at a given location with a given orientation.

This approach can be exemplified in Wood et al. (1985), where terms such as 'waveform morphology' and 'shape of scalp topography' are used to discuss the respective sources of MEG and EEG signals. This empirical approach to localization has considerably benefited from the constant increase in the number of sensors of MEG and EEG systems as exemplified in Figure 5–4.

Indeed, a surface representation of the field topographies on an approximation of the scalp surface – as a disc, a sphere or even as a realistic shape extracted from the subject's MRI – can be achieved using interpolation techniques of data between sensors that have gained considerable popularity in MEG and EEG research (Perrin et al., 1987). Wood et al. (1985) – like many others – used the distance between the minimum and maximum magnetic distribution of the dipolar-like field topography to infer the putative depth of a dipolar source model of the data.

There are Unknowns that are Not Known

Computational approaches to source localization attempt to mimic the talent of electrophysiologists, but with a more quantitative benefit. We have seen that the current dipole model has been adopted as the canonical equivalent

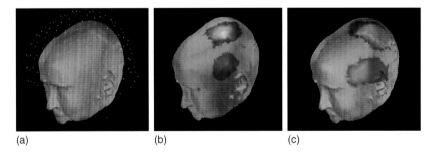

(a)   (b)   (c)

Figure 5–4. On the benefits of a larger number of sensors: (a) 3D rendering of a subject's scalp surface with crosshair markers representing the locations of 151 axial gradiometers as MEG sensors (coil locations are from the VSM MedTech 151 Omega System). (b) shows the interpolated field topography onto the scalp surface 50 ms following the electric stimulation of the right index finger. The fields reveal a strong and focal dipolar structure above the contralateral central cortex. (c) the number of channels has been evenly reduced to 27. Though the dipolar pattern is still detected, its spatial extension seems more spread out – hence the intrinsic spatial resolution of the measurements has been degraded – due to the effect of interpolation between sensors, which are now quite distant from the maxima of the evoked magnetic field pattern.

generator of the electrical activity of a brain region considered as a functional entity. Localizing a current dipole in the head implies that 6 unknown parameters be estimated from the data[2]. Therefore, characterizing the source model by a restricted number of parameters was considered as a possible solution to the ill-posed inverse problem, and has been attractive to many MEG scientists. Indeed, without additional prior information about the unknowns, the number of unknowns needs to be smaller than that of the instantaneous observations for the inverse problem to be well-posed in terms of unicity of a solution. Therefore, recent high-density systems with about 300 sensors would allow – theoretically – the unambiguous identification of 50 dipolar sources; a number that would probably satisfy the modeling of brain activity in many neuroscience questions.

It appears, though, that most recent research reports using MEG source localization show a more conservative profile by usually considering inverse source models with far fewer dipole sources (typically < 5). The reasons for this are both technical and proper to MEG brain signals, as we shall now discuss.

The Least-Squares Criterion

Numerical approaches to the estimation of unknown source parameters are generally based on the widely used least-squares (LS) technique which attempts to find the set of parameter values that minimizes the (square of the) difference between the observations and the predictions from the corresponding model. In other words, the LS approach is a pragmatic point of view on the evaluation of a model when facing experimental observations. Indeed, biosignals such as MEG traces are naturally contaminated by nuisance components (e.g., environmental noise and physiological artifacts) which should not be explained by the model of brain activity. Therefore, we need to add to the general systems equation (5–2) a nuisance term ε such that:

$$O = \mathrm{T}(I, \theta) + \varepsilon. \qquad (5–3)$$

This nuisance term has considerable impact on the evaluation of a source model, as we do not want an inverse model to account for perturbations induced by the reality of data acquisition. It is quite straightforward to understand that the noise components add some uncertainty to the estimation of the parameters: when noise components are independent and identically distributed (IID) on all sensors, one would theoretically need as many additional free parameters as the number of noise components to span the space occupied by all possible noisy observations. But we would then end up handling a problem with 300 additional unknowns, adding to the original 300 source parameters, for only 300 instantaneous data.

Hence, quite insidiously, this necessitates that the scientist understands what is of interest (signal: $\mathrm{T}(I, \theta)$) and what is perturbation (noise: ε) in the data.

Therefore – as in all other fields of experimental science – a selection of signal-processing manipulations from trial selection, averaging, filtering, etc. are necessary prior to any inverse modeling to reduce or reject the contribution of nuisance to observations.

This will lead us to solve the basic LS equation:

$$\hat{I} = \arg\min_{I} \left(\left\| O - T(I, \theta) \right\|^2 \right) = \arg\min_{I} \left(\left\| \varepsilon_{LS} \right\|^2 \right). \qquad (5\text{–}4)$$

and therefore consider that a relevant objective consists in minimizing the variance – or *power*, using the signal-processing glossary – of the deviation ε_{LS} of the model prediction from the data.

The Importance of Data Preprocessing

Hence, tuning the model parameters so that they perfectly fit the data would also result in explaining the remaining nuisance components; a general issue known as *overfitting* the observations. The LS approach defines a criterion to select the unknown parameters so that the resulting model is able to predict the signal part in the observations, without the nuisance contribution. This criterion assumes that ε is IID under normal distributions across sensors. This condition is violated for many types of perturbations such as physiological artifacts (e.g., cardiac and/or ocular), which produce highly correlated field patterns across a subset of head surface sensors (see Figure 5–5). Beyond artifact rejection and/or reduction techniques, careful preprocessing of the data may therefore also include a so-called pre-whitening procedure, which insures that the remaining perturbations are indeed IID (Kay, 1993).

From a statistical point of view, a LS fit of model parameters to data attempts to reduce the sample variance of the residuals – that is, the part in the observations left unexplained by the model – to some expected value; ideally the one of ε. In practice, this value may be estimated from the sample statistics of the MEG signals preceding the stimulation, or ideally from an acquisition run with the MEG recording only the environmental noise and/or with the subject resting quietly under the helmet (Huizenga et al., 2002; Jun et al., 2006).

The Techniques of LS Dipole Fitting

Estimating the 300 unknowns of a 50-dipole model from 300 observations would invariably result in overfitting any MEG data. This can be understood by first rewriting (5–2) as follows:

$$O = T(\theta)I. \qquad (5\text{–}5)$$

θ is the set of orientation and location parameters and I is the set of dipole amplitudes. (5–5) translates that the physics of MEG predicts that a current dipole produces magnetic fields that depend linearly on current amplitudes I, while they depend non-linearly on source orientations and locations θ (e.g., Baillet et al., 2001b). Let us now arbitrarily fix all values in θ at random. The resulting matrix $T(\theta)$ is *almost certainly* full-rank, i.e., invertible. This means that knowing θ, a solution $\hat{I}$ to (5–5) exists and is unique:

$$\hat{I} = T(\theta)^{-1} O. \tag{5–6}$$

If observations are from real – i.e., noisy – MEG data, then we have $O = T(\theta)I + \varepsilon$, which we replace in (5–6) to finally obtain:

$$\hat{I} = T(\theta)^{-1} \left(T(\theta)I + \varepsilon \right),$$
$$\hat{I} = I + T(\theta)^{-1} \varepsilon. \tag{5–7}$$

The fact that a random selection of θ can yield a perfect fit to arbitrary MEG observations is an illustration of the fundamental ill-posed nature of the MEG inverse problem which we have approached here using basic algebra.

Now let us suppose that we know the true source orientations and locations θ. By adding noise ε to this synthetic data set, we would still end up

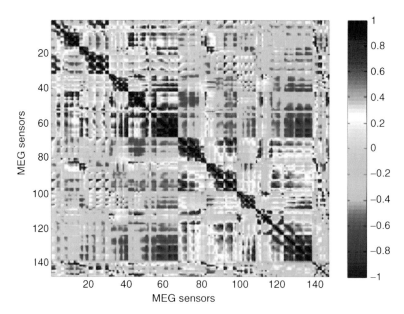

Figure 5–5. Matrix array of correlation coefficients across 147 MEG sensors during a 900 ms baseline recording of ongoing brain activity. Red and blue colors represent strong patterns of spatial correlation between MEG measurements, indicating – as expected – that supposed brain noise is not spatially independent.

overfitting the data by producing a model $\hat{I}$ in (5–7) that would also fully account for noise in the data (i.e. $\varepsilon_{LS} = 0$ in (5–4)), which is of course not desirable in practice.

Therefore, trying to fit as many parameters as there are unknowns does not lift the ill-posed nature or the modeling problem in real, noisy conditions. Here, although a solution to the inverse problem exists and is unique, it is highly dependent on the noise components in the data and ends up violating the third Hadamard condition to well-posedness (i.e., continuous dependency). Now let us suppose for the sake of further demonstration that the data is idealistically clean from any disturbance. Remember, we obtained the canonical inverse in (5–6) by estimating the amplitude parameters I after the other source parameters (orientations and locations) θ have been fixed. Now, if all 300 source parameters $\{I, \theta\}$ are left unconstrained, (5–5) is still linear in I but not in θ, as imposed by the forward model of the electromagnetics of MEG. Here, there are as many unknowns as there are instantaneous data, but the fact that some of them have a nonlinear dependency just makes them more difficult to estimate than in the situation where all unknowns linearly depend on the observations as in (5–6).

We need to solve the full LS optimization problem:

$$\left\{\hat{I}, \hat{\theta}\right\} = \operatorname*{arg\,min}_{I, \theta} \left(\left\| O - \mathrm{T}\left(I, \theta\right)\right\|^{2}\right). \tag{5–8}$$

However, (5–8) no longer reduces to a linear analytical solution for θ, as it did for I in (5–6). This implies the use of numerical optimization recipes based on automated search algorithms guided by, e.g., gradient descent (Press et al., 1986). Optimization will search for the minimum of (5–8), and there is no fundamental limitation to that endeavor, when the number of unknowns is kept below the number of observations. The minimum of ε_{LS} certainly exists and is theoretically unique when sources are constrained to be dipolar (see, e.g., Badia et al., 2004). The practice of non-linear optimization, however, may reveal that the landscape of $\| O - \mathrm{T}(I, \theta)\|^2$ in the dimensions of I and θ might be quite hilly; meaning that there are many sets of parameters $\{I, \theta\}$ leading to values of ε_{LS} which are *very close* to its global minimum. These values are naturally called *local minima*, and this is where the search for optimal parameter values might be trapped as illustrated Figure 5–6. Concretely, this will translate as a greater sensitivity of the search to its initial conditions, e.g., the values assigned to the unknown parameters to initiate the search.

In summary, even though localizing a number of elementary dipoles corresponding to the amount of instantaneous observations is theoretically well-posed, we are facing two issues that will drive us to reconsider the source-fitting problem in practice, as we shall see in the following section:

(1) Overfitting: meaning that the inverse model accounts for the noise components in the observations;

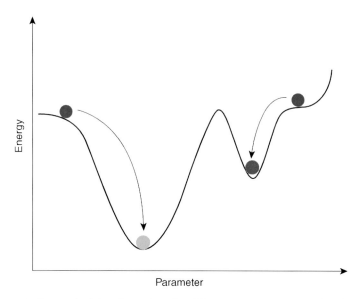

Figure 5–6. On optimizing functionals with non-convex energy landscapes. This is illustrated in this cartoon where the energy functional depends on a single parameter, which value can be altered along the x-axis. Two initial conditions are explored (blue disks). Initialization from the leftmost blue disk leads to the global minimum of energy (green disk). Optimization from the second initial condition (rightmost blue disk) ends up being trapped in a local minimum of the energy landscape (red disk).

(2) Non-linear searches that tend to be trapped in local minima of the LS cost which are all the more numerous as the inverse model contains more elementary sources.

"How Many Dipoles Should I Fit to My Data?"

A general rule of thumb when the data is noisy and the optimization principle is ruled by nonlinear dependency is to keep the complexity of the estimation as low as possible. Taming the complexity starts with bringing the number of unknowns to be estimated under the number of observations, thereby making (5–5) become overdetermined. Overdeterminacy should not be considered as big an issue in experimental sciences as underdeterminacy. Indeed, and very pragmatically speaking, the additional information brought by supplementary sensors just brings more information to the estimation problem, and might even give room to channel selection in case of noise or artifact contamination of a subset of sensors.

Early dipole fitters – as we have seen above – have naturally realized that fitting a single dipole to early-latency somatosensory data would be about the right way to start with computational source fitting (Okada et al., 1984). The somatotopy of primary somesthesic brain regions using single dipole models has been, and still is, yielding a flourishing literature, especially in clinical investigations (e.g., Meunier et al., 2003). This single equivalent dipole model (ECD) for supposedly isolated activations during the early stage of brain information processing was also conjectured and evaluated in auditory (Zimmerman et al., 1981) and visual (Lehmann et al., 1982) primary responses. Very early on, though, it appeared that most later components of evoked fields would necessitate more parameters to both 1) bring the LS-error ε_{LS} down to a level compatible with SNR, and 2) yield a source model with reasonable stability across successive observations on a time window compatible with the waveforms measured at the sensor level.

Scherg and von Cramon (1985) conceptualized the spatiotemporal (ST) dipole model, which also requires to solve a LS-optimization problem, but on a set of successive time samples. The ST dipole model was typically developed to localize the sources of scalp waveforms that were assumed to be generated by multiple and overlapping brain activations. The model therefore includes the *a priori* that a source in the inverse model is expected to be activated for a certain duration – with amplitude modulations – while staying at the same location with the same orientation. The ST model is typical of the introduction of further information in the tricky estimation problem confronting us.

Alternatively, the orientation constraint may be relaxed by considering that tiny displacements of the brain activity can be efficiently modeled by a rotating dipole source at some fixed location. This approach was extensively adopted in studies of the tonotopic organization of the auditory cortex (Zimmerman et al., 1981). In practice, a rotating dipole can be efficiently modeled by a triplet of orthogonal dipoles, which form a basis for a dipole with any orientation at the same location. Hence, the orientation parameters in θ can be reduced to the amplitude parameters of the dipoles in the equivalent triplet, i.e., parameters with linear dependency on the data.

When multiple sources are expected from the experiment, multiple-dipole models need to be fitted to the observations. As we have seen previously, fitting the entire set of parameters with too many dipoles is detrimental to the numerical stability and significance of the inverse model. Hence, the number of dipoles to be adjusted must also be estimated from the observations, and thereby constitutes some hidden parameter in the forward model.

Adding the number of sources to the LS error functional leads to intractable optimization. Other criteria based on information theory may be applied to automatically estimate the number of sources in the data, but have been of limited success in MEG because the statistics of the data do not match the methodological assumptions for which they were developed initially (Waldorp et al., 2005). Signal classification and spatial filtering techniques are efficient solutions to this problem as we shall see in the next section.

Let us conclude by stating that the localization approach, consisting in adjusting the parameters of a limited number of equivalent dipole sources, requires considerable expertise from users. Special care should be brought to the evaluation of the stability of the estimated sources with regards to changes in initial conditions of the optimization, so that reproducibility of the inverse model should not be questioned. With all that in mind, it has proven to be an efficient means to evaluate models of brain activity, even on complex paradigms (see Chapter 6).

Spatial Filters, Beamformers and Signal Classifiers

The inherent difficulties to source localization with generators of multiple origins and noisy data components have led signal processors to develop alternative approaches, most notably in the glorious field of radar and sonar in the 1970's. Rather than attempting to localize the sources by adjusting their tricky nonlinear parameters, scanning techniques have emerged and proceeded by systematically sifting through space to see how a predetermined source model would fit into the data at a specific region of space.

While doing so, the first approaches also attempted to block the contributions from the other parts of space, hence the nicknames of spatial filters and beamformers — just as if a virtual beam would be directed and listen exclusively at some region of space.

These approaches have triggered tremendous interest and applications in array signal processing, and have percolated the MEG community at several instances (e.g., Spencer et al., 1992 and more recently, Hillebrand et al., 2005).

In brief, spatial filters and beamformers are built on a source model defined *a priori*. This latter is usually a single or a triplet of current dipoles. At each point in a predefined 3D or surfacic grid, a narrow-band spatial filter is formed so that the contribution to data of the source model at this very point is estimated while the other brain regions are ideally muted – or at least attenuated – by the filter spatial block band. van Veen and Buckley (1988) have detailed a technical introduction to beamformers which is excellent further reading.

It is sometimes claimed that beamformers do not solve an inverse problem: this is a bit overstated. Indeed, spatial filters do require a source and a forward model, which will be both confronted to the observations. Instead of looking for *the* best solution (like, e.g., in the LS sense), beamformers scan the entire expected source space and systematically test the prediction of the source and forward models on the observations. This results in a model score map which should not be misinterpreted as a current density map, as in the imaging techniques we shall examine below. More technically – though with no details given here – the forward model is also somehow inverted as in (5–6), though iteratively on each source grid point to estimate the output of each narrow band filter, successively. Therefore, beamformers and spatial filters are truly avatars of inverse modeling.

Among all possible narrow-band spatial filters for MEG, linearly-constrained minimum variance (LCMV) beamformers (van Veen and Buckley,

1988) are by far the most popular, as they offer a reasonable tradeoff between the attenuating performances outside the pass-band and the degrees of freedom available from observations to build the filter coefficients.

Though beamformers are convenient in translating the source localization problem to a signal detection issue in a search space, they suffer from drawbacks that are important to bear in mind.

(1) They are built from a model of the covariance statistics of the data, which may be estimated from the data through sample statistics. However, even though a greater number of sensors is beneficial to the synoptic measurement of the brain magnetic fields, the more channels, the more data samples are necessary for robust – and numerically stable – estimation of the covariance statistics. This is the reason MEG beamformers have been evaluated on sweeps of ongoing, unaveraged data (see Chapter 9) in experimental conditions where behavioral stationarity was a means to ensure some stationarity in the data as well. In the context of evoked, time-locked activity, some recent developments suggest to consider samples across single trials to build the statistics (Cheyne et al., 2006).

(2) They are quite sensitive to errors in the head model. The filter outputs are usually normalized by local noise contributions evaluated from some baseline time window. However, SNR is not homogeneous everywhere in the source space, which results in sidelobe leakages from interfering sources nearby, which impedes the filter selectivity and, therefore, the specificity of source detection (Wax & Anu, 1996).

(3) They are fooled by simultaneous highly correlated activations that are interpreted by the beamformers as emerging from a single source, hence identified with an uncontrolled location bias.

Signal processors had long identified these issues, and consequently developed an alternative point of view on the data as being signal or noise, as an alternative technique to beamformers. Multiple signal classification (MUSIC) algorithm (Schmidt, 1986) starts by considering that the signal and noise components within observations are uncorrelated. Strong results in signal subspace theory show that these components live in separate subspaces which can be identified using, e.g., principal component analysis (PCA) of the data time series (Golub, 1996).

Mosher et al. (1999) gives an extensive review of signal classification approaches to MEG and EEG source localization. Their practice in various experimental conditions remains limited by their sensitivity in the definition of the signal vs. noise subspaces, which rules completely the subsequent classification and, therefore, the performances of source identification. Reasons for this come from the quite limited instrumental noise in EEG and MEG compared with the massive background brain activity which is very perturbing, because it is structured in a way very comparable with the signal of interest. An interesting application of MUSIC-like powerful discrimination ability, though, has been developed in epilepsy spike-sorting (Ossadtchi et al., 2004).

In summary, spatial filters, beamformers, and signal classification approaches bring us *closer* to a distributed representation of the brain electrical activity. As a caveat, the results generated by these techniques are not an estimation of the current density everywhere in the brain. It is rather a score map of a source model – generally a current dipole – which is evaluated at the points of a predefined spatial lattice, which sometimes leads to misinterpretations. The localization issue now becomes a signal-detection problem within the score map; and solutions to this issue are described in the literature (e.g., Mosher et al., 2003). Illustrations and examples of beamforming approaches are given in Chapter 9.

The imaging approaches we are about to introduce now, push this detection problem further by attempting to estimate the brain current density at once, and entirely from the MEG/EEG surface data.

The Imaging Approach

We have brought the inverse modeling problem from mere localization using point-like source models to a distributed score map of the same elementary source models as obtained from beamforming. The imaging approaches, which have developed quite in parallel, yield source models built from a distribution of elementary source currents as well, but with fixed locations – and usually orientations – and where amplitudes are estimated all at once.

Therefore, MEG source imaging yields an estimation of neural current intensity maps distributed within the brain volume or constrained at the cortical surface, just like pixels are distributed on a 2D image.

The Imaging Source Space

The imaging approach estimates the source amplitudes from the observations while constraining the locations and orientations to the brain volume or surface. In the volumic case, the brain is gridded using a 3D lattice of voxels, which might be either generic – e.g., inferred from an MRI template – or obtained directly from the subject's individual MRI and confined to a mask of the grey matter by using the appropriate software solution, e.g., SPM(http://www.fil.ion.ucl.ac.uk/spm/), brainVISA(http://brainvisa.info) or BrainSuite(http://neuroimage.usc.edu/brainsuite/).

The cortically-constrained image model derives from the assumption that MEG data originates essentially from large cortical assemblies of pyramidal cells, with currents from post-synaptic potentials (PSP) flowing orthogonally to the local cortical surface. The orientation constraint can either be strict (Dale and Sereno, 1993) or relaxed by authorizing some controlled deviation from the surface normal (Lin et al., 2006a).

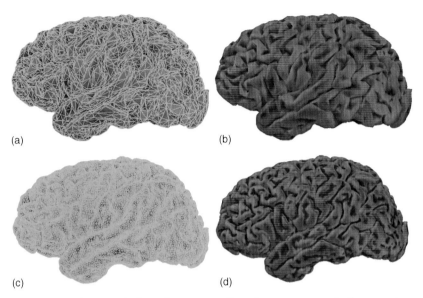

(a)   (b)

(c)   (d)

Figure 5–7. The cortical surface, tessellated at two resolutions, using: (a, b) 10,034 vertices (20,026 triangles with 10 mm² average surface area) and (c, d) 79,124 vertices (158,456 triangles with 1.3 mm² average surface area).

In both cases, reasonable spatial sampling of the image space requires an order of several thousands of elementary sources as depicted Figure 5–7. This number is very critical in the surfacic case, as the cortical mantle is severely convoluted. Consequently, though the imaging inverse modeling problem consists in estimating parameters of only linear-dependency in the data, it is dramatically underdetermined.

Just as in the context of source localization, where the number of sources is a restrictive prior as a remedy to ill-posedness, imaging models need to be complemented by *a priori* information. This is properly formulated with the mathematics of regularization, and we are now going to review and sort out the various priors which have been adopted in MEG source imaging so far.

Regularization With Priors on the Image Model

Adding priors to the imaging model can be adequately formalized in the context of Bayesian inference, where solutions to inverse modeling satisfy both the fit to observations – given some model of nuisances – and some additional priors. In the estimation perspective, where one is looking for a *best model* of some sort – and with the notations from the generic Equation (5–1) – it is possible to consider the mode of the *a posteriori* probability distribution of source intensity $p(I|O)$, given the observations as a mixture of the likelihood of the noisy data $p(O|I)$ – i.e., of the predictive power of a given source model – and the *a priori* probability of a given source model $p(I)$ following the Bayes rule that states.

$$p(I\,|\,O)\varpropto p(O\,|\,I)\,p(I).\qquad(5\text{–}9)$$

We do not want to detail the mathematics of Bayesian inference any further here, as this would reach outside the objectives of this chapter. Specific recommended further reading includes Demoment, (1989), for a Bayesian discussion on regularization and Baillet et al., (2001a), for an introduction to MEG imaging methods, also in the Bayesian framework.

Here, we will discuss pragmatically regularization from the restricted – but highly illustrative – perspective of the generalization of the least-squares criterion.

We may recall first the objective of LS, which consists in minimizing the error ε_{LS} between the observations and the prediction from the source model (Eq. (5–8)). Now our objective for source imaging would be that this prediction error be complemented by the adequation of the model parameters to some *a priori* information that could, e.g., be formulated literally as follows: "Among all possible solutions, favor those with spatial and temporal smoothness of the spatial distribution of neural currents and their time series (respectively); penalize models where currents have unrealistic, non-physiologically plausible amplitudes; favor adequation with an fMRI activation map; prefer source image models made of piecewise homogeneous activations; etc."

An important benefit of a well-chosen prior would be that there would exist **a unique solution** to the regularized inverse modeling problem, despite the original underdeterminacy. As relevant priors may take many faces, this explains the plethora of source imaging solutions, and the difficulty for newcomers to understand that these methods usually belong to the same technical background.

Concretely, we are moving from ordinary LS (OLS) to regularized-LS (RLS) by defining a new objective for the search of model parameters, that is, the amplitudes of all elementary source currents $\hat{I}_{RLS}$:

$$\hat{I}_{RLS} = \arg\min_{I}\left(\|O - TI\|^{2} + \lambda f(I)\right) = \arg\min_{I}\varepsilon_{RLS.}\qquad(5\text{–}10)$$

Note that we have removed the nonlinear parameters θ (e.g., the elementary source locations) from the optimization, as they are now all considered as fixed and predetermined. T is now entirely defined as the solution to the MEG forward problem for all elementary sources in the distributed model with arbitrary unit current amplitudes, and is generally referred to as the *gain matrix*; $f(I)$ is typically a positive monotonic function of source amplitudes, which takes large values when I deviates from the expected type of source distribution a priori; λ is a positive scalar that helps balance the parameter optimization between unregularized OLS prediction error $\varepsilon_{LS}(\lambda \ll 1)$ and

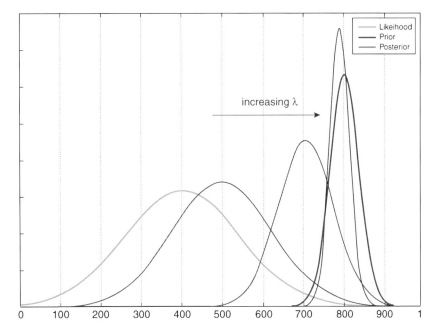

Figure 5–8. Influence of the regularization parameter λ on the profile of the posterior probability distribution. The prior (in blue) and likelihood (in green) are normally distributed with different modes and variances. As λ increases, the mode of the posterior probability distribution in red tends to the mode of the prior.

excessive trust in the priors regardless of the observations $(\lambda \gg 1)$ as illustrated Figure 5–8. For this reason ε_{LS} becomes a *data attachment term* in RLS.

Now it is obvious that the minimization of ε_{RLS}, and the existence of a unique solution to (5–10), strongly depends on the mathematical nature of $f(I)$.

A Collection of Priors

A widely used prior in the field of image reconstruction considers that the expected source amplitudes I be as small as possible on average. This is the well-described minimum-norm (MN) model where:

$$f(I) = \|I\|^2 . \tag{5–11}$$

Technically speaking, we are referring to the L2-norm. In that case, ε_{RLS} is quadratic in I, with a unique analytical solution which writes (Tarantola, 2004):

$$\hat{I}_{MN} - \mathrm{T}'\left(\mathrm{TT}' + \lambda \mathrm{I_d}\right)^{-1} O, \tag{5–12}$$

where T′ stands for the matrix transpose of T, and I_d the identity matrix. The computational simplicity of the MN estimate of distributed current amplitudes has been very attractive in MEG (Wang et al., 1992), because it demonstrated that a unique solution to the underdetermined MEG inverse problem could be elaborated.

The basic MN estimate has been demonstrated to be problematic, though, as it tends to favor the most superficial brain regions (e.g., gyral crowns) and underestimate the contribution of deeper source areas (such as sulcal fundi) (Fuchs et al., 1999) (Figure 5–9).

As a remedy, a slight alteration of the basic MN estimator consists in weighting each elementary source amplitude by the inverse of the norm of its contribution to sensors (i.e. of the corresponding column of the gain matrix (T)). This depth weighting yields a weighted MN (WMN) estimate which still benefits from unicity and linearity in the observations as the basic MN in (5–12) (Lin et al., 2006b).

Despite their robustness to noise and simple computation, it is relevant to question the neurophysiological validity of MN priors – though it would have been more rigorous to do so beforehand. Indeed – though reasonably intuitive - there is no evidence that neural currents would systematically match the principle of minimal energy. Some authors have speculated that a more physiologically relevant prior would be that the norm of spatial derivatives (e.g., gradient or Laplacian) of the current map be minimized (as in LORETA; Pascual-Marqui et al., 1994). As a general rule of thumb, however, all MN-based source imaging approaches greatly overestimate the smoothness of the spatial distribution of neural currents, while quantitative and qualitative empirical evidence demonstrate spatial discrimination of reasonable range at the sublobar brain scale (Darvas et al., 2004; Sergent et al., 2005). Refer to Chapters 7 and 8 for specific discussions on distributed-source modeling.

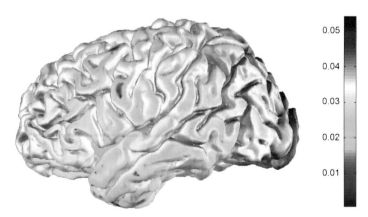

Figure 5–9. Sensitivity of MEG to cortical currents depends on their location and orientation. MEG signals are stronger on sulcus walls (yellow/red) than on the gyral crowns (green/blue).

Most of the recent literature in regularized imaging models for MEG consists in struggling to improve the spatial resolution of the MN-based models (see Baillet et al. (2001a) for a review), with notable increases in theoretical performances, but with limited impact on routine analysis in the MEG room so far, though, because of practical limitations due to the computational load of these techniques.

As a general principle, we are facing the dilemma of knowing that all priors about the source images are certainly abusive, hence that the inverse model is wrong, while hoping it is not *too* wrong for the sake of significance of the neuroscience question under scrutiny. This discussion is recurrent in the general context of estimation theory and model selection, and we shall return to this later.

At Last, a Word on Head Models: The Forward Problem

In previous sections, we have taken for granted that the forward model of MEG was solved prior to running into the questions of inverse modeling. We shall speak briefly of state-of-the-art approaches to modeling the neural currents and the magnetostatics first, always from a pragmatic perspective, and cite useful references for complete reading.

Modeling Starts at the Source

The solution to the forward problem in MEG (and, again, EEG) concerns the choice of two models that are bound to work together very complementarily: the source model and the prediction (modeling) of MEG/EEG surface measurements produced by such a model.

The canonical source model we have been using the all way through so far, is the electric current dipole. This model was initially motivated by the dipolar pattern of magnetic fields observed outside the scalp. Further, the depolarization process in neural cell assemblies is quite intuitively depicted as a current flow between a source and a sink over a limited distance, which is also well-accounted by an equivalent current dipole.

Indeed, most topographical patterns from evoked activity at the sensor level are essentially made of dipolar shapes of field distributions, thereby reinforcing the fitness of such a simple model for current density distribution in cell assemblies.

Some authors however, have questioned the predictive value of the dipolar model – especially in the context of ECD fits for source localization – when brain activity is susceptible to extending up to about $10cm^2$ to be detectable at the scalp surface, as evidenced by electrocorticographic (ECoG) recordings (Tao et al., 2005).

To understand this, we need to refer to the physics of magnetostatics, which state that the magnetic fields produced by any arbitrary current distribution may be decomposed as the sum of more elementary terms; the first being the dipolar contribution of the source, and the rest being built from the contributions of elementary multipolar current sources: this is called the 'multipolar expansion' of the field (Karp et al., 1980). When the source extension is small compared to its distance to sensors – e.g. from small ($\sim < 1cm^2$) shallow brain activations to deeper large source ($\sim > 10cm^2$), the multipolar contributions tend to be negligible compared with dipole's. However, when the extension of the local brain activity tends to increase, and/or when the distribution of neural currents within an active areas departs from uniformity – e.g., when local synchronization rate amongst cell assemblies is rather poor – multipolar components tend to become prominent in the measured field (Jerbi et al., 2002).

As a matter of fact, measures from simultaneous ECoG and EEG in epilepsy have shown that on the order of $10cm^2$ active brain surface is sometimes necessary, to be detected at the scalp level. Further, studies have shown that the ECD model in localization approaches for such large surface of brain activity, localize the source of the signals with a distance bias of few centimeters away from the patch centroid (Jerbi et al., 2004). Recently, federative efforts for compact multipolar modeling of large brain areas have been achieved (Jerbi et al., 2002) and triggered research on efficient localization using source models from multipolar expansions up to order 4 (quadrupole source model), which has shown very encouraging gain on localization bias (Jerbi et al., 2004). In the near future, this may be applied for further compact modeling in distributed source models and yield better-posed inverse modeling problems with more efficient numerical resolution.

Once a generic model of neural mass activity has been selected, the forward problem is further resolved by describing the source environment – i.e., the geometrical and the electromagnetic properties of head tissues – and the sensor array, both having influence on the fields produced by the source model.

Modeling the Sensor Array

The MEG sensor array is made of multiple pick-up coils (magnetometers), which are sometimes arranged in pairs or more, to form physical gradiometers (see Chapter 2). It is important that the sensing principles from which the data originate be modeled accurately prior to source estimation. If not, the model of data formation as in (5–2) would suffer from severe bias. We may note in passing that designing a model for the sensor array is quite straightforward in principle, but is subjected to practical caveats that one should bear in mind to avoid systematical errors.

The details of the sensor geometry are generally dependent on the manufacturer of the array, and the researcher needs to be aware of any possible options in solving for the sensor model. When the exact sensor geometry is not made available, the sensing coils are considered as point-like. This simplified sensor model is also the most common, and has limited impact on the accuracy of the forward model. If the geometrical details of the sensor coil are available, the computation of the total magnetic flux induction captured by the sensor can be more accurately modeled by integration within the sensor surface area. Gradiometer arrangements are readily modeled by applying the arithmetic operation they mimic by combining the fields modeled at each of its magnetometers.

Recent MEG systems include sophisticated noise-attenuation technology that may be routinely applied to the raw recordings. These include higher-order gradient corrections and signal-space projection techniques, which alter the basic data formation model and therefore need to be taken into account (Nolte & Curio, 1999). The researcher needs to be aware whether such correction procedure has been applied to the data. If yes, he/she will have to make sure that the software solution to the forward problem will be capable of altering the basic forward solution accordingly.

The most tricky part in the modeling of the MEG array consists of the accurate localization of the sensors relative to the head (i.e. the brain sources) of the subject. This general problem is known as the 'coregistration' issue and the bias in the estimation due to misspecification of the sensor locations may be quite dramatic. Fortunately, MEG system vendors have developed solutions to localize the sensors respectively to some coils attached to the subject's scalp, which are fully integrated to the acquisition software (see Chapter 2). As we shall discuss later, these solutions are satisfactory when the anatomy of the subject is not fully specified and source locations are interpreted qualitatively. However, when the individual cortical surface conditions the source distribution, as in the imaging approaches, or even when dipoles are secondarily projected into the MRI volume for further interpretation, the errors due to this registration procedure may also produce severe misinterpretation of the source solution (Schwartz et al., 1996).

Indeed, even though the MEG array is rigid, and therefore the relative distances between sensors are constant, the subject is likely to move during an acquisition run, thereby moving his head away from the initial position taken as a reference for the subsequent localization steps. Therefore, the head location has to be checked at least both at the beginning and at the end of a run. New MEG systems are now developed to monitor the head location online. This will greatly improve the quality check on the data and permit interruption of a run spoiled by head movements, or even allow a more precise offline correction of those movements (see, e.g., Uutela et al., 2001, and BrainStorm [http://neuroimage.usc.edu/brainstorm]).

Modeling of Head Tissues

Predicting the magnetic fields produced by an elementary source model at a given sensor array requires a last modeling step, which has occupied a large part of the MEG literature. This so-called *head modeling* is literally a model of the influence of the head geometry, and magnetostatic properties of head tissues, on magnetic fields measured outside the head.

In EEG for instance, it is quite intuitive that the skull would form a barrier of lower conductance that strongly distorts and attenuates the electric potentials at the scalp vs. at the cortical surface. This is also the case for MEG in an arbitrary head geometry, as the electric potentials and magnetic induction are coupled by the Maxwell's equations (Hämäläinen et al., 1993).

Simple geometrical models of the head have been extensively investigated; the most popular being concentric layers arranged in spheres, one sphere per major category of tissue (scalp, skull and brain). The reasons for this are both historical and pragmatic. From the historical point of view, the sphere was – again – initially investigated in MCG, and demonstrated an interesting trade-off between oversimplified models of body sources floating in an homogeneous medium, and the computationally-demanding numerical solutions required by realistic geometry, which basic computers could not handle routinely at the time.

From the pragmatic point of view, one can notice that most heads fit reasonably well inside a sphere centered about 5 cm above the plane defined by the usual anatomical fiducials used in MEG: the nasion, and both bilateral pre-auricular points.

The spherical geometry has demonstrated very attractive properties in MEG (Sarvas, 1987). Indeed, remarkably, MEG spherical solutions are absolutely insensitive to the number of shells, such that a single homogeneous sphere generates the same MEG fields as a set of concentric spheres of different conductivities. Therefore, for MEG purposes, only the center of symmetry, i.e., the common center of the concentric spheres, is important; the conductivity profile plays no role in the solution, nor do the radii of the spheres. Implicitly, it is assumed that the radius of the outermost sphere is smaller than the distance of any of the sensors from the center of symmetry. The sphere can be fit to the entire head, or restricted to regions of interest, such as parieto-occipital regions for visual studies.

Another remarkable consequence of the spherical symmetry is that the radial component of the magnetic field is not affected by the volume currents, and therefore only depends on the primary current source. However, this fact is of minor practical importance, since all field components can be easily computed from an analytical formula, which takes the contribution of the volume currents correctly into account (Sarvas, 1987). More importantly, however, radially oriented currents produce no magnetic field outside a spherically symmetric conductor. Therefore, signals from currents at the crests of the gyri and depth of the sulci are attenuated in the MEG data, whereas the contribution of the former is very prominent in EEG (see Figure 5.9, and Hillebrand & Barnes, 2002).

This has led researchers to investigate more realistic head geometries to enhance the sensitivity of MEG toward pseudo-radial sources. Boundary Element (BEM) and Finite Element (FEM) methods are generic numerical approaches to the resolution of continuous equations over discrete space, and have naturally been applied to MEG. Both approaches necessitate a geometric

tessellation of head tissues from the individual MRI, as a realistic approximation of their geometry (Figure 5–10).

In the case of BEM, the conductivity of tissues is supposed to be homogeneous and isotropic within each envelope. Therefore, each tissue envelope
is delimited using surface boundaries defined over a triangulation of each of
the segmented envelopes from the MRI.

FEM assumes that tissue conductivity may be anisotropic (such as the
skull and white matter), therefore the primary geometric element needs to be
volumic. Consequently, tetrahedra are elementary sample elements that will
fill the volume of each tissue compartment.

The main obstacle to a routine usage of BEM and, more pregnantly, in
FEM, is essentially the tessellation phase. Because the head geometry is intricate and not always well-defined from conventional MRI, automatic segmentation tools sometimes fail to identify robustly some tissue structures that
would justify the use of realistic head models by themselves. These include,

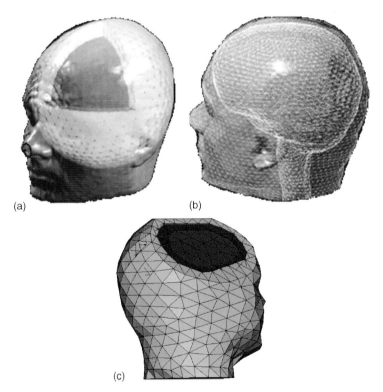

(a)   (b)

(c)

Figure 5–10. Three approaches to MEG head modeling: (a) Spherical
approximation of the geometry of head tissues; (b) Digitization of surface
envelopes using surfacic meshes with numerical solution using the BEM
approach; (c) An alternative to (b) using volumic meshes – here built from
tetrahedra – with numerical solution using the FEM approach.

e.g., the skull – which is invisible on conventional T1-weighted MRI (but see Dogdas et al., 2005) for an efficient estimation procedure).

The computational times also remain extremely long (several hours on a conventional workstation) and are detrimental to source localization methods where the source location is optimized, which necessitates the update of the corresponding forward model on the fly. Pragmatic solutions to this problem have been proposed recently. These include the interpolative approximation of the source lead-field from a dense precomputed volumic grid (Ermer et al., 2001), or from an atlas-based approach, which deforms a precomputed FEM tessellation to match the individual scalp of the subject (Darvas et al., 2006).

An alternative solution to these numerical approaches considers a set of overlapping spheres to compute the individual lead-fields at each sensor in the array (Huang et al., 1999) (Figure 5–11). In other words, a spherical head-model is designed locally to compute the led-field at each individual sensor location. If the tessellations of the three primary tissue layers are available, the initial decision is which layer to use for the fitting; practical experience is that the inner skull boundary is most useful for this fitting in the MEG case, since the currents are most affected by the inner skull boundary, and because the scalp layer in the inferior regions basically begins to flatten out as the scalp joins the neck regions. Fitting local spheres to these regions tends to create unrealistically large spheres, and fitting instead to the inner skull yields spheres that are more naturally fit to the brain regions (See BrainStorm).

Finally, let us close this section by mentioning that any realistic head model requires an estimation of the conductivity values of the tissues of the encephalon. Though solutions for impedance tomography using MRI (Tuch et al., 2001) and EEG (Goncalves et al., 2003) have been suggested, their practical impact is yet to be matured before entering the daily practice of

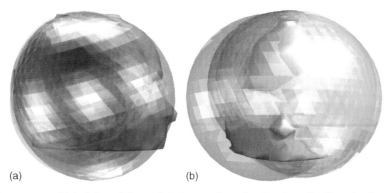

(a)   (b)

Figure 5–11. Side (a) and front (b) views of a selection locally-fitted spheres to the individual anatomy of a subject. Each sphere is adjusted to a given sensor location and the neighboring scalp surface to compute the corresponding lead field.

MEG researchers. So far, conductivity values from ex-vivo studies are conventionally integrated in all BEM and FEM models (Geddes & Baker, 1967).

Approaches to the Appraisal of MEG Inverse Models

Throughout this chapter, we have been dealing with modeling, and modeling implies dealing with uncertainty. MEG source estimation has uncertainty everywhere: data are complex and contaminated with various nuisances, source models are simplistic, head models have approximated geometries and conductivity properties that are poorly approached in vivo, priors are only priors, and can be considered as quite arbitrary, etc.

It is therefore reasonable to question how the numerical methods at stake may be sensitive to all these sources of errors and bias. This concerns the appraisal of the source model, which general methodology has been adapted to MEG just recently, and is now achieving a significant degree of maturity.

Confidence Intervals

We have seen before that fitting dipoles to a time chunk of data may be quite sensitive to their initial locations prior to the search. Similarly, imaging methods suggest that each brain location is active, potentially. It would be quite relevant to understand the confidence the researcher may have in the amplitudes suggested by the distributed source model.

In other words, we are now looking for error bars that would define a **confidence interval** about the estimated values of a source model.

Signal processors have long developed a systematic approach to what they have coined as 'detection and estimation theories' (Kay, 1993). The general stake consists in understanding how certain one can be about the estimated parameters of a model, given a model for the noise in the data. The basic approach consists in considering the estimated parameters (e.g., source location) as a random variable. The parametric approach to the estimation of error bounds on the source parameters consists in estimating their bias and variance.

Bias is an estimation of the distance between the true value and the expectancy of the average of a parameter due to perturbations. The definition of variance follows immediately. Cramer-Rao lower bounds (CRLB) on the estimator's variance can be explicitly computed using an analytical solution to the forward model, and given a model for perturbations (e.g., with distribution under a normal law). In a nutshell, the tighter the CRLB, the more confident one can be about the estimated values. Mosher et al. (1993) have investigated this approach using extensive Monte Carlo (MC) simulations, which evidenced a resolution of a few millimeters in single dipole models. These results were later confirmed by phantom studies (Baillet et al., 2001b; Leahy et al., 1998).

CRLB increased markedly for two-dipole models, thereby demonstrating their extreme sensitivity and the need for a careful usage in localization approaches.

Recently, nonparametric approaches to the determination of error bounds have greatly benefited from the commensurable increase in computational power. Jackknife, and more generally bootstrap-based approaches, proved to be efficient and powerful tools to estimate confidence intervals on MEG source parameter estimations without any explicit limitations on the nature of perturbations and head models.

These techniques are all based on data resampling approaches and have proven to be exact and efficient when a large-enough number of experimental replications are available (Davison & Hinkley, 1997). This is typically the case in MEG experiments where protocols are designed on multiple trials. If we are interested, e.g., in knowing about the confidence interval on a source location in a single-dipole model from evoked averaged data, the bootstrap will generate a large number (typically > 500) of averaged pseudo-data sets by randomly choosing trials from the original set of trials and averaging them all together. Because the trial selection is random, and systematically taken from the complete set of trials, the corresponding sample distribution of the estimated parameter values is proven to converge toward the true distribution.

A pragmatic approach to the definition of a confidence interval thereby consists in identifying the interval containing, e.g., 95% of the resampled estimates (see Figure 5–12; Baryshnikov et al., 2004; Darvas et al., 2005; McIntosh & Lobaugh, 2004).

These considerations naturally lead us to statistical inference, which questions hypothesis testing where the researcher is interested in addressing questions that are specific to the scientific hypothesis that motivated data acquisition, and which we shall review briefly in the next section.

Statistical Inference

Questions like: "How different is the dipole location between these two experimental conditions?" and "Are source amplitudes larger in such condition that in a control condition?" belong to statistical inference from experimental data. The basic problem of interest here is hypothesis testing, which is supposed to potentially invalidate a model under investigation. Here, the *model* must be understood at a higher hierarchical level than when talking about, e.g., a basic source model. It is supposed to address the neuroscience question that has motivated data acquisition and some experimental design (Guilford et al., 1978). Readers are also encouraged to refer to Chapter 10 in this book, which extensively documents this question.

In the context of MEG, population samples that will support the inference are either trials or subjects. Testing can therefore be run at the individual and group levels, respectively.

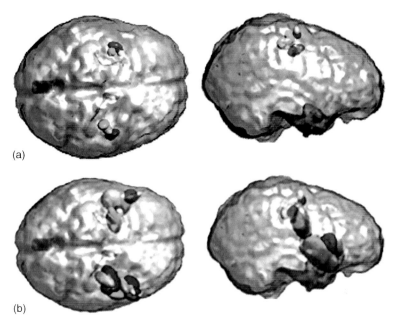

(a)

(b)

Figure 5–12. The bootstrap procedure yields nonparametric estimates of confidence intervals on source parameters. This is illustrated here with data from a study of the somatotopic cortical representation of hand fingers (Meunier et al., 2001). Ellipsoids represent the resulting 95% confidence intervals on the location of the ECD, as a model of the 40 ms (a) and 200 ms (b) brain response following hand finger stimulation. Colors encode for the stimulated fingers. While in (a) the respective confidence ellipsoids do not overlap between fingers, they considerably increase in volume for the secondary responses in (b), thereby demonstrating that a single ECD is not a proper model of brain currents at this later latency (adapted from Darvas et al., 2005). Note that similar evaluations may be drawn from imaging models using the same resampling methodology.

Brief Review of Tools for Statistical Inference

As for the estimation of confidence intervals, both parametric and non-parametric approaches to statistical inference can be considered. There is no space here for a comprehensive review of tools based on parametric models. They have been, and still are, extensively studied in the fMRI and PET communities – and recently adapted to EEG and MEG (Kiebel et al., 2005) – and popularized with software toolboxes such as SPM (Turner et al., 1998).

Nonparametric approaches like permutation tests are also emergent techniques for statistical inference applied to neuroimaging data (Nichols & Holmes, 2002; Pantazis et al., 2005). Rather than applying transformations to the data to secure the assumption of normally-distributed measures, nonparametric statistical tests take the data as they are, and are robust to departures from gaussianity.

In brief, hypothesis testing forms an assumption about the data that the researcher is interested in questioning. This basic hypothesis is called the null hypothesis, H0, and is traditionally formulated to translate no significant finding in the data, e.g., 'there are no differences in the source model in both experimental conditions'. The statistical test will express the significance of this hypothesis and evaluate the probability that the statistics in question would be obtained just by chance. In other words, the data from both conditions are interchangeable under the H0 hypothesis. This is literally what permutation testing is doing. It computes the sample distribution of estimated parameters under the null hypothesis, and verifies whether a statistics of the original parameter estimates was likely to be generated by this law.

We shall now review quickly the principle of multiple hypothesis testing from the same sample of measurements,which induces errors when multiple parameters are being tested at once. This issue pertains to statistical inference both at the individual and at the group levels. Samples will be therefore formed of repetitions (trials) of the same experiment in the same subject, or the results from the same experiment within a set of subjects, respectively.

This distinction is not crucial at this point. We shall, however, highlight the issue of spatial normalization of the brain across a sample of subjects either by applying normalization procedures (Ashburner & Friston, 1997) or by the definition of a generic coordinate system onto the cortical surface (Mangin et al., 2004; Fischl et al., 1999).

Controlling the Family-wise Error Rate

The outcome of a test will evaluate the probability p that the statistics computed from the data samples will be issued from complete chance as expressed by the null hypothesis. The researcher fixes a threshold on p, above which H0 cannot be *reasonably* rejected, thereby corroborating H0. Tests are designed to be computed once from the data sample so that the error – called the type I error – consisting in accepting H0, while it is invalid, stays below the predefined p-value.

If the same data sample is used several times for several tests, we multiply the chances that we commit a type I error. This is particularly critical when running tests in sensors or source amplitudes of an imaging model, as the number of tests is on the order of 100 and even 10,000, respectively. In this latter case, a 5% error over 10,000 tests is likely to generate 500 occurrences of false positives by wrongly rejecting H0. This is obviously not desirable, and this is the reason why this so-called family-wise error rate (FWER) should be kept under control.

Parametric approaches to address this issue have been elaborated using the theory of random fields, and have gained tremendous popularity through the SPM software. These techniques have been extended to electromagnetic source imaging, but are less robust to departure from normality than non-parametric solutions. The FWER in nonparametric testing can be controlled by using the statistics of the maximum over the entire source image, or topography at the sensor level – possibly across time (Pantazis et al., 2005).

The emergence of statistical inference solutions adapted to MEG has brought electromagnetic source localization and imaging to a considerable degree of maturity, quite comparable to other neuroimaging techniques (see Figure 5–13 for an example). Most software solutions now integrate sound solutions to statistical inference for MEG and EEG data, and this is a field that is still growing rapidly.

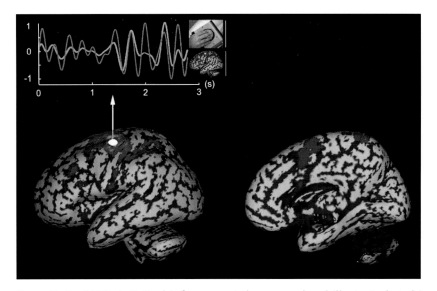

Figure 5–13. MEG statistical inference at the group level illustrated: Jerbi et al. (2007) have revealed a cortical functional network involved in hand movement coordination at low frequency (4Hz). The statistical group inference first consisted on fitting, for each trial in the experiment, a distributed source model constrained to the individual anatomy of each of 14 subjects involved. The brain area with maximum coherent activation with instantaneous hand speed was identified. The traces at the top illustrate excellent coherence in the [3,5]Hz range between these measurements (hand speed in green and M1 motor activity in blue). Secondly, the search for brain areas with activity in significant coherence with M1 revealed a larger distributed network of regions. All subjects were coregistered to a brain surface template in Talairach normalized space, with the corresponding activations interpolated onto the template surface. A nonparametric t-test contrast was completed using permutations between rest and task conditions (p < 0.01); adapted from (Jerbi et al., 2007).

Emergent Approaches for Model Selection

While there is a long tradition of considering inverse modeling as an optimization problem – i.e., designate *the* solution to an inverse problem as the source model corresponding to the putative global maximum of some adequacy functional – there are situations where, for empirical and/or theoretical reasons, the number of possible solutions is just too large to ensure this goal can be reached. This kind of situation calls for a paradigm shift in the approach to inverse modeling, which animates some discussion in the concerned scientific communities (Tarantola, 2006).

In MEG and EEG more specifically, we have admitted that picking a number of dipoles for localization purposes, or an imaging prior to insure unicity of the solution, has its (large) share of arbitrariness. Just like nonparametric statistical methods have benefited from the tremendous increase of cheap computational power, Monte Carlo simulation methods are powerful computational numerical approaches to the general problem of **model selection**. Indeed, a relevant question would be to let the data help the researcher decide whether any element from a general class of models would properly account for the data, with possibly predefined confidence intervals on the admissible model parameters.

These approaches are currently emerging from the MEG literature and have considerable potential (David et al., 2006; Mattout et al., 2006; Daunizeau et al., 2006). It is likely, however, that the critical ill-posedness of the source modeling problem will be detrimental to the efficiency of establishing tight bounds on the admissible model parameters. Further, these techniques are still extremely demanding in terms of computational resources.

Conclusions: "What am I supposed to do with my data?"

Throughout this chapter, we have stumbled across many pitfalls imposed by the ill-posed nature of the MEG source estimation problem. We have tried to offer a pragmatic point of view on these difficulties.

It is indeed quite striking that despite all these shortcomings, MEG source analysis might reveal exquisite relative spatial resolution when localization approaches are used appropriately, and – although being of relatively poor absolute spatial resolution – imaging models help the researchers tell a story on the cascade of brain events that have been occurring in controlled experimental conditions. From one millisecond to the next, it is often striking that imaging models reveal tiny alterations in the topography of brain activations at the millimeter scale.

An increasing number of groups from other neuroimaging modalities have come to realize that beyond mere cartography, the temporal and oscillatory brain responses are essential keys to the basic mechanisms of brain information processing at the neural mass level. The multiplicity of EEG systems installed in MR magnets, and the steady – though still slow – development of MEG equipments, reveal a lively scientific community with exciting perspectives for the future of multidisciplinary brain research.

Notes

1 To estimate retrospectively what was the distribution of temperature in a medium for instance.
2 3 for location *per se*, 2 for orientation and 1 for amplitude.

References

Arthur, R. M., & Geselowitz, D. B. (1970). Effect of inhomogeneities on the apparent location and magnitude of a cardiac current dipole source. *IEEE Trans Biomed Eng*, *17*(2), 141–146.

Ashburner, J., & Friston, K. (1997). Multimodal image coregistration and partitioning–a unified framework. *Neuroimage*, *6*(3), 209–217.

Badia, A. E. (2004). Summary of some results on an EEG inverse problem. *Neurol Clin Neurophysiol*, 2004, 102.

Baillet, S., Mosher, J.C., & Leahy, R.M. (2001a). Electromagnetic brain mapping. *IEEE Signal Processing Magazine*, *18*(6), 14–30.

Baillet, S., Riera, J. J., Marin, G., Mangin, J. F., Aubert, J., & Garnero, L. (2001b). Evaluation of inverse methods and head models for EEG source localization using a human skull phantom. *Phys Med Biol*, *46*(1), 77–96.

Baryshnikov, B. V., Van Veen, B. D., & Wakai, R. T. (2004). Maximum likelihood dipole fitting in spatially colored noise. *Neurol Clin Neurophysiol*, *2004*, 53.

Biomag. (1987). The biomagnetic inverse problem. The biomagnetic inverse problem conference proceedings. Milton Keynes, U.K., April 1986. In: *Phys Med Biol*, *32*(1), 1–146.

Cheyne, D., Bakhtazad, L., & Gaetz, W. (2006). Spatiotemporal mapping of cortical activity accompanying voluntary movements using an event-related beamforming approach. *Human Brain Mapping*, *27*(3), 213–229.

Cohen, D., & Hosaka, H. (1976). Part ii: magnetic field produced by a current dipole. *J Electrocardiol*, *9*(4), 409–417.

Cuffn, B. N., & Geselowitz, D. B. (1977). Computer model studies of the magnetocardiogram. *Ann Biomed Eng*, *5*(2), 164–178.

Dale, A. M., & Sereno, M. I. (1993). Improved localization of cortical activity by combining EEG and MEG with MRI cortical surface reconstruction: A linear approach. *Journal of Cognitive Neuroscience*, 5, 162–176.

Darvas, F., Pantazis, D., Kucukaltun-Yildirim, E., & Leahy, R. M. (2004). Mapping human brain function with MEG and EEG: methods and validation. *Neuroimage*, *23*, S289–S299.

Darvas, F., Rautiainen, M., Pantazis, D., Baillet, S., Benali, H., Mosher, J. C., et al. (2005). Investigations of dipole localization accuracy in MEG using the bootstrap. *Neuroimage*, *25*(2), 355–368.

Darvas, F., Ermer, J. J., Mosher, J. C., & Leahy, R. M. (2006). Generic head models for atlas-based eeg source analysis. *Hum Brain Mapp*, *27*(2), 129–143.

Daunizeau, J., Mattout, J., Clonda, D., Goulard, D., Benali, H., & Lina, J-M. (2006). Bayesian spatio-temporal approach for eeg source reconstruction: conciliating ecd and distributed models. *IEEE Trans Biomed Eng*, *53*(3), 503–516.

David, O., Kiebel, S. J., Harrison, L. M., Mattout, J., Kilner, J. M., & Friston, K. J. (2006) Dynamic causal modeling of evoked responses in EEG and MEG. *Neuroimage*, *30*(4), 1255–1272.

Davison, A. C., & Hinkley, D. V. (1997). *Bootstrap methods and their application*. Cambridge series on statistical and probabilistic mathematics. Cambridge: Cambridge University Press.

Demoment, G. (1989). Image reconstruction and restoration: overview of common estimation structures and problems. *IEEE Transactions on Signal Processing*, *37*(12), 2024–2036.

Dogdas, V., Shattuck, D. W., & Leahy, R. M. (2005). Segmentation of skull and scalp in 3-d human MRI using mathematical morphology. *Hum Brain Mapp*, *26*(4), 273–285.

Ermer, J. J., Mosher, J. C., Baillet, S., & Leahy, R. M. (2001). Rapidly recomputable EEG forward models for realistic head shapes. *Phys Med Biol*, *46*(4), 1265–1281.

Feynman, R. P. *The Feynman Lectures on Physics.* (Volume 2). Reading, Massachusetts: Addison-Wesley.

Fischl, B., Sereno, M. I., & Dale, A. M. (1999). Cortical surface-based analysis. ii: Inflation, flattening, and a surface-based coordinate system. *Neuroimage*, *9*(2), 195–207.

Fuchs, M., Wagner, M., Köhler, T., & Wischmann, H. A. (1999). Linear and nonlinear current density reconstructions. *J Clin Neurophysiol*, *16*(3), 267–295.

Geddes, L. A., & Baker, L. E. (1967). The specific resistance of biological material–a compendium of data for the biomedical engineer and physiologist. *Med Biol Eng*, *5*(3), 271–293.

Geselowitz, D. B. (1963). The concept of an equivalent cardiac generator. *Biomed Sci Instrum*, *1*, 325–330.

Geselowitz, D. B. (1964). Dipole theory in electrocardiography. *Am J Cardiol*, *14*, 301–306.

Geselowitz, D. B. (1973). Electric and magnetic field of the heart. *Annu Rev Biophys Bioeng*, *2*, 37–64.

Golub, C. F., & van Loan, G. H. (1996). *Matrix Computations.* (3rd ed.). Baltimore: Johns Hopkins University Press.

Goncalves, S. I., de Munck, J. C., Verbunt, J. P. A., Bijma, F., Heethaar, R. M., & Lopes da Silva, F. (2003). In vivo measurement of the brain and skull resistivities using an EIT-based method and realistic models for the head. *IEEE Transactions On Biomedical Engineering*, *50*(6), 754–767.

Guilford, J. P., & Fruchter, B. (1978). *Fundamental Statistics in Psychology and Education.* (6th ed.). New York: McGraw-Hill.

Hadamard, J. (1902). *Sur les problemes aux derivees partielles et leur signification physique.* Princeton University Bulletin, pp. 49–52.

Hämäläinen, M., Hari, R., Ilmoniemi, R., Knuutila, J., and Lounasmaa, O. (1993). Magnetoencephalography: Theory, instrumentation and applications to the non-invasive study of human brain function. *Rev Mod Phys*, *65*, 413–497.

Hillebrand, A., & Barnes, G. R. (2002). A quantitative assessment of the sensitivity of whole-head MEG to activity in the adult human cortex. *NeuroImage*, *16*, 638–50.

Hillebrand, A. Singh, K. D., Holliday, I. E., Furlong, P. L., & Barnes, G. R. (2005). A new approach to neuroimaging with magnetoencephalography. *Hum Brain Mapp*, *25*(2), 199–211.

Hosaka, H., & Cohen, D. (1976). Part iv: visual determination of generators of the magnetocardiogram. *J Electrocardiol*, *9*(4), 426–432.

Huang, M. X., Mosher, J. C., & Leahy, R. M. (1999). A sensor-weighted overlapping-sphere head model and exhaustive head model comparison for meg. *Phys Med Biol*, *44*(2), 423–440.

Huizenga, H. H., de Munck, J. C., Waldorp, L. J., & Grasman, R. P. (2002). Spatiotemporal eeg/meg source analysis based on a parametric noise covariance model. *IEEE Trans Biomed Eng*, *49*(6), 533–539.

Jerbi, K., Mosher, J. C., Baillet, S., & Leahy, R. M. (2002). On MEG forward modelling using multipolar expansions. *Phys Med Biol*, *47*(4), 523–555.

Jerbi, K., Baillet, S., Mosher, J. C., Nolte, G., Garnero, L., & Leahy, R. M. (2004). Localization of realistic cortical activity in MEG using current multipoles. *Neuroimage*, *22*(2), 779–793.

Jerbi, K., Lachaux, J.P., NDiaye, K., Pantazis, D., Leahy, R.M., Garnero, L., et al. (2007). Coherent neural representation of hand speed in humans revealed by MEG imaging. *Proc Natl Acad Sci USA*, *104*(18), 7676–7681.

Jun, S. C., Plis, S. M., Ranken, D. M., & Schmidt, D. M. (2006). Spa tiotemporal noise covariance estimation from limited empirical magnetoencephalographic data. *Phys Med Biol*, *51*(21), 5549–5564.

Karp, P. J., Katila, T. E., Saarinen, M., Siltanen, P., & Varpula, T. T. (1980). The normal human magnetocardiogram. ii. a multipole analysis. *Circ Res*, *47*(7), 117–130.

Kay, S. M. (1993). *Fundamentals of Statistical Signal Processing: Estimation Theory.* Englewood Cliffs, NJ: Prentice Hall.

Kiebel, S. J., Tallon-Baudry, C., & Friston, K. J. (2005). Parametric analysis of oscillatory activity as measured with eeg/meg. *Hum Brain Mapp*, *26*(3), 170–177.

Kooi, K. A., Holland-Moritz, E. K., & Marshall, R. E. (1969). Oscillatory motion of a dipole as a model for the generation of cerebral rhythms having asymmetrical wave forms including the "14 and 6/sec" pattern. *Electroencephalogr Clin Neurophysiol*, *26*(1), 116.

RLeahy, M., Mosher, J. C., Spencer, M. E., Huang, M. X., & Lewine, J. D. (1998). A study of dipole localization accuracy for MEG and EEG using a human skull phantom. *Electroencephalogr Clin Neurophysiol*, *107*(2), 159–173.

Lehmann, D., Darcey, T. M. & Skrandies, W. (1982). Intracerebral and scalp fields evoked by hemiretinal checkerboard reversal, and modeling of their dipole generators. *Adv Neurol*, *32*, 41–48.

Lin, F. H., Belliveau, J. W., Dale, A. M., & Hämäläinen, M. S. (2006a). Distributed current estimates using cortical orientation constraints. *Human brain mapping*, *27*(1), 1–13.

Lin, F. H., Witzel, T., Ahlfors, S. P., Stuffebeam, S. M., Belliveau, J. W., & Hämäläinen, M. S. (2006b). Assessing and improving the spatial accuracy in meg source localization by depth-weighted minimum-norm estimates. *Neuroimage*, *31*(1), 160–171.

Mangin, J-F., Rivière, D., Coulon, O., Poupon, C., Cachia, A., Cointepas, Y., Poline, J-B., et al. (2004). Coordinate-based versus structural approaches to brain image analysis. *Artif Intell Med*, *30*(2), 177–197.

Mattout, J., Phillips, C., Penny, W. D., Rugg, M. D., & Friston, K. J. (2006). Meg source localization under multiple constraints: an extended bayesian framework. *Neuroimage*, *30*(3), 753–767.

McIntosh, A. R. & Lobaugh, N. J. (2004). Partial least squares analysis of neuroimaging data: applications and advances. *Neuroimage*, *23* Suppl 1, S250–S263.

Meunier, S., Garnero, L., Ducorps, A., Mazières, L., Lehéricy, S., du Montcel, S. T., et al. (2001). Human brain mapping in dystonia reveals both endophenotypic traits and adaptive reorganization. *Ann Neurol*, *50*(4), 521–527.

Meunier, S., Lehéricy, S., Garnero, L., & Vidailhet, M. (2003). Dystonia: lessons from brain mapping. *Neuroscientist*, *9*(1), 76–81.

Miller, W. T., & Geselowitz, D. B. (1974). Use of electric and magnetic data to obtain a multiple dipole inverse cardiac generator: a spherical model study. *Ann Biomed Eng*, *2*(4), 343–360.

Mosher, J. C., Spencer, M. E., Leahy, R. M., & Lewis, P. S. (1993). Error bounds for eeg and meg dipole source localization. *Electroencephalogr Clin Neurophysiol*, *86*(5), 303–321.

Mosher, J. C., Baillet, S., & Leahy, R. M. (1999). EEG source localization and imaging using multiple signal classification approaches. *J Clin Neurophysiol*, *16*(3), 225–238.

Mosher, J.C., Baillet, S., Leahy, & R.M. (2003). Equivalence of linear approaches in bioelectromagnetic inverse solutions. In: *Proceedings of the 2003 IEEE Workshop on Statistical Signal Processing*, pp. 294–7.

Nichols, T. E., & Holmes, A. P. (2002). Nonparametric permutation tests for functional neuroimaging: a primer with examples. *Hum Brain Mapp*, *15*(1), 1–25.

Nolte, G., & Curio, G. (1999). The effect of artifact rejection by signal-space projection on source localization accuracy in meg measurements. *IEEE Trans Biomed Eng*, *46*(4), 400–408.

Okada, Y. C., Tanenbaum, R., Williamson, S. J., & Kaufman, L. (1984). Somatotopic organization of the human somatosensory cortex revealed by neuromagnetic measurements. *Exp Brain Res*, *56*(2), 197–205.

Ossadtchi, A., Baillet, S., Mosher, J. C., Thyerlei, D., Sutherling, W., & Leahy, R. M. (2004). Automated interictal spike detection and source localization in magnetoencephalography using independent components analysis and spatiotemporal clustering. *Clin Neurophysiol*, *115*(3), 508–522.

Pantazis, D., Nichols, T. E., Baillet, S., & Leahy, R. M. (2005). A comparison of random field theory and permutation methods for the statistical analysis of MEG data. *Neuroimage*, *25*(2), 383–394.

Pascual-Marqui, R. D., Michel, C. M., & Lehmann, D. (1994). Low resolution electromagnetic tomography: a new method for localizing electrical activity in the brain. *Int J Psychophysiol*, *18*(1), 49–65.

Penfield, W. G., & Boldrey, E. (1937). Somatic motor and sensory representation in the cerebral cortex of man as studied by electrical stimulation. *Brain*, *60*, 389–443.

Perrin, F., Pernier, J., Bertrand, O., Giard, M. H., & Echallier, J. F. (1987). Mapping of scalp potentials by surface spline interpolation. *Electroencephalogr Clin Neurophysiol*, *66*(1), 75–81.

Petit-Dutaillis, D., Fischgold, H., & Rougerie, J. (1952). Progress made at the Neurosurgical Clinic of the Hôpital de la pitié from 1949 to 1952 in the localization and diagnosis of cerebral tumors by electroencephalography and arteriography. *Bull Acad Natl Med*, *136*(24-26), 444–448.

Popper, K. R. (1959) *The Logic of Scientific Discovery*. New York: Basic Books.

Press, W. H., Flannery, B. P., Teukolsky, S. A., & Vetterling, W. T. (1986). *Numerical Recipes: The Art of Scientific Computing*. Cambridge: Cambridge University Press.

Sarvas, J. (1987). Basic mathematical and electromagnetic concepts of the biomagnetic inverse problem. *Phys Med Biol, 32*(1), 11–22.

Scherg, M. & von Cramon, D. (1985). Two bilateral sources of the late aep as identified by a spatio-temporal dipole model. *Electroencephalogr Clin Neurophysiol, 62*(1), 32–44.

Schmidt, R. O. (1986). Multiple emitter location and signal parameter estimation. *IEEE Transactions on Antennas and Propagation, 34*, 276–280.

Schwartz, D., Poiseau, E., Lemoine, D., & Barillot, C. (1996). Registration of MEG/EEG data with MRI: Methodology and precision issues. *Brain Topography, 9*, 101–116.

Sergent, C., Baillet, S., & Dehaene, S. (2005). Timing of the brain events underlying access to consciousness during the attentional blink. *Nature Neuroscience, 8*(10), 1391–1400.

Spencer, M.E., Leahy, R.M., Mosher, J.C., & Lewis, P.S. (1992). Adaptive filters for monitoring localized brain activity from surface potential time series. In: IEEE, ed., *Conference Record of The Twenty-Sixth Asilomar Conference on Signals, Systems and Computers*, Vol. 1, pp. 156–161.

Tao, J. X., Ray, A., Hawes-Ebersole, S., & Ebersole, J. S. (2005). In tracranial eeg substrates of scalp eeg interictal spikes. *Epilepsia, 46*(5), 669–676.

Tarantola, A. (2004). *Inverse Problem Theory and Methods for Model Parameter Estimation*. Philadelphia: SIAM Books.

Tarantola, A. (2006). Popper, Bayes and the inverse problem. *Nat Phys, 2*(8), 92–494.

Tikhonov, A., & Arsenin, V. (1977). *Solutions of Ill-Posed Problems*. Washington, D.C.: Winston & Sons.

Tuch, D. S., Wedeen, V. J., Dale, A. M., George, J. S., & Belliveau, J. W. (2001). Conductivity tensor mapping of the human brain using diffusion tensor MRI. *Proc Natl Acad Sci USA, 98*(20), 11697–11701.

Turner, R., Howseman, A., Rees, G. E., Josephs, O., & Friston, K. (1998). Functional magnetic resonance imaging of the human brain: Data acquisition and analysis. *Exp Brain Res, 1-2*(123), 5–12.

U.S. National Library of Medicine. The pubmed online database. Retrieved from: http://www.ncbi.nlm.nih.gov/entrez/query.fcgi?db=PubMed.

Uutela, K. Taulu, S., & Hämäläinen, M. (2001). Detecting and correcting for head movements in neuromagnetic measurements. *Neuroimage, 14*(6), 1424–1431.

van Veen, D., & Buckley, K. M. (1988). Beamforming: a versatile approach to spatial filtering. *ASSP Magazine, IEEE Signal Processing Magazine, 5*, 4–24.

Waldorp, L. J., Huizenga, H. M., Nehorai, A., Grasman, R. P., & Molenaar, P. C. M. (2005). Model selection in spatio-temporal electromagnetic source analysis. *IEEE Trans Biomed Eng, 52*(3), 414–420.

Wang, J. Z., Williamson, S. J., & Kaufman, L. (1992). Magnetic source images determined by a lead-field analysis: the unique minimum-norm least-squares estimation. *IEEE Trans Biomed Eng, 39*(7), 665–675.

Wax, M., & Y. Anu, Y. (1996). Performance analysis of the minimum variance beamformer. *IEEE Transactions on Signal Processing, 44*, 928–937.

Wood, C. C., Cohen, D., Cuffn, B. N., Yarita, M., & Allison, T. (1985). Electrical sources in human somatosensory cortex: identification by combined magnetic and potential recordings. *Science, 227*(4690), 1051–1053.

Zimmerman, J. T., Reite, M., & Zimmerman, J. E. (1981). Magnetic auditory evoked fields: dipole orientation. *Electroencephalogr Clin Neurophysiol, 52*, 151–156.

6

Multi-Dipole Modeling in MEG

Riitta Salmelin

- MEG data are usually not ambiguous; it is mostly obvious where the active areas are located
- Diligence in identifying clear dipolar field patterns yields well-behaved models
- Parametric variation of stimuli is essential for functional localization and helpful in source modeling
- The proposed solution should be obvious also in the original sensor signals – always check

Introduction

The types of information one would typically like to extract from MEG data are approximate location of active brain areas, time course of activation in those areas, and effect of task or stimulus category on the neural timing and/ or strength of activation. The Equivalent Current Dipole (ECD) model is an excellent tool in this endeavor. It is simple, well defined, and robust, as it requires the minimum number of assumptions and, importantly, these assumptions are entirely transparent to the user.

As an example of a neuroscience question with multiple experimental conditions, let us consider silent reading of words and nonwords. Figure 6–1 displays MEG responses in one subject to short and long words, and nonwords.

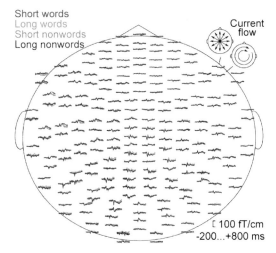

Figure 6–1. MEG signals to short and long words and nonwords, in one subject. The measurement helmet is viewed from above, flattened onto the plane, with the nose pointing upwards. In this Vectorview™ system, sensors are arranged in 102 locations along the helmet. In each location, there are two planar gradiometers that are most sensitive to orthogonal orientations of current flow (see schematic heads in the upper right corner) and one magnetometer (data not shown). Time runs along the horizontal axis, from 200 ms before stimulus onset to 800 ms after it. Variation of magnetic field is shown on the vertical axis.

The displayed time interval extends from 200 ms before stimulus presentation to 800 ms after it. Each curve shows the signal recorded by one MEG sensor. This particular MEG system (Vectorview™, Elekta-Neuromag Ltd.) uses two orthogonally oriented planar gradiometers at each recording site, which detect the maximum signal directly above an active cortical area. There are deflections in the curves essentially everywhere over the helmet, reflecting multiple active areas in the brain. In a number of sensors, the responses vary by stimulus type.

By using ECDs one can identify the multiple areas that generate these signals and their time courses of activation. In this experiment, there were four experimental conditions and eight subjects. The analysis proceeds through a number of steps, and we will start with single-subject analysis. First, we focus on each experimental condition separately, and construct a source model. Then, in order to compare the stimuli, we form a single, combined source model that works for all conditions in this subject. Based on this common model, we can identify cortical areas and time windows that show significant differences between conditions. Then we move onto group analysis. We first group the individual source areas according to function, location, direction of current flow, and/or timing, and then test for significant effects at the group level.

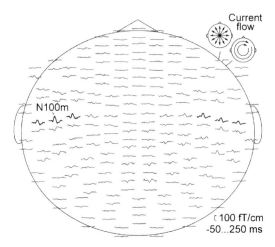

Figure 6–2. MEG responses to right-sided auditory stimulation (1-kHz tones, duration 50 ms) in one subject. The time window extends from 50 ms before tone onset to 250 ms after it.

This is a straightforward but not trivial task. In this chapter we will begin with simpler paradigms in order to illustrate the basics of ECD source modeling, then work our way to increasingly complex data sets, and eventually return to the question of reading words and nonwords. In addition, we will touch upon the issue of mouth movements in an MEG experiment. Finally, we will briefly discuss the use of ECD modeling in the analysis of cortical rhythms and their task-related modulation.

Basic Auditory Responses

Here, subjects listened to brief tones given alternately to the left and right ear, approximately once per second (e.g., Mäkelä et al., 1993; Pantev et al., 1998; Salmelin et al., 1999). Figure 6–2 depicts MEG signals averaged with respect to tones given to the right ear, in one subject. A clear deflection at about 100 ms after stimulus onset (N100m) shows that there is a sudden change in the magnetic field, that is, transient current flow in the brain underneath those sensors. A very similar response is seen over both hemispheres.

Figure 6–3 depicts the magnetic field pattern over the left hemisphere when moving through the strong N100m response. At about 60 ms, there is very little signal. Around the peak response, there is a clearly dipolar (symmetric) field pattern. At about 150 ms after stimulus onset, there is another strongly dipolar field pattern, but anterior and inferior to the earlier pattern. Although highly informative, these maps only provide coarse information on source loci. Next, one needs to determine the underlying source areas in the brain.

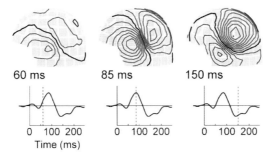

60 ms   85 ms   150 ms

0 100 200   0 100 200   0 100 200
Time (ms)

Figure 6–3. Distribution of magnetic field over the course of the auditory response. The red area indicates magnetic field emerging from the brain, and the blue area the reentering field. Electric current flows in the middle, along the zero line (black curve).

As the fields are clearly dipolar, it seems reasonable to model the underlying sources with Equivalent Current Dipoles that represent the center of an active cortical patch, and the direction and magnitude of electric current therein (Hämäläinen et al., 1993). By scanning through the N100m response, we find a time point at which the field is as closely dipolar as possible (Figure 6–4a). The density curves should then be fairly symmetrical, and the line connecting the maxima should be perpendicular to the zero field line, indicated by the black curve. The center of the dipole should fall on the crossing of these two lines. In this way, one should already have a feeling of what to expect before computing the ECD solution.

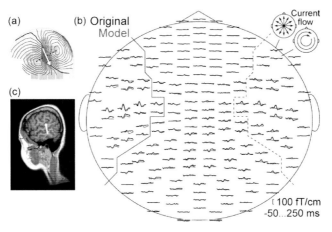

Figure 6–4. Source localization at 100 ms post-stimulus. (a) Optimally dipolar field pattern during the N100m response. (b) Selection of MEG sensors for calculation of ECD parameters. (c) Source of the left-hemisphere N100m response in the lower lip of the Sylvian fissure, with current flow perpendicular to the course of the sulcus.

To find the source of the left N100m response, we select a subset of sensors, covering the local field maxima (Figure 6–4b, solid line). The selection is also depicted on the helmet as light gray squares. The source is located in the lower lip of the Sylvian fissure, with the current flowing downwards, away from the cortical surface (Figure 6–4c). As there is only one clear field pattern in the left hemisphere, the exact selection of MEG sensors is not critical.

A model using this one source, plotted in purple in Figure 6–4b, allows comparison with the original signals, which are plotted in black. This source accounts adequately for the N100m in the left hemisphere but less so for the later component, which had a clearly different field pattern (cf. Figure 6–3). The right-hemisphere N100m remains unexplained, as it should. One can determine the right-hemisphere N100m source in the same way, by finding a clear dipolar field pattern and using another subset of sensors, as shown by the dashed line in Figure 6–4b.

If we only use the left-hemisphere N100m source to account for the data recorded by all MEG sensors, we will find that the waveform depicted in Figure 6–5a describes the time course of activation in the left auditory cortex. The overall level of explanation for the whole helmet, the goodness-of-fit value, remains quite low, as one would expect. When we only include the right-hemisphere N100m source (Figure 6–5b), the result is very similar, with a clear time course of activation locally but poor explanation overall. When we include both left and right N100m sources (Figure 6–5c), the explanation rises dramatically and exceeds 80% around the peak of activation. Importantly,

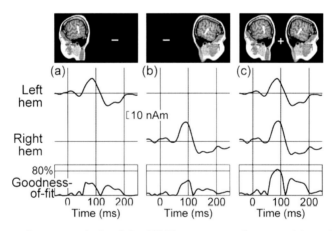

Figure 6–5. Source analysis of the N100m response in one subject. (a) Time course of activation in the left auditory cortex (source waveform) and goodness-of-fit over the whole helmet when only one ECD in the left auditory cortex was included. (b) Time course of activation in the right auditory cortex when only one ECD in the right auditory cortex was included. (c) Time courses of activation in the bilateral auditory cortex when two ECDs were included, one in each hemisphere.

the source waveforms remain exactly the same, regardless of whether we include only one or both sources in the model. This is exactly how it should be if our source models are good, and represent independent source areas. We can conclude that there is no interaction between these two sources and, according to this criterion, our model is adequate for the N100m deflection.

However, the later deflection at around 200 ms was not well explained by the N100m source. In this subject, the later so-called P200m sources (from EEG literature) were located slightly anterior to the N100m sources, apparently in the upper lip of the superior temporal sulcus (Figure 6–6). The N100m and P200m sources are spatially rather close to each other and have fairly similar orientations (but opposite directions) of current flow. However, we can still try to include them all in the multidipole model. The 4-dipole model (thick solid curves) shows how the N100m sources are active first, and then return to the base level when the P200m sources become active. The goodness-of-fit value now exceeds 80% for most of the measurement interval.

For comparison, Figure 6–6 also includes the previous 2-dipole model with only the N100m sources, plotted as dashed lines. The N100m waveforms are slightly affected by the inclusion of the P200m dipoles, because of the closeness of the sources, and the effect is obviously strongest in the later time window. Importantly, the unphysiological change of polarity in the waveforms of the 2-dipole model is removed in the more realistic 4-dipole model. Eventually, we have a well-behaved 4-dipole model that accounts for most of the activity recorded by all the sensors. This so-called source analysis is done individually for each subject.

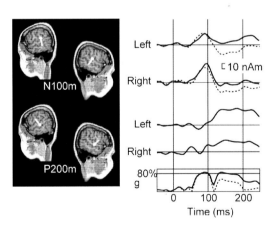

Figure 6–6. Complete source analysis of auditory responses in one subject, including both the N100m and P200m ECDs in both hemispheres (solid lines). For comparison, the time courses of activation in the auditory cortex are also plotted for the model with only the bilateral N100m sources included (dashed lines). The abbreviation 'g' stands for goodness-of-fit.

Somatosensory Responses

Let us now move on to a slightly more complex data set. Figure 6–7 displays responses to right median nerve stimulation (e.g., Forss et al., 1994; Schnitzler et al., 1995). Again, the displayed time interval is 300 ms. Obviously, there is plenty of activity, with different time behaviors: early components are observed medially over the left central sulcus, and later components medially in the left hemisphere and more laterally in both hemispheres.

Also in this case, by scanning through the field patterns one can recognize the different source areas at distinct time points (Figure 6–8). At about 20 ms after stimulus onset, there is a dipolar field pattern forming over the left hand area in the central sulcus. The picture becomes even clearer at about 30 ms, but the current now flows in the opposite direction. Until about 50 ms, the field pattern remains fairly unchanged. At about 80 ms, the left parietal cortex produces a pronounced dipolar field pattern. At around 100 ms, it is accompanied by activations laterally in the left and right hemisphere. The location is very similar to that of the auditory responses, but the opposite direction of current flow now indicates activation in the upper lip of the Sylvian fissure.

When several source areas are active rather simultaneously, one has to put some effort into selecting the subsets of sensors used for source localization. For the early sources in the upper row of Figure 6–8, almost any selection will do, as there is no other simultaneous activation. For the parietal source, one should exclude the left frontal sensors, which detect the lateral activation. Conversely, for the left lateral source, the sensor selection should avoid the parietal region. As in the auditory responses, the question here is

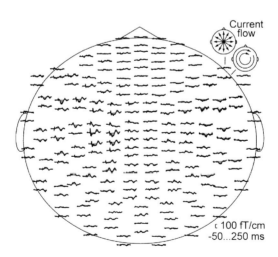

Figure 6–7. MEG responses to electric stimulation of the right median nerve at the wrist in one subject. The time window extends from 50 ms before stimulus onset to 250 ms after it.

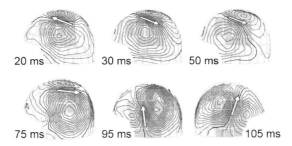

Figure 6–8. Magnetic field patterns at different times after right median nerve stimulation. The arrows represent the ECDs that best account for each field pattern.

not where the active areas are, but how to find such unequivocal field patterns that it is possible to reliably localize the sources. It is important to find the time point at which each field pattern is optimally dipolar. It is worth noting that this optimal time point may, or may not, coincide with a peak in the signal.

In Figure 6–9, the sources are shown on the subject's MR images. The 20-ms and 30-ms responses are generated by slightly different sources in the hand area. However, they are so similar in location and orientation that both cannot be included in the multidipole model because they interact too much. Therefore, the strong 30-ms source in the primary somatosensory cortex, SI,

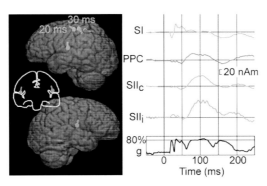

Figure 6–9. Final source model for right median nerve stimulation in the same subject for whom original MEG data was displayed in Figures 6–7 and 6–8. *Left:* Locations and directions of the ECDs displayed on the subject's MRI. *Right:* Time courses of activation in the brain. SI = primary somatosensory cortex, PPC = posterior parietal cortex, SII = second somatosensory cortex contralateral (c) and ipsilateral (i) to stimulation. Because of the close similarity of the ECDs determined at 20 ms and 30 ms, they are both represented in the SI waveform (negative deflection at 20 ms, positive deflection at 30 ms).

represents the hand area activation in the model. In the source waveform, the peak at 30 ms is preceded by a small negative deflection at 20 ms. Note that this is not deactivation but simply reflects the opposite direction of current flow in almost the same cortical location. Usually, one would be concerned about a waveform that shows both positive and negative values, but here we know that this is a real effect.

The other sources are located in the posterior parietal cortex (PPC) and in the left and right second somatosensory cortices in the upper lip of the Sylvian fissure (SII). We now have a sequence from SI to posterior parietal, and further to the ipsi- and contralateral SII cortices, with all activations partly overlapping in time. Again, one may check for possible interactions between sources by leaving out one source at a time and observing whether it affects the other waveforms.

For this high-quality data set, other analysis approaches will provide essentially the same sequence of activation. The active areas can also be visualized using so-called distributed models, which produce probability maps of current distribution (e.g., Dale et al., 2000; Lin et al., 2004; Uutela et al., 1999). Figure 6–10 displays Minimum Current Estimate (MCE; Uutela et al., 1999) of this data set. From 20–50 ms, activity is concentrated to the SI cortex. At about 80 ms, both the posterior parietal cortex and the contralateral SII show activation. At about 100 ms, the SII activations have reached their maximum in both hemispheres.

It is important to realize that the focal ECDs and the distributed probability maps produce exactly the same electromagnetic field outside of the head, so both are equally correct. The appearance of the result is determined by the choice of analysis method (model), not by the structure of active areas in the brain. The bottom line is that MEG (or EEG) gives an estimate of the center of an active area but—at least in typical experimental setups and signal-to-noise ratios—no direct information about its spatial extent.

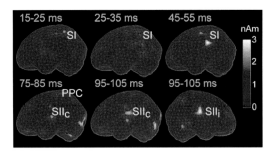

Figure 6–10. Minimum Current Estimate (MCE) of the data displayed in Figure 6–7. The current distribution is projected on a triangle mesh representing the brain surface and integrated over the time intervals of interest, corresponding to those in the ECD analysis. The color represents the estimated current strength.

The localization accuracy is best when perpendicular to the current flow (where small changes in location result in large changes in the magnetic field distribution) and worst along the current and in depth. The uncertainty in source depth is particularly relevant when comparing activation strengths. If a particular source is localized deeper in experimental condition A than in B, systematically across subjects, then it is likely that the active area is, indeed, centered at a slightly different depth in the two conditions. However, a more typical finding is that there are some differences within individual subjects but no systematic ordering at the group level. In this case, it is likely that the noise in the data (including the influence of other active sources nearby) has resulted in some error in source localization. If a source is localized too deep with respect to its true location, its activation will appear stronger than it actually is; if it is localized too superficially, it will appear weaker than in reality. Accordingly, when comparing experimental conditions that suggest sources in the same general brain area, but with some variability in source depth, it is reasonable to equate the source locations, i.e., to use the same source to model activity in all conditions before comparing the activation strengths between the conditions. For the same reason, comparison of activation strength in the left vs. right hemisphere is always somewhat problematic, as there may be actual or artifactual differences in source depths that affect the apparent activation strength. The comparison can be argued best if the sources are centered approximately at the same depth in homologuous areas of the left and right hemisphere.

The localization accuracy varies from ~1 mm to ~1 cm, depending on the signal-to-noise ratio and the overall distribution of activation in the brain. The orientation of current flow, perpendicular to the course of the sulcus where the current is generated, is a very accurate and useful measure.

Reading Words and Nonwords

Let us now return to the reading task (Figure 6–1). The Dual-Route Model of reading (Figure 6–11; Coltheart et al., 1993) assumes that when we see a familiar word, like 'brain', the visual features must be processed first before the analysis can proceed to the content—apparently first at the level of single letters, and then as a whole word, which further activates the word's meaning and its sound form. However, when we see an unfamiliar word or a nonword, we cannot use the lexical route because there is no representation for these letter-strings in our mental lexicon. Instead, we are supposed to process the letter-strings letter by letter, and convert each letter to its corresponding sound in order to obtain a sound form for the letter-string, which again may lead to some type of semantic association.

In this MEG experiment on word vs. nonword reading (Wydell et al., 2003) the stimuli were short and long real Finnish words (e.g., 'talo' = house, 'lautanen' = plate), and short and long pronounceable nonwords (e.g., 'roki',

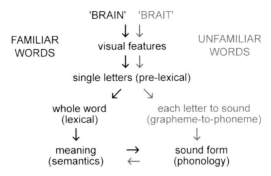

Figure 6–11. Outline of the dual-route model of reading. Modified from Coltheart et al. (1993).

'soijinto'). For real words, the lexical route should dominate, and length should have little effect. Processing of nonwords, on the other hand, would rely on the letter-level grapheme-to-phoneme conversion, and letter-string length should have a strong effect. There were 100 stimuli of each type, shown in a randomized sequence. The letter-strings were presented for 400 ms, and each stimulus was followed by a blank interval of 2.6 s. The subjects were reading the letter-strings silently, but, occasionally, a question mark prompted them to read aloud the preceding word (4% of trials). The task coerced the subjects to process the words until pronunciation. Movement artifacts were avoided by performing the analysis on the silent trials (96%).

Figure 6–12 displays enlarged views of MEG signals recorded by three sensors over the left temporal, parietal, and occipital areas. There are some interesting effects. Over the left temporal area, the response is markedly different to long nonwords than to the other word types. In the posterior parietal cortex, on the other hand, there is a particularly strong response to long real words. The early posterior visual response is similar for all stimuli.

Figure 6–13 illustrates the field patterns that produce the occipital and left temporal signals in the different experimental conditions: short words, long words, short nonwords, and long nonwords. The occipital field pattern at about 200 ms after stimulus onset is very similar for all stimulus types. Therefore, it is easy to represent these field patterns by a single ECD that works well for all experimental conditions. It is worth noting that there are small differences in location and orientation, which may result from noise in the data or reflect real variability between the conditions. For example, there may be a slight inferior–superior shift in location for long vs. short letter-strings. However, the difference is so small that the sources would not appear as separate ECDs in multidipole modeling (cf. discussion of auditory and somatosensory data above). The same is true for the field pattern over the left temporal cortex at 400–500 ms. The pattern is essentially the same for all conditions, except that it is particularly strong for the long nonwords, and most difficult to identify for long real words when, at the same time, there is

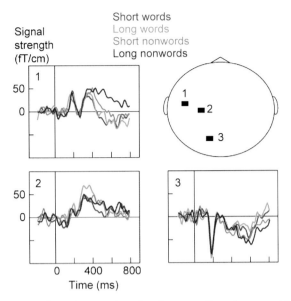

Figure 6–12. Examples of MEG signals when reading short and long words, and nonwords. Enlarged views of three sensors. The complete data set of this subject is displayed in Figure 6–1.

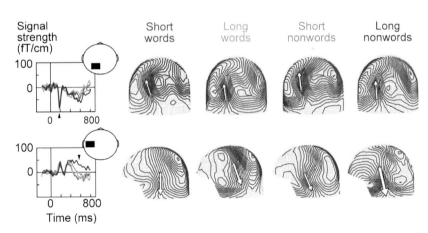

Figure 6–13. Field patterns and the best-fitting ECDs (arrows) corresponding to the MEG signals recorded over the occipital and left temporal areas (cf. Figure 6–12) in the different experimental conditions.

another field pattern nearby in the parietal cortex. How should one proceed with the analysis?

Constructing the Source Model

Just as for the auditory and somatosensory data above, source areas generating these signals are determined one by one. The localization is done by scanning through the response to identify time points at which each distinct field pattern is as closely dipolar as possible, selecting a subset of sensors that covers the local field maximum, and computing the ECD that best accounts for the signal measured by these sensors. The resulting ECDs are then brought into a multidipole model where the locations and orientations of the ECDs are kept fixed, while their amplitudes are allowed to vary in order to best account for the data recorded by all MEG sensors over the time interval of interest. The resulting source waveforms are then used for estimating cortical dynamics within and across experimental conditions.

There are at least two possible approaches:

(i) Analyze each experimental condition independently, and then combine the sources into a single multidipole model that works for all conditions.
  - Start, e.g., from the most prominent response pattern or from the earliest systematic response and then work through the data to find the weaker/later sources.
  - For the combined model, choose the sources (or sets of nearby sources) with clearest field patterns and/or best confidence values. Check that the combined model accounts for the data in each experimental condition as adequately, and in the same way, as the models constructed specifically for those conditions.
(ii) Equally well, one can start from one experimental condition, use those sources as a starting point when one sets off to analyze the next condition, and add and modify the sources while one works through the data sets.

In fact, it would be best to analyze the data (at least) two or three times, using different approaches. It is important that one learns to know the data. Separate sets of sources for each condition are useful if one expects to find small but systematic differences in location or orientation of current flow—say, for short vs. long words (cf. Figure 6–13). However, for controlled comparison of activation strengths and timing between conditions, one will want to compose a single set of ECDs (if possible). The minimum number of sources should be used that can explain the data. It may take some effort to find the time points and experimental conditions in which a consistently observed field pattern is most dipolar, i.e., where the signal is strong and interference from other source areas is minimal. However, the endeavor is worth the effort, as clean dipolar field patterns facilitate reliable identification of the underlying sources that normally account both adequately and robustly for the entire data set.

In the reading experiment, we may start to look for sources in the long nonword condition where there was an exceptionally strong left temporal activation (Figure 6–13). By selecting the frontotemporal sensors painted in light gray (Figure 6–14a) we can avoid the unwanted effect of other active areas. The source is located in the superior temporal cortex (Figure 6–14b). A model that only includes this one source accounts well for the sustained left temporal signals (Figure 6–14c,d). Characterization of one clear dipolar field pattern also helps to further recognize systematic unexplained signals in other areas. The word 'systematic' here refers to appearance of the same waveform on several adjacent sensors. For example, the same unexplained waveform is seen on three neighboring sensors over the right occipitotemporal cortex (Figure 6–14c,e).

In cognitive data sets, signals are often weaker overall than for basic sensory/motor responses, and the large number of active brain areas that are

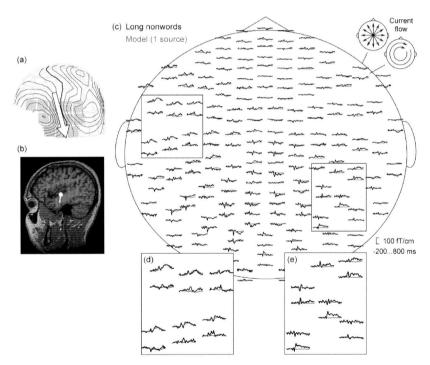

Figure 6–14. Localization of left temporal activation in the reading task (long nonwords) in one subject. (a) Field pattern and the best-fitting ECD over the left hemisphere. (b) ECD displayed on the MR image of the subject's brain. (c) Whole-head view of the MEG signals, with measured signals plotted in black and the explanation, using the one ECD in the left temporal cortex, plotted in purple. (d) Enlarged view of left temporal sensors. (e) Enlarged view of right occipitotemporal sensors.

spatially and temporally quite close to each other appear as additional 'noise' when localizing the sources. Accordingly, one must often tolerate focal field patterns that are not perfectly dipolar. The emerging and re-entering field patterns may not be fully symmetrical and the resulting ECD will, therefore, not fall exactly on the zero field line. Nevertheless, when one makes the effort to find time points at which the different field patterns are as dipolar as possible, ECD modeling is entirely feasible for cognitive data sets as well.

An effective decrease in signal-to-noise ratio will increase the potential risk of mislocalizing the source unphysiologically deep. Normally, the localization can be improved by testing other time points and sensor selections, in order to minimize the effect of other nearby sources. Occasionally, a spatially extended field pattern may seem to be generated by an unphysiologically deep ECD when, in reality, it is generated by two source areas that are active at the same time. Such sources could be located quite close to each other, with fairly similar directions of current flow, yet separable in space (e.g., distance within 2–3 cm, difference in direction less than 20–30 deg; see Helenius et al., 1999, for an example of superior temporal activation). This type of situation can usually be solved by scanning through the different experimental conditions and identifying the sources at time points where one or the other field pattern is emphasized.

After the 2–3 analysis rounds, with different approaches, we have a model composed of 9 ECDs in this subject, with sources in the occipital lobe, left temporal and parietal, and right occipitotemporal cortex (Figure 6–15a). One should always check that each individual source makes sense, by comparing the source waveforms with the original signals. As an example, we could focus on the left temporal area (Figure 6–15b). The signals in the upper and lower row of the sensor pairs display quite different stimulus dependence. This device has two orthogonal sensors in each measurement location. Therefore, we would expect to see these differential effects on the sensors map onto two different source areas in the brain that are fairly close to each other but have almost orthogonal directions of current flow. Indeed, our solution suggests that sources 5 and 9 produce these signals. The long nonwords differ from the other stimuli in source 9 in the superior temporal cortex, while in the more inferior, rather horizontally oriented source 5, the response is strongest for the short nonwords, in agreement with the original measured signals.

In order to check that the model is really meaningful, it is very useful to compare two stimulus conditions at a time. Figure 6–16 depicts responses to long words and long nonwords. There are at least two very obvious differences in the original waveforms—one over the left temporal and the other over the posterior parietal cortex (Figure 6–16b). These areas apparently correspond to sources 9 and 8, respectively (Figure 6–16a). Indeed, source 9 shows the strong response to nonwords, whereas source 8 displays the stronger activation to real words, with the time behavior matching that of the original sensor waveforms. Accordingly, we can be reasonably satisfied with this model.

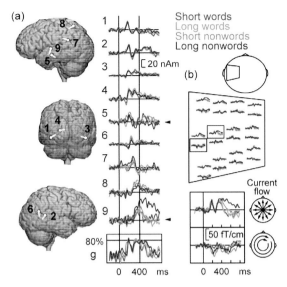

Figure 6–15. Source analysis in the reading task in one subject. (a) ECDs shown on the surface rendering of the subject's MRI and time courses of activation in those areas for the different stimulus types. The sources are ordered according to latency of activation. Goodness-of-fit value (g) is plotted at the bottom. (b) Selection of MEG sensors over the left temporo-parietal cortex. Enlarged view of two orthogonally oriented sensors is plotted below.

Testing for Differences Between Experimental Conditions

After an acceptable source model has been compiled, one may collect any descriptive values from the waveforms (e.g., onset/offset/peak timing, peak amplitude, mean amplitude, or integral over specific time intervals) and test them for significant stimulus/task effects.

Here, as an example, we will describe one possible approach for the data set on word/nonword reading. Behaviorally, it has been reported that naming latencies are shorter for short than long words, and that this length effect is markedly stronger for naming nonwords than real words (Weekes, 1997). A comparison between short words and long nonwords should encompass all these effects: length effect, lexicality effect, and their interaction.

First, we search for significant differences in individual subjects. Figure 6–17 displays the time course of activation in the left temporal cortex for those two conditions, in one subject. The signal variation in the prestimulus baseline interval carries information about the noise level in this area, in this specific source model and in these experimental conditions. A rather conservative approach is to estimate, for example, the level of 2.58 times standard deviation (corresponding to $p < 0.01$), represented by the gray box, and only accept as significant those differences between the two waveforms that exceed this

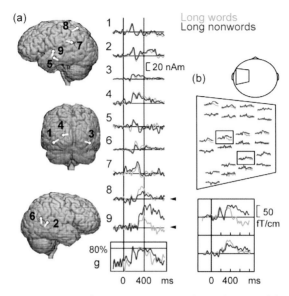

Figure 6–16. Comparison of two experimental conditions. (a) ECDs shown on the surface rendering of the subject's MRI and time courses of activation in the source areas for the two stimulus types. Goodness-of-fit value (g) is plotted at the bottom. (b) Selection of MEG sensors over the left temporoparietal cortex. Enlarged view of two sensors is plotted below.

level (cf. Tarkiainen et al., 1999). In this case, we would identify a significantly stronger activation to long nonwords than short words in the left superior temporal cortex at about 400 to 700 ms after stimulus onset.

Cortical areas with stimulus effects were identified in the same way in all subjects. Figure 6–18 collects the subsets of source areas that showed significant differences between the extreme conditions of long nonwords and short real words. The source clusters are presented separately for differences detected within the first 200 ms after stimulus onset (Figure 6–18a) and after 200 ms (Figure 6–18b). Within 200 ms after stimulus, differences in the peak

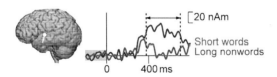

Figure 6–17. Within-subject test for significant differences between experimental conditions in the left superior temporal cortex. The height of the gray box represents 2.58 times standard deviation within the prestimulus baseline interval (-200...0 ms). The dashed lines indicate the borders of the interval during which activation was significantly (p<0.01) stronger to long nonwords than short real words.

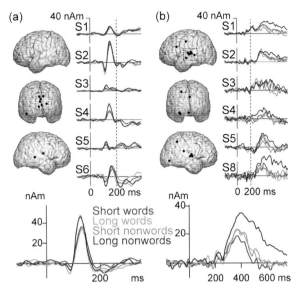

Figure 6–18. Source areas showing significantly stronger activation to long nonwords than short real words. (a) Differences detected within 200 ms after stimulus onset in the occipital cortex (6 subjects). (b) Differences detected after 200 ms following stimulus onset. Source waveforms are plotted for the left temporal cluster (6 subjects). The individual source waveforms are plotted on top and the grand mean waveform below. Abbreviations S1 to S8 refer to individual subjects.
Modified from Wydell et al. (2003).

amplitude were found in 6 of 8 subjects, with the sources clustered around the occipital midline. After 200 ms, the most salient cluster of such sources (6 of 8 subjects) was found in the left superior temporal cortex.

Here, we used functional criteria combined with location information to identify sources that were observed consistently across subjects. Within these occipital and left temporal clusters, we now test for group-level statistical effects between all four stimulus categories. The strength of the early occipital activation (Figure 6–19a) showed a pure length effect, and most probably reflects basic visual feature analysis within the first 200 ms (cf. Tarkiainen et al., 1999). In the left temporal cortex, the duration of activation showed interesting behavior—namely, a weak effect of length for real words but a marked effect for nonwords; the duration for the 8-letter nonwords was twice that for the 4-letter nonwords (Figure 6–19b). The peak amplitude and mean signal strength also showed the same interaction between length and lexicality. This pattern parallels that reported for reaction times in word and nonword reading (Weekes, 1997). If we accept the dual-route model of reading, this pattern should be interpreted as reflecting phonological analysis. Considering that activation of the left superior temporal cortex in this very

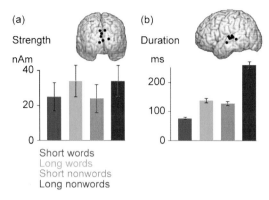

Figure 6–19. Significant stimulus effects at the group level. (a) Maximum amplitude (mean ± SEM) of the early occipital activation was significantly stronger to long than short letter-strings, regardless of lexicality. (b) Duration of the left temporal activation was also influenced by letter-string length but significantly more for nonwords than real words.
Modified from Wydell et al. (2003).

same time window has been consistently associated with lexical-semantic analysis (e.g., Halgren et al., 2002; Helenius et al., 1999) this finding would seem to suggest considerable spatiotemporal overlap between analysis of meaning and sound-form of written words.

Instead of identifying source clusters by functional criteria, one could have performed the clustering solely on the basis of source locations and directions of current flow. The result would have been essentially the same, only somewhat more noisy (see, e.g., Cornelissen et al., 2003).

Reading Words Aloud

When words are read overtly, mouth movement artifacts come into play. Figure 6–20 illustrates such an experiment. A word was presented for 300 ms. Then there was a blank interval of 500 ms. A question mark then appeared for 2 s, prompting the subject to read the word out loud. A blank screen was again shown for 2 s before a new word was presented. EMG was recorded across the opposite corners of the mouth. Microphone signal was registered to determine the timing of lip movement and speech onset. The purpose of this experiment was to compare speech production in fluent speakers and developmental stutterers (Salmelin et al., 2000).

Mouth movement artifacts are an obvious problem, as they cause strong signals that mask the cortical activity. Fortunately, those disturbing field patterns can usually be removed from the MEG data. Figure 6–21 depicts examples of mouth EMG and microphone signals in five single trials during

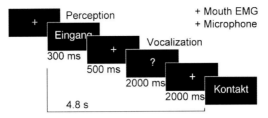

Figure 6–20. Experimental setup for comparing speech production in fluent speakers and stutterers. The delayed reading paradigm was used to focus separately on preparation and actual production.
Modified from Salmelin et al. (2000).

the experiment. The signals are aligned to the stimulus onset, which is shown by the continuous vertical line. The mouth movement and speech onset vary by about 100 to 200 ms from trial to trial, both with respect to the stimulus onset and with respect to each other. This jitter makes it possible to dissociate the artifact signal from the cortical activity of interest.

In Figure 6–22, the original MEG data were averaged with respect to speech onset, recorded with a microphone. The speech artifact is usually quite accurately time-locked to microphone onset and, therefore, one can get a very clean artifact pattern with this averaging procedure. The signal concentrates along the rim of the helmet. Task-related cortical activity has faded out because of the jitter with respect to stimulus onset. By emphasizing the artifact this way, one can then remove the disturbing field pattern from the responses. This can be done with the help of, e.g., the Signal Space Projection (SSP) method (Uusitalo and Ilmoniemi, 1997).

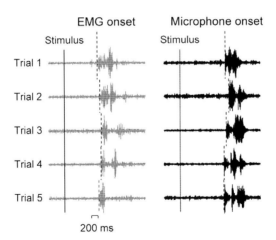

Figure 6–21. Intertrial variability of EMG onset (mouth movement) and microphone onset (speech production) with respect to stimulus presentation, illustrated for five trials in one subject.

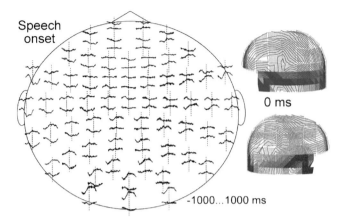

Figure 6–22. MEG data averaged with respect to speech onset, determined from the microphone record. The helmet views illustrate the magnetic field pattern at speech onset (t = 0 ms).

The same data can also be averaged with respect to the EMG signal, that is, mouth movement onset (Figure 6–23). This procedure allows focus on the motor control of speech production. The speech artifact field (Figure 6–22) has been removed from the averaged signals. Clear dipolar field patterns emerge over the left and right frontal lobes, approximately at the time when the mouth movement starts. The sources of these field patterns are readily localized to the bilateral face motor cortex.

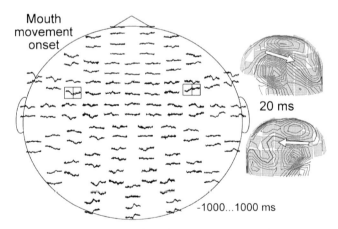

Figure 6–23. MEG data averaged with respect to mouth movement onset, determined from the EMG record. The helmet views illustrate the magnetic field pattern approximately at mouth movement onset (t = 20 ms) and the arrows the best-fitting ECDs. The planar gradiometers that are maximally sensitive to activation in these source areas are marked with rectangles.

Figure 6–24 displays the same data finally averaged in the typical fashion, with respect to the stimulus onset. Again, the speech artifact field has been removed. In this data set, bilateral frontal activations are observed best at about 500 ms after word presentation. Over the left hemisphere the field pattern is clearly dipolar, and the source in the face motor cortex can be determined reliably. However, in the right hemisphere, the field pattern points to activation of the motor cortex but the underlying source area is practically impossible to localize; the helmet view in Figure 6–24 represents the most dipolar field pattern one can detect. Activation of the right motor cortex in this subject thus seems to be more strongly time-locked to mouth movement onset than to stimulus onset. A reasonable approach would be to determine this source from the signals averaged with respect to mouth movement onset (Figure 6–23) and then use that ECD to account for activity in the signals averaged with respect to stimulus onset (Figure 6–24).

Figure 6–25 illustrates the cortical activation sequence at the group level. In this experiment there was no systematic functional variation in the stimuli or task. The main aim was to compare fluent speakers and stutterers in the basic task of overt reading of single words. The source areas from individual subjects were grouped together primarily by similarity in location. The curves give the mean time course of activation in those areas, averaged across fluently speaking subjects. The first vertical line indicates the word presentation and the second vertical line the appearance of the vocalization prompt (question mark).

The occipital and the left and right inferior occipitotemporal cortices were active within the first 200 ms. Next, there was activation in the left superior

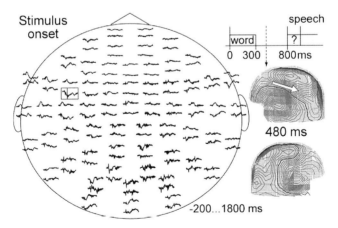

Figure 6–24. MEG data averaged with respect to stimulus onset. The helmet views illustrate the magnetic field pattern when the subject is waiting for the vocalization prompt (t = 480 ms) and the arrow the best-fitting ECD in the left hemisphere. The planar gradiometer that is maximally sensitive to activation in this source area is marked with a rectangle.

temporal and inferior parietal cortices, starting about 200 ms after word onset and reaching the maximum at about 400 ms. The left inferior frontal cortex, approximately Broca's area, showed activation in the same time window. The sources assigned to the temporal cluster are spatially quite close to those assigned to the inferior frontal cluster, on the one hand, and sources belonging to the inferior parietal cluster, on the other hand. Here, the orientation of current flow was used as an additional criterion (white bars plotted on the three source clusters in Figure 6–25, middle column) which clearly distinguished between the adjacent clusters.

All the activations listed in the two left-most columns return to baseline before the vocalization prompt. The signals depicted in the right-most column begin at about 200 ms after word onset, and persist until actual vocalization and even beyond it. This is quite reasonable, as those signals arise from the left and right sensorimotor and premotor cortices and, apparently, from the supplementary motor area.

Differences between the time courses of activation in fluently speaking individuals and stutterers are collected in Figure 6–26. There were group differences in three brain areas and time windows. Within the first 400 ms, while preparing for vocalization the fluent speakers first activated Broca's area, and then the left motor/premotor cortex, which appears to be a natural order of events. In the stutterers, however, the sequence was reversed. They showed exceptionally early activation in the left sensorimotor/premotor area, already within the first 200 ms, whereas activation of Broca's area was delayed with

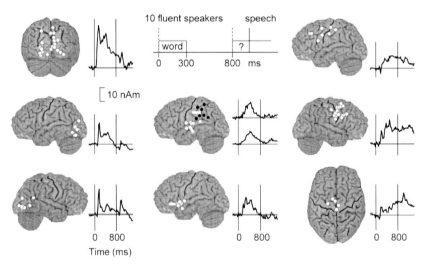

Figure 6–25. Group-level clusters of active cortical areas and their mean time courses of activation across 10 fluently speaking subjects. In the middle column, the mean orientation of current flow in the source clusters is shown as well (white bars).
Modified from Salmelin (2007).

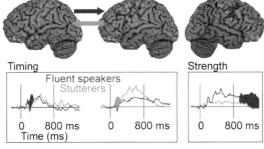

Figure 6–26. Source areas in which differences were found between groups of fluent speakers and stutterers. The time courses of activation are depicted below. Differences in timing were found within 400 ms after word presentation and differences in activation strength during speech production.

respect to that observed in fluent speakers. After the vocalization prompt, the right motor cortex showed significantly stronger activation in fluent speakers than in stutterers. The combination of MEG data and ECD analysis thus made it possible to compare the groups at three different levels: the locations of the active areas were fairly similar, but differences emerged in timing within the first 400 ms and in activation strength during overt vocalization.

ECD Analysis of Cortical Rhythmic Activity

At rest, cortical neurons generate spontaneous oscillatory activity. Figure 6–27 shows an 8-s interval of MEG signals recorded over the left and right sensorimotor cortex, and over the posterior visual areas. The subject was sitting relaxed, with his eyes closed. The spectra show the typical frequency distribution in a healthy adult subject. The parieto-occipital activity is mainly in the 10-Hz range, called alpha rhythm, whereas the sensorimotor activity has both 10- and 20-Hz components, and is known as the mu rhythm. The mu rhythm is suppressed by moving the hand, as shown by the black curve, and the alpha rhythm by opening the eyes—that is, broadly speaking, when those brain areas are involved in actual task performance (Hari & Salmelin, 1997; Pfurtscheller & Lopes da Silva, 1999). In this section, we will consider ECD analysis when localizing sources of cortical rhythms and quantifying their event-related modulation. The focus is on the spatially well-defined sensorimotor mu rhythm, for which ECD analysis is particularly suitable.

For ECD modeling, the data is bandpass filtered to the desired frequency range. For example, Figure 6–28 shows a stretch of data filtered to 16–24 Hz. During the bursts of 20-Hz activity, a clear dipolar field pattern is formed over the central sulcus. In principle, the procedure of ECD localization is similar to that described for the analysis of evoked responses above. However, localization

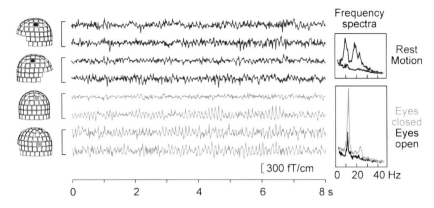

Figure 6–27. Stretch of non-averaged MEG data recorded by the sensors plotted in color on the helmets. On the right side, power spectra of signals recorded by sensors over the central sulcus (top) and over the parieto-occipital area (below).

of cortical rhythms is done from non-averaged data with signal-to-noise ratio far inferior to that of averaged evoked responses. Accordingly, one needs to collect a large number of samples and identify reliable clusters of ECDs. For example, one could randomly pick 10 samples of 30-s stretches of data and determine the best-fitting ECD every 10 ms (corresponding to 5 data points per each period of a signal oscillating at 20 Hz), resulting in 30,000 ECDs. An obvious baseline interval can usually not be defined; instead, one may estimate the base level of rhythmic activity as the mean signal level over the entire data set.

The subset of sensors used in the ECD calculation (cf. Figures 6–4 and 6–8 in analysis of evoked responses) can be selected with the help of the spatial distribution of the frequency spectra, and by visual evaluation of the field patterns (Figure 6–28, left). A visual check of the field patterns, combined

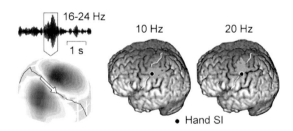

Figure 6–28. Localization of spontaneous rhythms to the central sulcus. *Left:* Stretch of non-averaged MEG data filtered to 16–24 Hz. Typical field pattern during peaks of the strong 20-Hz oscillations. *Right:* Source clusters along the central sulcus for oscillations in the 10-Hz and 20-Hz range, in one subject. The course of the central sulcus is depicted (white curve).

with test calculation of ECDs for a number of time points, provides an estimate for setting acceptance criteria (e.g., goodness-of-fit value, confidence values for localization) for the large set of ECDs obtained with automatic localization over long stretches of data. Typically less than 5% of the original ECDs represent reliable dipolar sources within the brain region covered by the selection of sensors (Salmelin & Hari, 1994a; Salmelin et al., 1995).

Figure 6–28 gives examples of source clusters along the central sulcus in one subject, obtained from data filtered around 10 Hz and around 20 Hz. The clusters may also be conveniently displayed as dipole density plots (e.g., Lehtelä et al., 1997; Liljeström et al., 2005; Vieth et al., 1996). In the resting brain, the sources of mu rhythm are concentrated in and around the hand representation area in the central sulcus. The 10-Hz component originates largely in the somatosensory cortex—but also precentrally—whereas the 20-Hz component seems to be predominantly a motor cortical rhythm (Salenius et al., 1997; Salmelin & Hari, 1994b; Salmelin et al., 1995).

In voluntary movements the 20-Hz activity shows somatotopic organization. Figure 6–29 illustrates the results of a study in which subjects made self-paced movements of the left and right toes, index fingers, and mouth. The colored dots show foot, hand, and mouth representation areas along the central sulcus, determined with electric stimulation of the tibial and median nerve and the lower lip, respectively. The colored blobs are sources of 20-Hz oscillations. For movement of left and right toes, the sources were concentrated close to the foot area; for left and right index finger flexion, close to the contralateral hand area; and for mouth movements, sources extended laterally to the mouth area—in this subject, mainly in the right hemisphere. Note that the sources again cluster frontally with respect to the central sulcus. This result

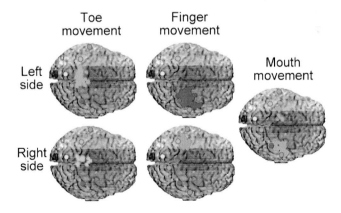

Figure 6–29. Localization of sources of 20-Hz activity when the subject made voluntary movements of the left and right toes or fingers, or opened the jaw. The colored dots represent the foot, hand, and mouth areas in the somatosensory cortex, determined with electrical stimulation. Modified from Salmelin et al. (1995).

implies that one may use 20-Hz activity to evaluate functionality of different parts of the motor cortex, not only the hand area.

Figure 6–30 presents the whole-head view of one subject when he was reading words aloud. The curves display the mean amplitude of 20-Hz oscillations from 1 second before word onset to 5 seconds after it (Salmelin et al., 2000). The MEG signals were filtered to 16–24 Hz, their absolute value taken, and the resulting signals averaged with respect to word onset (TSE, Temporal Spectral Evolution; Salmelin & Hari, 1994b). This approach reveals modulation of activity that occurs systematically, but not exactly at the same time, from trial to trial (event-related vs. phase-locked activity). There is a clear suppression of 20-Hz activity quite locally over the lateral areas, but also more medially, with different time behaviors.

Figure 6–31a illustrates the localization of the 20-Hz oscillations—a general pattern, here illustrated in one (typical) subject—to the hand and mouth areas of the right and left hemispheres. With these candidate source areas one may proceed, in principle, through the same steps as in the multidipole analysis of evoked responses described above. One can estimate the time course of activity in the proposed ECDs in the left and right hand and mouth areas (Figure 6–31b). In order to evaluate, in individual subjects, how well the sources account for the MEG signals measured over the whole head, we can perform a forward calculation to map the estimated source activity onto the MEG sensors (model signals). In this study, the interest was in localizing the sources of the 20-Hz modulation. Accordingly, TSE curves of modeled MEG signals were compared with TSE curves of the original measured MEG signals. The four sources (Figure 6–31a) were found to account well for the event-related modulation of 20-Hz activity (Figure 6–30).

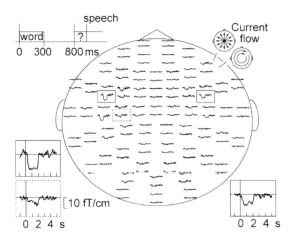

Figure 6–30. Mean amplitude of 20-Hz oscillations recorded by MEG sensors when the subject was reading words aloud. The time window extends from 1 s before word onset to 5 s after it.
Modified from Salmelin et al. (2000).

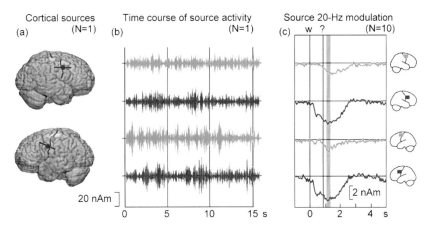

Figure 6–31. Source analysis of 20-Hz activity. (a) ECDs in the left and right hand and mouth areas along the central sulcus in one subject. (b) Time course of 20-Hz activation in those areas. Vertical lines denote a new trial (word presentation). (c) Grand average time course of 20-Hz modulation, calculated across 10 subjects.
Modified from Salmelin et al. (2000).

From the continuous source activity (Figure 6–31b), one can compute the mean level of activity (TSE) in those brain areas. Figure 6–31c displays grand-averaged source-level TSE curves (10 subjects) in the right hand and mouth, and left hand and mouth areas. The first vertical line indicates word presentation, and the second line indicates the vocalization prompt. The gray bar indicates actual speech production. Just as in the analysis of phase-locked evoked responses, it is important to check that the ECDs included in the multidipole model do not interact—i.e., that they are not too close to each other, and that the orientation of current flow in those areas is not too similar. In the case of rhythmic activity, possible interaction is harder to evaluate from the source waveforms than it is in the case of evoked responses. However, clearly different time behaviors, like those between the hand and mouth areas within each hemisphere in this data set, speak in favor of independence of the ECDs. One may, for example, estimate the space angle between the magnetic field distributions produced by the ECDs (should exceed 30–40 degrees), or simulate activity in those areas and evaluate how much of the signal generated by one ECD is accounted for by the other ECD. In reality, the possible interactions are not determined only by pairs of sources but by all sources included in the model. Nevertheless, comparison of the most suspicious pairs of ECDs provides a good approximation of the potential risks.

Equipped with reasonable source models, one may proceed to comparison of different experimental conditions or subject groups, in the same way as for phase-locked evoked responses. Figure 6–31c shows that in the mouth motor cortex the 20-Hz rhythm was strongly suppressed well before vocalization.

Further research has demonstrated that this suppression is correlated with timing of the visual instruction rather than mouth movement onset—clearly pointing to involvement of motor cortex in cognitive processing, not simply motor control (Saarinen et al. 2006). Interestingly enough, the hand areas seem to be involved in speech production as well, although obviously much less than the mouth areas, and only during the actual movement. It has been shown that the mouth vs. hand area segregation in the motor cortex is stronger for verbal than nonverbal mouth movements, independent of sequence length or complexity. The main factor appears to be the verbal vs. nonverbal contrast; that is, the hand areas are more involved in producing nonverbal than verbal mouth movements (Saarinen et al., 2006; Salmelin & Sams, 2002). The segregation between hand and mouth area involvement in speech production is significantly weaker in stutterers than fluently speaking individuals (Salmelin et al., 2000).

ECD localization of rhythmic activity is fast and accurate, and allows one to take full advantage of the changes of rhythmic activity at different times. For example, using ECD analysis, one only needs short intervals of clear dipolar signals to obtain good candidates for source analysis. However, when there are multiple source areas generating the rhythmic activity, as in the case of parieto-occipital 10-Hz rhythm, ECD analysis and testing of the explanatory power of the sources may become very time-consuming. Furthermore, selection of optimal subsets of sensors for source localization may require considerable expertise. A potentially more serious limitation of the ECD modeling is that it can only be done for time intervals in which there is clear signal. Accordingly, brain areas in which rhythmic activity is suppressed can only be identified indirectly, by first localizing the sources in the time windows during which there is discernible activity, and then testing whether those sources also account for the suppression. In the case of the central mu rhythm, suppression and enhancement of rhythmic activity normally occur in the same general area, at least in terms of the spatial accuracy available with MEG. Alternative methods using distributed modeling or beamformer techniques (with their own limitations) have been proposed (see Chapters 7, 8, and 9) and compared with ECD modeling (Liljeström et al., 2005).

Discussion

This chapter has, hopefully, emphasized to the reader that MEG data are usually not ambiguous. It is mostly quite obvious which areas are active. In that sense, the infamous inverse problem is not really the problem in MEG data analysis. It is more a question of identifying the clear field patterns, localizing the sources that generate them, and constructing a clean, well-behaved model with those sources.

Careful experimental design and high-quality data are the prerequisite for successful data analysis. The experimenter should make sure that the data are of highest quality. No analysis method can redeem data of poor quality. The first step is to decide what one really needs to find out, and choose the paradigm accordingly. For example, accurate localization is certainly needed for presurgical mapping of the central sulcus. The early somatosensory evoked fields are well suited for this purpose, as there is little activity in other cortical areas than the primary somatosensory cortex. However, if one studies differences in timing, e.g., during language tasks, extremely accurate localization is not really the issue to push. Parametric variation of stimuli or tasks is essential for functional localization (e.g., Tarkiainen et al., 1999) and very useful in source modeling.

One has to learn to read the MEG signals. That is the sound basis for all analysis. It is essential to know the data throughout. It may be a good idea to use different analysis methods to look at the same data; it also makes one spend more time scrutinizing the signals and thus become thoroughly familiar with them. This makes it possible to fully understand the solutions one gets.

Finally, when a solution or model is ready, one should be able to recognize it also in the original signals. Everything should make sense in the end. The analysis tools must provide visual control of the model and what it explains.

A major advantage of the ECD approach is that there are no hidden assumptions in mapping the field pattern to activation in the brain. The main criticism that has been raised against ECD modeling is that the user makes (or can make) subjective choices about the total number of active areas and the subset of sensors to be included in source localization. However, fundamentally this is no different from the subjective choices of thresholding one needs to make when using distributed analysis methods, or in PET/fMRI analysis. When ECD analysis is performed on the same MEG data set by different, experienced researchers, the same major sources emerge; variability, if any, appears in the inclusion of the weakest sources. The unparalleled asset of ECD analysis is that, having full visual control of the process, the user knows exactly why certain areas are found to be active and others not. It is advisable to carry out an ECD analysis, at least in a cursory fashion, before using more automatic analysis or visualization tools.

Basic sensory or motor processes often involve a relatively small number of brain areas that can be readily distinguished by location and/or direction of current flow and that show clear dipolar field patterns, at least at specific time intervals. When studying cognitive functions, the overall activation tends to be weaker, the time intervals of interest longer, and the effective signal-to-ratio lower because of the large number of sources that are spatially close and show considerable temporal overlap. Because of that, one often has to accept less perfect dipolarity of the field patterns than for functionally simpler tasks. Otherwise, the general procedures and considerations are similar for all types of data sets.

When using the ECD approach, one obviously seeks to identify the distinct dipolar field patterns in the data. In principle, one could argue that such an assumption ignores active areas that do not show dipolar signal distribution. However, at the distance MEG signals are recorded (at least 3 cm from the source currents) cortical activity appears dipolar as higher terms are reduced, relatively more rapidly, with distance. Most importantly, when a set of ECDs, determined from clearly dipolar field patterns, suffice to account for the data recorded by all sensors without leaving any systematic group of signals unexplained—and that is normally the case—it is hard to argue that alternative accounts of source structure would be critically needed.

Obviously, there are no miracle tools that would be more correct than others—and this is, of course, the real inverse problem in MEG (or EEG) analysis. User-independent tools should be particularly suitable for comparison across sites and users; nevertheless, one should not assume that such methods are more correct than others. For clear, good-quality data, any analysis tool should work well and give very similar results. Whichever tool one uses, one should be cautious in the interpretations—but that is true for all imaging techniques.

References

Coltheart, M., Curtis, B., Atkins, P., & Haller, M. (1993). Models of reading aloud: dual-route and parallel-distributed-processing approaches. *Psychological Review, 100,* 589–608.

Cornelissen, P., Tarkiainen, A., Helenius, P., & Salmelin, R. (2003). Cortical effects of shifting letter-position in letter-strings of varying length. *Journal of Cognitive Neuroscience 15,* 731–746.

Dale, A. M., Liu, A. K., Fischl, B. R., Buckner, R. L., Belliveau, J. W., Lewine, J. D., et al. (2000). Dynamic statistical parametric mapping: Combining fMRI and MEG for high-resolution imaging of cortical activity. *Neuron, 26,* 55–67.

Forss, N., Hari, R., Salmelin, R., Ahonen, A., Hämäläinen, M., Kajola, M., et al. (1994). Activation of the human posterior parietal cortex by median nerve stimulation. *Experimental Brain Research, 99,* 309–315.

Halgren, E., Dhond, R. P., Christensen, N., Van Petten, C., Marinkovic, K., Lewine, J. D., et al. (2002). N400-like magnetoencephalography responses modulated by semantic context, word frequency, and lexical class in sentences. *Neuroimage, 17,* 1101–1116.

Hari, R. & Salmelin, R. (1997). Human cortical oscillations: a neuromagnetic view through the skull. *Trends in Neurosciences 20,* 44–49.

Helenius, P., Salmelin, R., Service, E., & Connolly, J. F. (1999). Semantic cortical activation in dyslexic readers. *Journal of Cognitive Neuroscience, 11,* 535–550.

Hämäläinen, M., Hari, R., Ilmoniemi, R. J., Knuutila, J., & Lounasmaa, O. V. (1993). Magnetoencephalography – theory, instrumentation, and applications to noninvasive studies of the working human brain. *Reviews of Modern Physics, 65,* 413–497.

Lehtelä, L., Salmelin, R., & Hari, R. (1997). Evidence for reactive magnetic 10-Hz rhythm in the human auditory cortex. *Neuroscience Letters, 222,* 111–114.

Liljeström, M., Kujala, J., Jensen, O., & Salmelin, R (2005). Neuromagnetic localization of rhythmic activity in the human brain: a comparison of three methods. *Neuroimage, 25,* 734–745.

Lin, F. H., Witzel T., Hämäläinen, M. S., Dale, A. M., Belliveau, J. W., & Stufflebeam, S. M. (2004). Spectral spatiotemporal imaging of cortical oscillations and interactions in the human brain. *Neuroimage, 23,* 582–595.

Mäkelä, J., Ahonen, A., Hämäläinen, M., Hari, R., Ilmoniemi, R., Kajola, M., et al. (1993). Functional differences between auditory cortices of the two hemispheres revealed by whole-head neuromagnetic recordings. *Human Brain Mapping, 1,* 48–56.

Pantev, C., Ross, B., Berg, P., Elbert, T., & Rockstroh, B. (1998). Study of the human auditory cortices using a whole-head magnetometer: left vs. right hemisphere and ipsilateral vs. contralateral stimulation. *Audiology and Neurootology, 3,* 183–190.

Pfurtscheller, G., & Lopes da Silva, F. H. (1999). Event-related EEG/MEG synchronization and desynchronization: basic principles. *Clinical Neurophysiology, 110,* 1842–1857.

Saarinen, T., Laaksonen, H., Parviainen, T., & Salmelin, R. (2006). Motor Cortex Dynamics in Visuomotor Production of Speech and Non-speech Mouth Movements. *Cerebral Cortex, 16,* 212–222.

Salenius, S., Schnitzler, A., Salmelin, R., Jousmäki, V., & Hari, R. (1997). Modulation of human cortical rolandic rhythms during natural sensorimotor tasks. *Neuroimage, 5,* 221–228.

Salmelin, R. (2007). Clinical neurophysiology of language: the MEG approach. *Clinical Neurophysiology, 118,* 237–254.

Salmelin, R., & Hari, R. (1994a). Characterization of spontaneous MEG rhythms in healthy adults. *Electroencephalography and clinical Neurophysiology, 91,* 237–248.

Salmelin, R., & Hari, R. (1994b). Spatiotemporal characteristics of sensorimotor MEG rhythms related to thumb movement. *Neuroscience, 60,* 537–550.

Salmelin, R., Hämäläinen, M., Kajola, M., & Hari, R. (1995). Functional segregation of movement-related rhythmic activity in the human brain. *Neuroimage, 2,* 237–243.

Salmelin, R., & Sams, M. (2002). Motor cortex involvement during verbal versus nonverbal lip and tongue movements. *Human Brain Mapping, 16,* 81–91.

Salmelin, R., Schnitzler, A., Parkkonen, L., Biermann, K., Helenius, P., Kiviniemi, K., et al. (1999). Native language, gender, and functional organization of the auditory cortex. *Proceedings of the National Academy of Sciences USA, 96,* 10460–10465.

Salmelin, R., Schnitzler, A., Schmitz, F., & Freund, H.-J. (2000). Single word reading in developmental stutterers and fluent speakers. *Brain, 123,* 1184–1202.

Schnitzler, A., Salmelin, R., Salenius, S., Jousmäki, V., & Hari, R. (1995). Tactile information from the human hand reaches the ipsilateral primary sometosensory cortex. *Neuroscience Letters, 200,* 25–28.

Tarkiainen, A., Helenius, P., Hansen, P. C., Cornelissen, P. L., & Salmelin, R. (1999). Dynamics of letter string perception in the human occipitotemporal cortex. *Brain, 122,* 2119–2131.

Uusitalo, M. A., & Ilmoniemi, R. J. (1997). Signal-Space Projection method for separating MEG and EEG signals into components. *Medical & Biological Engineering & Computing, 35,* 135–140.

Uutela, K., Hämäläinen, M., & Somersalo, E. (1999). Visualization of magnetoencephalographic data using minimum current estimates. *Neuroimage, 10,* 173–180.

Vieth, J. B., Kober, H., & Grummich, P. (1996). Sources of spontaneous slow waves associated with brain lesions, localized by using the MEG. *Brain Topography, 8,* 215–221.

Weekes, B. S. (1997). Differential effects of number of letters on word and nonword latency. *Quarterly Journal of Experimental Psychology, 50A,* 439–456.

Wydell, TN., Vuorinen, T., Helenius, P., & Salmelin, R. (2003). Neural correlates of letter-string length and lexicality during reading in a regular orthography. *Journal of Cognitive Neuroscience, 15,* 1052–1062.

7

Estimating Distributed Representations of Evoked Responses and Oscillatory Brain Activity

Ole Jensen and Christian Hesse

- Distributed representations of electrophysiological activity are typically done using current estimates and beamforming techniques
- Distributed representations allow for spatial normalization and group averages
- Minimization constraints are applied when calculating distributed current estimates, resulting in spatially smooth solutions
- Both event-related responses and oscillatory brain activity can be modeled by distributed current estimates
- Beamforming approaches are best suited for longer lasting brain responses such as modulations of oscillatory activity

Introduction

Several techniques have been developed to construct source models accounting for electrophysiological brain activity measured by EEG and MEG. Rather than modeling the measured signal using only a small number of (discrete) dipole sources, the approaches considered in this chapter essentially estimate the contribution of all sources within the entire brain volume to the observed MEG or EEG, and thereby provide a distributed representation of the underlying neuronal activity. A major advantage is that such distributed representations can be spatially normalized to a standardized brain, and averaged over multiple subjects. This has become a crucial requirement in modern-day cognitive neuroimaging research.

From a practical point of view, there are two commonly used approaches to calculating distributed neuronal activation, both of which involve discretizing the brain volume onto a three-dimensional grid. The first approach is based on a distributed source model, and seeks to simultaneously estimate the current at all grid locations by fitting this model to the data, which involves inversion of an overdetermined set of linear equations. The second approach uses so-called "beamformers," which are adaptive spatial filters, to separately and sequentially estimate the contribution of sources at each grid location to the overall signal at the sensors. While beamforming does not assume a distributed source model, the technique also results in a distributed representation of brain activity.

MEG and EEG data are typically analyzed with respect to event-related responses or modulations in oscillatory brain activity. From a theoretical perspective there are no differences between the source models of these two types of brain responses. However, from a practical perspective there are important considerations when estimating the distribution of brain activation for event-related responses compared to oscillatory brain activity.

In this chapter we will discuss the relative advantages and disadvantages of distributed representations of source activity. After covering some theoretical considerations, a discussion follows on how to apply the technique in practice to event-related fields and oscillatory activity.

Theory

Basics of Source Modeling

The aim of biophysical source modeling is to account for the measured MEG/EEG signal in terms of a set of underlying current sources located within the brain volume. Equivalent current dipoles are a widely used model (Fig. 7–1) for approximately describing the spatial and temporal characteristics (orientation and magnitude) of the local current flow within a small volume of brain tissue, caused by the synchronized activation (post-synaptic currents) of many neurons (pyramidal cells). More formally, the N measured signals $\mathbf{b}(t) = [b_1(t), b_2(t),\ldots, d_N(t)]^T$ reflecting the time-varying magnetic field (or electric potential) patterns at the scalp are assumed to have been generated by the summed field patterns of a set of M (unobserved) current dipole sources

$$\mathbf{b}(t) = \mathbf{G}\mathbf{q}(t) + \mathbf{n}(t) \qquad (7\text{–}1)$$

Each column of the N-by-M leadfield matrix $\mathbf{G}$ contains the projection weights that reflect the spatial attenuation pattern at the sensors of the field,

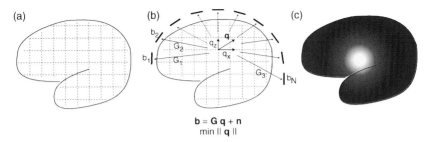

$$b = G\,q + n$$
$$\min \|\, q \,\|$$

Figure 7–1. The principle of current estimates. (b) The brain volume is modeled by a three-dimensional grid. (b) The full current distribution is approximated by the current dipoles, q, at each grid point. The aim is to find the current distribution that produces a field that matches the field measured by the sensors, **b**. The forward model **G** relates the current distribution to the measured field. (b) For visualization, the magnitudes of the current dipoles are projected to the brain surface and represented by a color code.

generated by a (unit magnitude) current dipole at a certain grid location, whose time-varying current strength (magnitude) is given by the corresponding row of $\mathbf{q}(t) = [q_1(t), q_2(t),\ldots, q_M(t)]^T$. The additive noise term $\mathbf{n}(t) = [n_1(t), n_2(t),\ldots, n_N(t)]^T$ is intended to account for any residual variance not explained in terms of the current sources within the brain.

The weights in the leadfield matrix **G** are determined independently of the measured signal, using an electromagnetic volume conductor model (i.e., the forward model) whose geometry is often a simple approximation of the anatomy of the head, e.g., a spherical multi-shell or boundary element model. Moreover, a triplet of dipoles at the same (grid) location, having orthogonal orientations in x, y, and z directions, can be used to explain the activity of any current dipole source at this location. Thus, in practice, the total number of current dipole sources M is three times the number of grid points. The (average) orientation of a dipole at each grid location can be determined from the current magnitude time courses $\mathbf{q}(t)$ in the x, y and z directions.

The fundamental aim of the source modeling approaches discussed in this chapter is to estimate the current magnitudes $\mathbf{q}(t)$ at all locations of the grid covering the brain volume, given a predetermined leadfield matrix **G**, and assuming that noise is negligible or at least sufficiently reduced, e.g., by averaging over trials. The difference between the methods is that distributed source modeling seeks to estimate the elements of $\mathbf{q}(t)$ all at once, whereas beamforming estimates the elements $\mathbf{q}(t)$ of at each grid location separately. As we will see subsequently, these source/current estimation approaches can be applied to MEG/EEG signals both in the time-domain (e.g., to model event-related fields) and in the frequency domain (e.g., to model ongoing or induced oscillatory activity).

Basics of Distributed Current Estimates

If the noise term is disregarded, and we consider a single time instant **t**, Equation (7–1) essentially describes a system of simultaneous linear equations, where **b** and **G** are known (either observed or specified) and where the vector **q** is the unknown quantity. Distributed source modeling approaches essentially try to estimate the currents by solving Equation (7–1) for **q** by inverting the system of equations, which can be loosely thought of as "dividing" both sides by **G**. However, since the number of grid points is much larger than the number of sensors—there are usually several thousand dipoles compared with only a few hundred sensors—the system of equations is underdetermined, which means that the solution for **q** cannot be uniquely determined unless additional constraints on **q** are applied. A typical constraint is to minimize the total current:

$$\min \| \mathbf{q} \| \qquad (7\text{–}2)$$

From a practical perspective, the current minimization constraint results in source estimates that are biased toward spatially smooth solutions. This is illustrated in Figure 7–2A, where current distributions producing similar fields are shown. The solutions to the right will be chosen, given that they result in the smallest absolute current. The minimization constraint in Equation (7–2) can be applied with respect to different norms. The L2–norm minimizes the sum of the squared current values, whereas the L1–norm minimizes the sum of the absolute current values. Current estimates obtained with respect to the L2–norm are referred to as Minimum Norm Estimates (MNE), (Dale & Sereno, 1993; Hamalainen & Ilmoniemi, 1994; Matsuura &

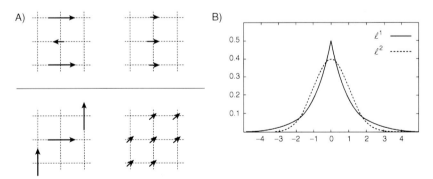

Figure 7–2. (A) The current distributions to the left and the right produce very similar fields. However, when applying the minimum current constraint the distributions to the right are chosen. (B) The *a priori* distributions of current magnitudes when applying the L1- and the L2-norm estimates. Reproduced from Uutela et al. (1999).

Okabe, 1995) whereas estimates obtained using the L1–norm are referred to as Minimum Current Estimates (MCEs) (Matsuura & Okabe, 1995; Uutela et al., 1999). The L2–norm implicitly assumes a Gaussian *a priori* current distribution, whereas the L1–norm assumes a Laplacian (double exponential) distribution (Figure 7–2B). Consequently, the MNE results in more spatially smeared current distributions compared to the MCE. Thus, when selecting between the L1– and the L2–norm, an implicit choice is being made in terms of spatial smoothness of the current distributions. From a theoretical point of view there are no well-motivated reasons for choosing one approach over the other. From a physiological perspective we do not have sufficient information to judge which approach is more appropriate. Minimization procedures with additional smoothness constraints have been implemented in the LORETA method (Pascual-Marqui et al., 1994). As for MNE, the LORETA approach results in quite smeared source estimates.

One practical problem that arises when calculating current estimates is that superficial sources are overestimated at the expense of deeper sources. This is a consequence of deep focal sources producing fields very similar to extended superficial sources (Figure 7–3). Since the MEG sensors are more sensitive to nearby sources, the current-estimate methods become biased toward the superficial sources when applying the minimization constraint. In order to reduce this bias, a weighted norm is often applied to reduce the contribution of the superficial currents (Ioannides et al., 1990; Liu et al., 1998; Uutela et al., 1999). It is important to keep in mind that when selecting a specific approach to reduce the depth bias, a choice is implicitly being made that has consequences for the final current distribution. The minimum norm estimate using the L2–norm can be derived directly by inverting Equation (7–1), but this is not the case for the minimum current estimate, since it involves the L1–norm. Uutela et al. (1999) used linear programming in order to solve

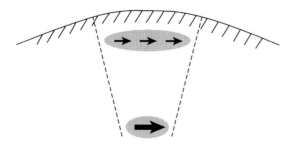

Figure 7–3. Deep focal and superficial distributed sources produce very similar fields. Since magnetic fields decrease with distance, the deeper sources must be stronger in magnitude compared to superficial sources in order to produce the same field. Thus, the minimization constraint biases the solution toward superficially distributed sources.

the L1 optimization problem. For reasons of computational efficiency they proposed first to calculate the current orientations using the L2–norm, and subsequently calculate the current amplitudes using the L1–norm for the fixed current orientations.

There are several methods of visualizing the current estimates. The method used by Uutela et al. (1999) visualizes the estimated solutions by projecting the current distribution onto a triangular mesh representing the brain surface. The current magnitudes are then interpolated and color coded. Subsequently the sources of interest can be manually identified by means of a graphical user interface. The coordinates of the sources of interest can be mapped onto the anatomical MRI of the individual subjects. As for dipole modeling, the coordinates of the head model are aligned to the structural MRI of the subjects with reference to anatomical landmarks (see, e.g., Dale et al., 2000; Lin et al., 2004).

It should be noted that current estimates for groups of subjects typically are performed differently for EEG and MEG data. ERPs from EEG data are often averaged across subjects at the sensor level. This can be done, since the electrodes in different subjects have approximately the same position with respect to the brain. In the case of MEG, different subjects will have different positions inside the helmet. As a consequence, individual brains are positioned differently with respect to the sensor array. Thus, it is preferable to average the estimated current distributions across subjects. Scaling to a normalized brain (e.g., the MNI or a Talairach brain) or morphing is typically done prior to averaging.

Basics of Beamforming

An alternative way of estimating the contribution of each source in the brain volume to the MEG/EEG signal measured at the scalp is to use the so-called beamforming approach. Instead of trying to solve a system of equations with more unknown than known parameters using norm constraints on the solution, the activation time-course at each source location (and in each direction) can be determined independently of all other locations, by means of spatial filters. Adaptive spatial filtering is a general technique in multichannel signal processing, which was initially developed for radar and antenna array processing (e.g., Capon, 1969; Van Veen & Buckley, 1988; Van Veen, 1992). Early applications of different versions of this signal estimation technique, in conjunction with MEG/EEG source analysis, have been described by Van Veen (1997), Robinson and Vrba (1999), and by Gross et al. (2001). For reviews of beamforming applied to MEG, see Hillebrand and Barnes (2005) and Hillebrand et al. (2005).

A spatial filter comprises a set of coefficients or weights ($\mathbf{w} = [w_1, w_2,..., w_N]^T$) that essentially define a linear combination (weighted sum) of the signals at all sensors is supposed to selectively enhance activity at the target location (source) while suppressing interfering activity from sources at all other locations.[1] Thus, an estimate of the activation time course of a source at a given source (grid) location i is estimated as

$$\hat{q}_i(t) = \mathbf{w}_i^T \mathbf{b}(t) \tag{7-3}$$

To obtain a distributed representation of source activity using this approach in practice, one "scans" through the brain volume and constructs a separate set of spatial filter weights (beamformers) $\mathbf{w}_j$ for each point (and orientation) of the grid, which are then used to obtain a current estimate for that source using Equation (7–3). The resulting distributed representation of source activity can then be visualized and further analyzed in much the same manner as the current estimates obtained using the MNE and MCE methods.

How are the weights of the spatial filter determined? Mathematically, it can be shown (see, e.g., Haykin, 2002) that the spatial filter weights that provide the best linear estimate (in the least square-error sense) of the activation time course of a source $q_i(t)$ at a given location $\mathbf{G}_i$ are determined by

$$\mathbf{w}_i = \frac{\mathbf{C}^{-1}\mathbf{G}_i}{\mathbf{G}_i^T\mathbf{C}^{-1}\mathbf{G}_i} \tag{7-4}$$

where $\mathbf{C}^{-1}$ is the inverse of the cross-covariance matrix of the measured signal $\mathbf{C} = \mathbf{b}(t)\mathbf{b}(t)^T/(T\text{-}1)$, where T is the number of time.

The expression for the spatial filter weights in Equation (7–4) is variously known as *Capon's beamformer*, the *linearly constrained minimum variance* (LCMV) beamformer, and the *minimum mean square error* (MMSE) estimator (e.g., Haykin, 2002). It is the use of the cross-covariance matrix of the data that makes this type of filter "adaptive" and accounts for its spatially selective enhancement and interference-suppression characteristics. When applied to frequency-domain data, the cross-covariance matrix $\mathbf{C}$ is replaced by a matrix reflecting the cross spectrum (or cross-spectral density) at a particular frequency, or over a frequency band of interest. In the context of MEG/EEG neuroimaging, frequency-domain beamforming is also known as the *dynamic imaging of coherent sources* (DICS) method (e.g., Gross et al., 2001; Chapter 9). Alternatively, LCMV beamforming can also be applied to bandpass-filtered data, which, in MEG neuroimaging, is also referred to as *synthetic aperture magnetometry* (SAM) analysis (Robinson & Vrba, 1999).

Beamforming relies on two key assumptions, namely: a) that the activation time courses of all sources are mutually uncorrelated; and b) that the forward model describing the field patterns of the sources is correct, or at least sufficiently accurate.[2] The mathematical exposition required to explain in detail why these assumptions are necessary—and what happens when they are violated—is beyond the scope of this introductory chapter. However, a relative intuitive account would be the following: The cross-covariance matrix **C** captures the dependency structure of the MEG/EEG signals at the sensor level, and reflects *both* correlations due to the projection of the same source signal onto each of the sensors, as well as correlations between different source signals. In the ideal case, where the waveforms of all sources are uncorrelated, then the spatial filter only has to suppress interference between sources with spatially correlated field patterns. In this case, the cross-correlation matrix only contains spatial correlations, and the multiplication by its inverse essentially removes these correlations. Correlated source-activation time courses constitute an additional source of cross-covariance, which cannot be disambiguated from the cross-covariance due to spatially correlated field patterns, and hence are not effectively cancelled by the inverse covariance matrix. In effect, the beamformer is trying to simultaneously maximize and suppress (parts of) the same signal, and this can lead to large errors in the source estimate (e.g., Van Veen, 1997).

In cognitive neuroscience, beamforming is used mainly to estimate the power of oscillatory activity. Beamforming is (by mathematical construction) not optimally suited for providing "good" estimates of sources with correlated activation time courses. Thus, it is not clear when applications of this method (i.e., based on separately scanning individual locations within the brain volume) are appropriate for visualizing or localizing networks of coherent cortical sources—whose activations are, by definition, correlated to some degree, dependent on the phase angle—but see, e.g., Gross et al. (2001) and Kujala et al. (2007) for successful applications. Attempts to overcome this problem by simultaneously scanning at several grid locations have been made (Brookes et al., 2007).

A further practical requirement is that the estimate of the cross-covariance matrix of the data is accurate, and that the cross-covariance matrix is invertible. These are the problems often encountered when applying beamforming for source analysis of event-related fields (ERFs). The cross-covariance matrix can become rank-deficient (and hence not invertible) in two circumstances: if the epoch of interest contains fewer time samples than sensors, or (at least theoretically) if the time-locked, averaged MEG signal reflects the activity of only a very small number of neuronal sources, and any background activity and noise effectively disappears by averaging an extremely large number of trials. In practice, rank-deficient cross-covariance matrices can be made invertible by regularization, which effectively involves injecting additional noise into the signal—this, in turn, tends to spatially smear the neuronal activity. For this reason, beamforming is not widely used in MEG/EEG source analysis of evoked activity.

Since the adaptive spatial filters computed using Equation (7–3) are dependent on the leadfield matrix **G**, beamforming—like the MNE/MCE methods for distributed source modeling—does not provide accurate estimates of deep sources. This is essentially due to the fact that the field patterns at the scalp of neighboring dipole sources approaching the center of the head are generally more similar to each other (i.e., more spatially correlated) than the fields of neighboring dipoles close to the surface. Particularly in the presence of noise, this leads to larger localization errors. Primarily because of this "spatial leakage," beamformers tend to overestimate the signal power of deeplying sources, which makes it difficult to interpret the "raw" beamformer signal amplitude estimates. Two approaches have been proposed to circumvent this problem. A normalization approach based on the *neural activity index* (NAI), put forward by Van Veen (1997), scales (divides) the projected power at each source location by the corresponding projected noise power, using a suitably accurate model estimate of the signal noise.[3] A practical alternative for comparisons of source activity between two experimental conditions is to simply use the ratio of source power between conditions. The latter approach assumes an implicit signal model in which the noise characteristics (regardless of interpretation) are identical in both conditions, and is more widely used in cognitive neuroscience (e.g., Nieuwenhuis et al., 2008).

Finally, it should be noted that beamforming, or adaptive spatial filtering as such, is *not* a source localization technique, but rather a method for estimating (extracting) a signal at a known location. Nevertheless, the location of important or dominant sources can be determined by appropriate postprocessing of the distributed representation of source activity obtained by beamforming, e.g., thresholding or detection of local peaks in activation/power.

Characterizing Spontaneous Oscillatory Activity by Power Spectra

The approaches so far pertain to current estimates of event-related fields, which reflect transient time-locked changes in brain activity. However, it is clear that the brain also produces oscillatory activity, which is not phase-locked to stimuli or responses (Hari & Salmelin, 1997; Tallon-Baudry & Bertrand, 1999). It is useful to distinguish between two types of oscillatory activity: spontaneous, and induced. Spontaneous oscillatory activity occurs in the absence of stimuli or overt behavior, but can be modulated by various conditions. An example of spontaneous oscillations is posterior alpha activity (7–13 Hz), which emerges when subjects are resting (Niedermeyer & Lopes da Silva, 1999). For instance, the power of the posterior alpha activity is much higher when the eyes are closed than when the eyes are open. Induced oscillatory activity is measured in response to repeated stimuli. These oscillations are not necessarily phase-locked to the stimuli (Figure 7–4). An example of induced oscillatory activity is the "beta rebound," which are ~20 Hz oscillations that emerge after median nerve stimulation (Salmelin & Hari, 1994). Given that these oscillations are not phase-locked to the stimuli, it is not possible to average the measured traces and then calculate the source estimates. We will here discuss various approaches used to identify the sources of oscillatory activity by means of current estimates.

Several studies have investigated power in various frequency bands. For instance, power differences in the delta, theta and alpha band have been compared in different patient groups (Niedermeyer & Lopes da Silva, 1999).

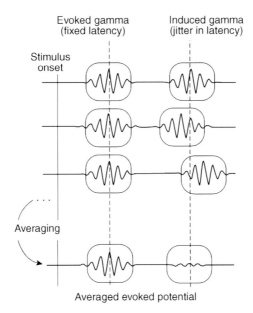

Figure 7–4. Evoked responses are phase-locked to the stimulus and will subsequently be presented in the averaged data. Induced responses are not necessarily phase-locked, and are attenuated by averaging. Reproduced from Tallon-Baudry and Bertand (1999).

It should be pointed out that just because there are differences in a given frequency band when comparing two groups of subjects, it does not necessarily mean that there is spontaneous oscillatory activity with a magnitude strong enough for the sources to be modeled. In order to be able to assess whether the sources of spontaneous oscillatory activity can be identified, it is recommended to perform a spectral analysis of power at the sensor level. Such an analysis serves several purposes. If a "clear" peak in the spectra can be identified, it suggests that oscillatory activity is present, rather than a broad band signal. Second, spectral analysis will allow for identifying the frequency peak and range. Given that the peak frequency of alpha oscillations varies among subjects, the optimal approach when identifying oscillatory sources is to target the peak frequency in individual subjects (Posthuma et al., 2001). A common approach to spectral analysis of spontaneous oscillatory activity is to apply Fourier transforms to the ongoing data. We will here describe in detail how this is done, given that this insight is important for understanding how to calculate MCEs/MNEs in the frequency domain. The power spectrum is calculated from the modulus of the Fourier transform squared as a function of frequency. Typically, the fast Fourier transform (FFT) algorithm is applied. Using this approach directly for power estimation has one drawback: the variance of the power spectra estimates does not decrease with increasing data length. This problem can be solved using Welch's method by dividing the data into segments of equal length ("windowing"). The power spectra calculated for each segment are then averaged, thus reducing the variance of the spectral estimate with increasing number of segments (Welch, 1967; Challis & Kitney, 1991). Frequency smoothing can be controlled by changing the length of the data segments, i.e., the frequency resolution decreases as the length of the data segments becomes shorter. Some frequency smoothing might be advantageous, given the frequency fluctuations in cortical rhythms. For instance, in a typical subject the alpha activity might fluctuate between 10 and 12 Hz. Practical experience has shown that adjusting the length of the time window yielding a frequency resolution of 0.5–1 Hz results in sensible power spectra for activity in the alpha and beta range. Another concern that arises when segmenting data prior to spectral estimates, is spectral leakage emerging due to edge effects of the segments. The spectral leakage can be reduced by applying a windowing function, i.e., a taper, to each segment. Often a Hanning taper is applied (Challis & Kitney, 1991). To compensate for the data loss due to the taper at the edges of the segment, overlapping segments are applied—e.g., 50% overlapping segments are typically used for Hanning tapers. Figure 7–5A shows an example where the power spectra have been calculated using Welch's method for a subject resetting with eyes closed. Note that the dominant frequencies of both alpha and beta activity can be identified in the spectra. While Welch's method for power spectra estimation is commonly used, multitaper techniques provide a better control of the frequency smoothing, and are becoming increasingly popular (Percival, 1993; Mitra & Pesaran, 1999).

Current Estimates of Spontaneous Oscillatory Activity

The main complication when identifying sources of oscillatory activity is that the phases of the oscillatory signals are not time-locked to events. This precludes averaging the signals directly in order to improve the signal-to-noise ratio. One approach is to identify the sources in the frequency domain by using dipole modeling (Lutkenhoner, 1992; Tesche & Kajola, 1993) or current estimates (Gomez & Thatcher, 2001; Jensen & Vanni, 2002). Current estimates in the frequency domain are done by calculating the Fourier transforms for the frequency of interest within the magnetic fields measured by the sensors. The current estimates (L1, L2 or LORETA) are then calculated for the complex representations. As when calculating power spectra (see previous section) it is advantageous to apply a time window that divides the data into epochs, in order to control the frequency resolution and increase the signal-to-noise ratio (see Figure 7–6). The current estimates of the complex Fourier transform are then calculated for each time window and combined. Selecting short time windows results in a relatively high signal-to-noise ratio, but low frequency resolution; selecting long time windows increases the frequency resolution at the expense of a lower signal-to-noise ratio. As for Welch's

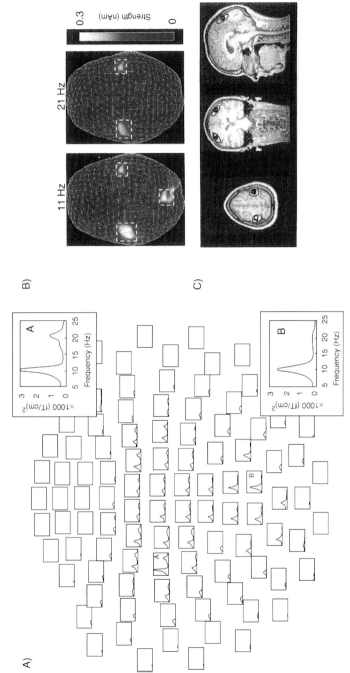

Figure 7–5. Power spectra and MCEs calculated from MEG data recorded from a subject resetting with eyes closed. (A) The power spectra were calculated using Welch's method. The window length was 1.7 s. (B) The frequency domain MCEs were calculated for the peak frequencies (11 and 21 Hz) identified in the power spectra. (C) The sources of the peak frequencies were co-registered on the subject's MRI. Reproduced from Jensen and Vanni (2002).

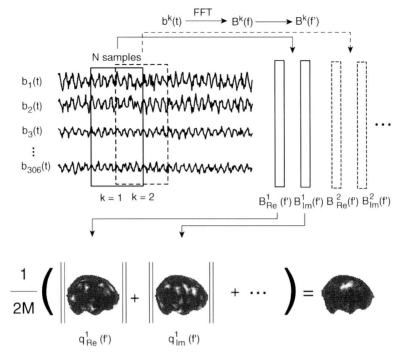

Figure 7–6. Calculating MCEs in the frequency domain. The Fourier transform is calculated for the each time window (epoch) for the frequency of interest. The current estimates for the real and imaginary parts of the Fourier-transformed data are combined for each time window. Finally, the current estimates are averaged.
Reproduced from Jensen and Vanni (2002).

methods for power spectra estimation, applying a Hanning taper to each window will reduce the spectral leakage. Windowing the data poses one problem: the complex current estimates for each time window will have different phases. This problem is solved by calculating the current estimates for the real and imaginary parts of the Fourier-transformed data. The real and imaginary parts of the current estimates are then combined, leaving only the magnitude of the current estimate (Jensen & Vanni, 2002). These magnitudes are then averaged over time windows. As a result, the phase information and thus the source orientation are lost. While this method has been implemented for MCEs (Jensen & Vanni, 2002), it should be mentioned that the same approach can be used for MNE and LORETA. The implications for the estimated source distributions are the same as those for event-related fields: the MNE source distributions will be more spatially smeared as compared to those calculated by MCE. Figure 7–5 shows an example where the sources of spontaneous oscillatory activity in alpha and beta band have been estimated. First, the power spectra were calculated in order to identify the frequency peaks at ~11 and

~21 Hz. The current distributions for those frequencies were then estimated and subsequently mapped onto the subject's anatomical MRI.

Time-frequency Representations of Induced Oscillatory Activity

Prior to performing source modeling of induced oscillatory activity, it is important to characterize when in time, and at which frequency bands, a given effect occurs. While power spectra are convenient for determining the frequency band of interest for spontaneous activity, more elaborate methods are required in order to characterize changes in oscillatory activity in response to a given stimulus. One commonly applied method is based on filtering the data in the frequency band of interest (Kalcher & Pfurtscheller, 1995). After each trial has been bandpass filtered, it is rectified and smoothed over time. The resulting representations are then averaged over trials, thus preserving activity that is not phase-locked to the stimulus. Subsequently, the amplitude representations are normalized with respect to a baseline interval, in order to express amplitude changes in percent. Amplitude increases are termed "event-related synchronization" (ERS), and decreases are termed "event-related desynchronization" (ERD). The terminology ERD/ERS has not been generally adopted since it assigns a physiological interpretation to changes in amplitude. Another much-related approach is termed "temporal spectral evolution" (TSE) which characterizes absolute rather than relative power changes with respect to a baseline (Salmelin & Hari, 1994). The TSE and ERD/ERS methods have been used to characterize oscillatory activity in specific frequency bands. As computer power over the years has increased, methods are nowadays applied that simultaneously investigate a range of frequencies. Wavelet techniques and spectrograms are typically applied (Tallon-Baudry & Bertrand, 1999). With respect to the wavelets technique, a *wavelet family* for the frequencies of interest is constructed. The complex Morlet wavelet is often applied:

$$w(t,f) = A \exp(\frac{-t^2}{2\sigma_t^2}) \exp\left(2i\pi\ f_0 t\right) \qquad (7\text{--}5)$$

where $A = \dfrac{1}{\sigma_t \sqrt{2\pi}}$. The time-frequency representation (TFR) of power $P(t, f_0)$ for a given signal at time (t) and frequency (f) is given by the squared norm of the convolution of a Morlet wavelet to the signal $s(t)$:

$$P(t, f_0) = |\, w(t, f_0) \times s(t)|^2 \qquad (7\text{--}6)$$

The "band width" of the wavelet measured in numbers of cycles is determined by $m - \dfrac{f_0}{\sigma_f}$, where $\sigma_f = 1/2\pi\sigma_t$. The wavelet balances the time and frequency

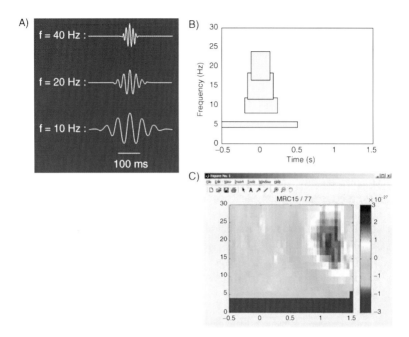

Figure 7–7. Complex wavelets applied in the analysis of induced oscillatory activity. (A) The real part of a complex Morlet wavelet (m = 7) shown for different frequencies. (B) The 'tiles' illustrate the time-frequency tradeoff of the wavelets transformations with increasing frequencies. (C) An example of a time-frequency presentation of induced beta activity calculated using Morlet wavelets. The induced beta is strongest in the time interval 0.8–1.3 s and at frequencies 13–25 Hz.

resolution of the representations over different frequency bands. As the frequency increases the wavelets become shorter, thus increasing the time resolution (Figure 7–7A). Longer wavelets (a larger m) will result in a better frequency resolution at the expense of the time resolution; the contrary is the case for shorter wavelets. Typically, wavelets of width m = 7 provide a good compromise between time and frequency resolution. Figure 7–7B shows an example in which the TFR has been calculated for an induced oscillatory signal in the beta band. The TFRs of power are useful for determining the time intervals and frequency bands in which the induced amplitude modulation of ongoing oscillatory activity occurs. This is crucial information when localizing the sources reflecting the induced changes in oscillatory activity, using both distributed source modeling (MNE/MCE) and beamforming methods.

Current Estimates of Induced Oscillatory Activity

When localizing induced oscillatory activity, the aim is to calculate the time course of oscillatory sources. This is different from localizing the sources of event-related fields, since the single trial signals cannot be assumed to be phase-locked to the stimuli. Thus, the current estimates must be calculated for each trial and then averaged in an appropriate manner. In principle it is possible to extend the method of Jensen and Vanni (2002) in order to identify sources of induced oscillatory activity, by applying a sliding time window to each trial. The power values of the current estimates for each time window, with respect to the same delay in relation to the stimuli, are then averaged. Lin et al. (2004) have proposed such an approach based on the complex wavelet transform. Like the Fourier transform, the complex wavelet transform yields real and imaginary representations for which the current estimates can be calculated. The current estimate's real and imaginary parts are then summed, averaged over trials, and represented as a function of time (Figure 7–8). Lin et al. applied this method to MNEs, but it can also be used in conjunction with MCEs. As always, when characterizing induced activity it is convenient to study changes in power of induced oscillatory activity with respect to a baseline period, since this attenuates noise due to slow drifts in signal power. Lin et al. (2004) proposed to use an F–test to compare stimulus power to baseline power in the current estimates, thus effectively producing a signal-to-noise estimate of the induced activity. Only a few applied neuroscience studies so far have been published using MNEs/MCEs to identify induced oscillatory activity. However, given the growing interest in oscillatory activity, more studies on this subject are bound to emerge in the near future.

Applications

Applications of Current Estimates to Event-Related Fields

How well do the current-estimate techniques compare to other methods? This question cannot be answered unequivocally, given that the various methods are based on different assumptions. We will here address one study that directly attempted to compare MCE to dipole modeling. In order to compare the different approaches, Stenbacka et al. (2002) designed several data sets and asked 10 trained researchers to localize the sources by means of dipole modeling and MCE. The data sets varied in difficulty with respect to number of dipoles and temporal overlap between the source activations. In general, the researchers were able to identify sources equally well using MCE and dipole modeling. Independent of the method it was problematic to identify deep sources and sources with close-to-radial orientations. For both methods, source localization became difficult if the degree of temporal overlap between the activated sources was increased.

A)

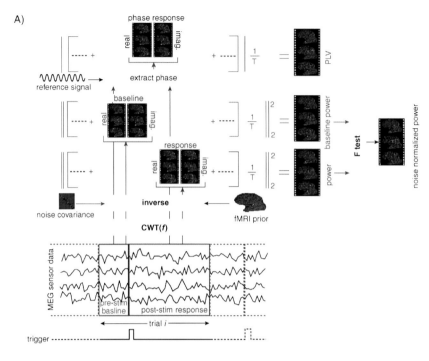

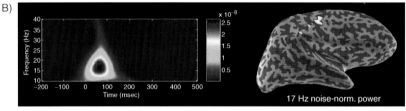

Figure 7–8. Wavelets and MNE applied to study the temporal development of induced oscillatory activity. (A) CWT denotes complex wavelet transformations applied to the data. The MNEs are calculated for the real and imaginary parts of the wavelet transformations and summed. The current estimates are then averaged over trials and an F-test is applied to normalize the data with respect to noise. (B) Early activity (40–100 ms) in the beta band (~17 Hz) was identified using the wavelet approach and MNE. The beta activity was induced by median nerve stimulation. The resulting MNE is represented on the subject's inflated brain. As expected, the sources are localized around sensorimotor cortex.

Reproduced from Lin et al. (2004).

Typically, both methods produced sensible solutions; however, MCE was found to systematically underestimate the source amplitudes of the identified sources. This was due to the spatial spread of the sources arising from the current estimates. Additionally, more false sources were found using the MCE approach, since the researchers tended to confound noise with real sources. It should be mentioned that no distributed sources were included in the test data sets. The advantage, that current estimates can be easily averaged over data sets from several subjects was not accessed, either. Averaging over subjects would have most likely removed the falsely identified sources for the MCEs. In conclusion, MCE is likely to perform as well as dipole modeling when localizing sources of event-related fields. However, MCE is inferior compared to dipole modeling when estimating the true strength of highly focal sources.

The first MEG study we will address uses MCE to investigate how brain activation is modulated by visual attention. The experimental question is as follows: are there brain regions where the activation to peripheral stimuli is modulated by foveal attention? If yes, when in time does this modulation occur? To address this question, Vanni and Uutela (2000) designed a study in which subjects were supposed to detect luminance changes in a foveally presented fixation square. Since these changes occurred unpredictably, they required the subjects to attend intensively (Figure 7–9A). Occasionally, a square was flashed in the right or the left peripheral hemisphere. Event-related fields in response to the peripheral stimuli were measured. Control conditions (passive viewing, intertrial) were similar, except that there was no detection task. The MCEs were calculated for the individual subjects with respect to a spherical head model. The head models were fitted to the brain surface in each subject. Subsequently, the MCEs were averaged across subjects. The current estimates were then projected to the surface of a geometry obtained from a standard brain. In the time window, a 100–160 ms difference was found between attended and control conditions. Stronger activity was found for the attended compared to the control condition (passive viewing) in right precentral areas (Figure 7–7B). Using this region of interest, the time course of the precentral area was identified from time resolved MCEs (Figure 7–9C). Note that the attention modulation of the right precentral activity is present for both left and right peripheral visual field stimulation. Figure 7–9D shows an example from a single subject in which the activity from the precentral region was mapped to the segmented brain surface. Note the overlap in the regions identified for left and right stimulation (indicated by white and black outlines). The region modulated by attention corresponds to the frontal eye field (FEF). Beyond identifying the FEF, the study also showed that the effect of attention occurred 130 ms after the onset of the peripheral stimuli. The findings show that focusing attention to a fixation point enhances responses in the FEF to non-attended peripheral stimuli. This is consistent with monkey studies showing that the FEF is an important note in the parietofrontal network involved in planning and execution of saccades.

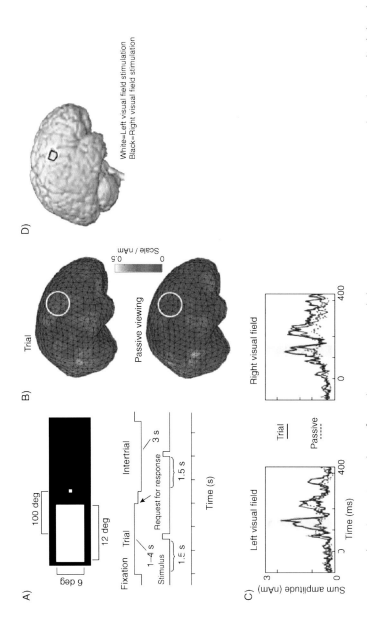

Figure 7–9. MCEs used to investigate how foveal attention modulates MEG responses to peripheral stimuli. (A) When the luminance of the foveal fixation square changed, subjects were supposed to respond by button-press. The ERFs were calculated from the MEG data time-locked to peripheral squares flashing in the right or left visual fields. The ERFs were calculated during passive viewing as well, and the intertrial intervals were used as control conditions. (B) Grand average of the MCEs in the 100-160 ms time period. The white circles indicate the regions of interest where the attention effect was identified. (C) The time course of the regions of interest shown for stimulation in the left and right visual fields. (D) The regions of interest mapped onto the segmented brain of a single subject. Reproduced from Vanni & Uutela (2000).

The second example is an MEG study in which the MNE rather than MCE approach has been applied to investigate the N400m effect. The N400 component has been intensively studied using EEG, and refers to a negative detection in the ERPs occurring ~400 ms post-stimulus. The N400 component increases in magnitude in response to semantic violations (i.e., a word in the sentence that does not make sense)—this is referred to as the N400 effect (Kutas & Hillyard, 1980). Using MEG, the dominant sources of the N400 effect have been identified in the left and right superior temporal cortex by dipole modeling (Helenius et al., 1998). MNE has also been applied in order to identify the sources of the N400 effect (Halgren et al., 2002). The study was designed as a standard N400 paradigm in which 240 sentences were presented visually. Half of the sentences ended with a word that was semantically incongruent with respect to the sentence context; the other half of the sentences had congruent endings. Figure 7–10A shows a typical ERF from one sensor over the left temporal region. Note the stronger N400m component for the incongruent sentences. Field distributions are shown in Figure 7–10B after subtracting the two conditions.[4] The field distribution over the left hemisphere is well described by a dipole in the superior temporal cortex. Additionally, the MNE approach was applied to account for the N400 effect. The MNEs were calculated in time-steps of 5 ms and converted to a dynamic statistical parametric map (dSPM). These maps represent the MNE results in terms of signal-to-noise ratios rather than baseline-subtracted current distributions

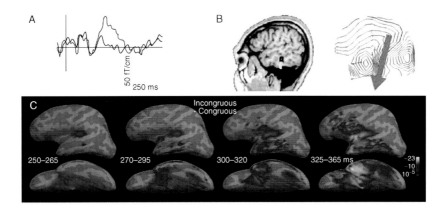

Figure 7–10. The MNE applied to the N400 effect. (A) The ERFs for congruent (black) and incongruent (red) sentence-endings for a single subject. (B) A dipole model accounting for the subtracted ERFs for a single subject. (C) The MNEs of the subtracted conditions represented as dSPMs. The source distributions in each subject were mapped to inflated brain representations, and morphed prior to grand averaging.
Reproduced from Halgren et al. (2002).

(for details see Liu et al., 1998; and Dale et al., 2000). The noise used in dSPM is estimated from the measured data. As shown in Dale et al. (2000), the MNEs become more focal after noise normalization and thresholding. Source distributions were mapped to the segmented brain surface for the two conditions subtracted. The brain surfaces were then morphed according to gyri and sulci and a grand average over 8 subjects was performed (Figure 7–10C). At about 250 ms, the first activity emerges in Wernicke's area. It then spreads and, after 300 ms, prefrontal activity can be observed, which eventually includes Broca's areas. It should also be mentioned that the threshold applied to the dSPMs is somewhat arbitrary. In conclusion, the MNE approach applied to the N400 effect allows for visualizing the spatiotemporal development of event-related activity. Compared to the dipole model, MNE does produce source distributions that are fairly smeared.

Applications of Current Estimates to Spontaneous Oscillatory Activity

In an attempt to compare different techniques developed to localize oscillatory sources, Liljestrom et al. (2005) tested three different methods using simulated and measured data. The methods tested were dipole models of bandpass-filtered data, MCE in the frequency domain, and Dynamica Imaging of Coherent Sources (DICS, see Chapter 9). The study showed that all three methods performed well when identifying the sources of the dominant spontaneous rhythms (the alpha and mu rhythms). As for modeling event-related fields, dipole modeling had the disadvantage in that during the fitting procedure, operations such as manually selecting a group of sensors had to be performed. DICS proved better than MCE when separating nearby sources.

The following example addresses the modulation of oscillations in the beta band by benzodiazepines. From clinical EEG research it is well known that beta oscillations increase in power if a patient has been administered benzodiazepine. The pharmacologically induced beta oscillations have a frontal EEG distribution; however, it is not known where the sources accounting for the beta increase are localized. In a study by Jensen et al. (2005), spontaneous MEG data were measured before and after administration of benzodiazepine in 8 subjects. Figure 7–11A shows the spontaneous power spectra for sensors over the central band. Note that (1) the power in the beta band increased dramatically with benzodiazepine, and (2) the beta power decreased in frequency. Given that the frequency peaks in the 8 subjects varied from 13 to 23 Hz, it was essential to calculate the current estimates in each subject with respect to the individually dominant beta frequency peaks. Figure 7–11B shows the grand average of the MCEs before and after the administration of benzodiazepine. The MCEs were calculated in each subject with respect to a spherical head model fitted to the individual brain surfaces. The current estimates were then projected onto the surface of a standard brain, and averaged across subjects. The identified sources were also mapped to structural MRI in

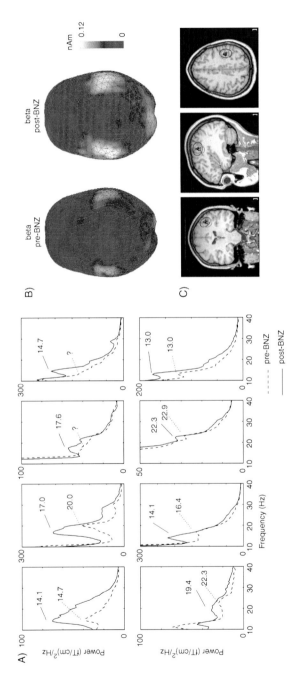

Figure 7–11. Sources accounting for the increase in beta oscillations with benzodiazepine. (A) The power spectra from sensors over the central band before and after the administration of benzodiazepine. Data from 8 subjects. (B) The grand average of the MCEs calculated in the frequency domain. (C) The sources of the beta activity mapped onto the MRI. Example from a single subject.

Reproduced from Jensen et al. (2005).

the individual subjects. As seen in the example in Figure 7–11C, the beta sources were located in the sensorimotor cortex around the central sulcus. In conclusion, this study shows that the increase in beta-band oscillations with benzodiazepine can be accounted for by sources in sensorimotor cortex. Prior to performing the MCE analysis, it was essential to first calculate the power spectra in each subject in order to identify the peak frequency of the beta oscillations.

Beamforming Techniques Applied to Induced and Prestimulus Oscillatory Activity

The beamforming approach has proven successful in localizing oscillatory brain activity in numerous studies (Hillebrand & Barnes, 2005; Bauer et al., 2006; Gaetz & Cheyne, 2006; Medendorp et al., 2006; Osipova et al., 2006; Jokisch & Jensen, 2007; van Dijk et al., 2008). We will here present a few examples demonstrating the capabilities of the method. The first study is on gamma activity induced by long-term memory recall (Nieuwenhuis et al., 2008). The participants learned to associate a face to one of eight locations, in two types of training schemes. In the first scheme (stabilized), the training was distributed over a week. In the second scheme (labile) the training was done in one block on the day of the recall session (Figure 7–12a). During the recall session, only the faces were presented and subjects were asked to move each face to the remembered location with a joystick. Figure 7–12b demonstrates that strong posterior gamma activity was elicited in response to the presentation of the face. Using the beamforming approach, subjected to data from a 100 ms sliding time window, it was possible to track spatiotemporal progression of the gamma activity. The DICS approach was used, calculating the induced power in the frequency domain. The gamma activity was mapped onto the individual subject's structural MRI. The individual brains were then morphed to a standard brain, and the induced activity averaged across subjects. As seen, the gamma activity was first induced in early visual areas and then progressed to higher order areas, including parietal cortex. When comparing the labile to the stabilized condition, stronger gamma activity was observed in visual areas (Figure 7–12c). Note that Figure 7–12c represents a statistical map of the difference: using a randomization cluster technique, the statistically significant activity across subjects was identified and illustrated. This approach corrects for multiple comparisons over the grid points.

The beamforming approach also allows for identifying prestimulus induced oscillatory activity. In the example in Figure 7–13, visual stimuli were presented at detection threshold (van Dijk et al., 2008). The prestimulus activity that was present just prior to the onset of the visual stimuli was then analyzed. It was found that stronger alpha activity was associated with a decrease in detection performance (Figure 7–13b). The beamforming approach allowed for identifying the alpha activity to the parieto-occipital cortex. As mentioned in the theory section, the beamforming approach is

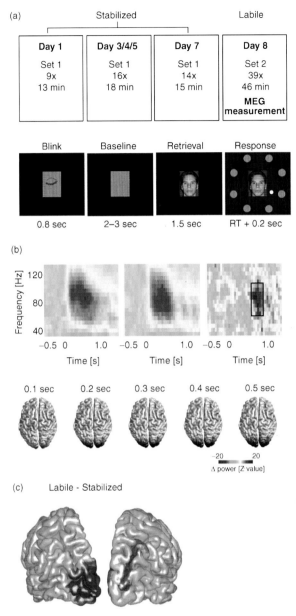

Figure 7–12. The beamforming approach applied to localize sources of gamma activity during long-term memory recall. (a) Subjects were trained on associating a face to one of eight locations. Two training schemes were applied. In the 'stabilized' scheme, associations were training over a week, and in the 'labile' scheme, training was done at the day of recall. (b) Strong induced oscillatory gamma activity was observed over posterior brain regions. The activity could be tracked to start in early visual areas, and then it progressed to parietal regions. (c) The sources representing the difference in gamma activity were localized to early visual areas. The colored regions indicate statistically significant differences, corrected for multiple comparisons using a cluster-randomization approach.
Reproduced from Nieuwenhuis et al. (2008).

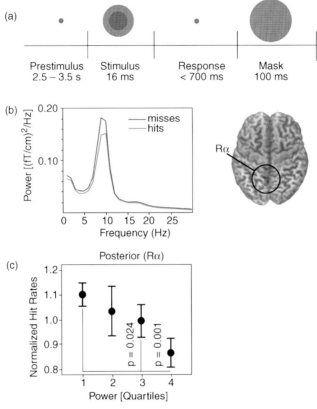

Figure 7–13. The beamforming approach used to localize oscillatory pre-stimulus activity. (a) For the visual stimuli, a smaller disc was superimposed on a larger disc with a slightly different gray level. Subjects were asked to detect if there was a difference in gray level or not. (b) Posterior pre-stimulus alpha activity was stronger for the detected stimuli. The sources representing the difference were identified to parieto-occipital cortex. (c) A spatial filter also based on beamforming was used to extract the single trial alpha power. The trials were sorted in four bins according to alpha power, and the hit rates were calculated for each bin. The hit rate decreased systematically with alpha power.
Reproduced from van Dijk et al. (2008).

based on constructing spatial filters for each grid point of the discretized brain volume. These filters can also be used to extract the activity from individual trials. This is done in Figure 7–13c, in which the signal trial, alpha power, was derived for the parieto-occipital region. The trials were then sorted in four bins according to alpha power, and the hit rates were calculated for each bin. These findings confirm that hit rate decreases with an increased alpha power produced in the parieto-occipital sulcus.

Practical Concerns

There are both commercial and free software packages available for calculating current estimates and beamformer. Below, find Table 7–1 summarizing the various software packages. It should be mentioned that each package has different features, making if difficult to directly compare the different methods. Nevertheless, when choosing a software package users are encouraged to read publications related to the experiment(s) in which the actual the software has been applied. This will provide insight into whether the software is suitable to answer a given question.

Summary

In this chapter we have described several approaches for constructing distributed representations of source activity. A common advantage of the different estimation methods is that the resulting distributed representations can be morphed onto a standard brain, and subsequently averaged across subjects.

Table 7–1 An overview of the software packages available for performing current estimates and beamforming. Please refer to the respective software web pages for further information.

	Current estimates			Beam former			Systems				
	MNE (L2)	MCE (L1)	Loreta	LCMV/ SAM	DICS	Elektra/ Neuromag	4-D Neuroimaging	VSM-CTF	Free	Open source
Fieldtrip				X	X	X	X	X	X	X
Loreta			X						X	
MNE- software	X					X	X	X	X	
NUTMEG				X				X	X	
SAM (VSM/CTF)				X				X		
MCE (Elek/Neu)						X	X			
BESA	X				X	X	X	X		
Curry	X	X	X			X	X	X		

This makes the approaches convenient for modern-day cognitive neuroimaging studies, which typically rely on grand averages across 10 to 30 subjects. When it comes to the modeling of event-related fields, MCE or MNE estimates of distributed source models are typically the favored approach. The current estimates allow for tracking the evoked activity over time. For the modeling of oscillatory brain activity, the beamforming approach has been shown to produce robust results, and has proven successful for characterizing induced oscillatory activity in numerous studies. In practice, beamforming requires a good estimate of the data cross-covariance or cross-spectral density matrix, and is typically less suitable for analyzing evoked responses. While beamforming so far works reasonably well for characterizing activation differences between conditions, both the underlying spatial filtering method and the subsequently applied statistical techniques could benefit from further refinement (Sekihara et al., 2004 and 2008). In particular, statistical comparisons of the difference in activity distributions could be improved, in order to appropriately deal with type–1 statistical errors over grid points in relation to the spatial correlations stemming from the source estimation.

Notes

1 It is important to point out that in the context of beamforming, the terms "spatial" and "location" do not in the first instance refer to the 3-dimensional space of the brain volume and the points within. What is meant is the N-dimensional measurement space defined by the sensor array, in which the vector representations of the scalp field patterns of all sources within the brain volume happen to define a point.

2 Here, the term "accuracy" does not exclusively refer to the quality of the electromagnetic volume conductor model used to compute the columns of the leadfield matrix **G**. The field patterns of spatially extended sources (e.g., locally or bilaterally synchronized neuronal activity), which effectively comprise dipole sources at several grid locations (and orientations) with essentially the same—and hence highly correlated—activation time courses, are not accurately described by the fields of source at individual grid locations. Thus, spatially extended sources, in fact, violate both of the fundamental assumptions underlying the beamforming approach.

3 This is not a trivial problem, since it requires not only a concrete and precise definition of what the noise term refers to in Equation (7–1), and what are its statistical properties, but also necessitates the use of ancillary methods for estimating the (brain) signal and noise-subspace-component contributions to the cross-covariance matrix. Poor choices or estimates of the noise model invariably distort the amplitude estimates for neuronal sources.

4 Alternatively, the noise-normalized current distributions for the conditions could have been calculated and then subtracted.

References

Bauer, M., Oostenveld, R., Peeters, M., & Fries, P. (2006). Tactile spatial attention enhances gamma-band activity in somatosensory cortex and reduces low-frequency activity in parieto-occipital areas. *J Neurosci, 26*, 490–501.

Brookes, M. J., Stevenson, C. M., Barnes, G. R., Hillebrand, A., Simpson, M. I., Francis, S. T., et al. (2007). Beamformer reconstruction of correlated sources using a modified source model. *Neuroimage, 34*, 1454–1465.

Capon, J. (1969). High-resolution frequency-wavenumber spectrum analysis. *Proceedings of the IEEE, 57*, 1408–1418.

Challis, R. E., & Kitney, R. I. (1991). Biomedical signal processing (in four parts). Part 2. The frequency transforms and their inter-relationships. *Med Biol Eng Comput, 29*, 1–17.

Dale, A., & Sereno, M. (1993). Improved localization of cortical activity by combining EEG and MEG with MRI cortical surface reconstruction: a linear approach. *J Cogn Neurosci, 5*, 162–176.

Dale, A. M., Liu, A. K., Fischl, B. R., Buckner, R. L., Belliveau, J. W., Lewine, J. D., et al. (2000). Dynamic statistical parametric mapping: combining fMRI and MEG for high-resolution imaging of cortical activity. *Neuron, 26*, 55–67.

Gaetz, W., & Cheyne, D. (2006). Localization of sensorimotor cortical rhythms induced by tactile stimulation using spatially filtered MEG. *Neuroimage, 30*, 899–908.

Gomez, J. F., & Thatcher, R. W. (2001). Frequency domain equivalence between potentials and currents using LORETA. *Int J Neurosci, 107*, 161–171.

Gross, J., Kujala, J., Hämäläinen, M., Timmermann, L., Schnitzler, A., & Salmelin, R. (2001). Dynamic imaging of coherent sources: Studying neural interactions in the human brain. *Proc Natl Acad Sci USA, 98*, 694–699.

Halgren, E., Dhond, R P., Christensen, N., Van Petten, C., Marinkovic, K., Lewine, J. D., et al. (2002). N400-like magnetoencephalography responses modulated by semantic context, word frequency, and lexical class in sentences. *Neuroimage, 17*, 1101–1116.

Hämäläinen, M. S., & Ilmoniemi, R. J. (1994). Interpreting magnetic fields of the brain: minimum norm estimates. *Med Biol Eng Comput, 32*, 35–42.

Hari, R., & Salmelin, R. (1997). Human cortical oscillations: a neuromagnetic view through the skull. *Trends Neurosci, 20*, 44–49.

Haykin, S. (2002). *Adaptive filter theory.* (4th ed.). Upper Saddle River, New Jersey: Prentice Hall.

Helenius, P., Salmelin, R., Service, E., & Connolly, J. F. (1998). Distinct time courses of word and context comprehension in the left temporal cortex. *Brain, 121* (Pt 6), 1133–1142.

Hillebrand, A., & Barnes. G. R. (2005). Beamformer analysis of MEG data. *Int Rev Neurobiol, 68*, 149–171.

Hillebrand, A., Singh, K. D., Holliday, I. E., Furlong, P. L., & Barnes, G. R. (2005). A new approach to neuroimaging with magnetoencephalography. *Hum Brain Mapp, 25*, 199–211.

Ioannides, A., Bolton, J., & Clarke, C. (1990), Continuous probabilistic solutions to the biomagnetic inverse problem. *Inverse Problems, 6*, 523–542.

Jensen, O., & Vanni, S. (2002). A new method to identify multiple sources of oscillatory activity from magnetoencephalographic data. *Neuroimage. 15*. 568–574.

Jensen, O., Goel, P., Kopell, N., Pohja, M., Hari, R., & Ermentrout, B. (2005). On the human sensorimotor-cortex beta rhythm: sources and modeling. *Neuroimage, 26,* 347–355.

Jokisch, D., & Jensen, O. (2007). Modulation of gamma and alpha activity during a working memory task engaging the dorsal or ventral stream. *J Neurosci, 27,* 3244–3251.

Kalcher, J., & Pfurtscheller, G. (1995). Discrimination between phase-locked and non-phase-locked event-related EEG activity. *Electroencephalogr Clin Neurophysiol, 94,* 381–384.

Kujala, J., Pammer, K., Cornelissen, P., Roebroeck, A., Formisano, E., & Salmelin, R. (2007). Phase coupling in a cerebro-cerebellar network at 8-13 Hz during reading. *Cereb Cortex, 17,* 1476–1485.

Kutas, M., & Hillyard, S. A. (1980). Reading senseless sentences: brain potentials reflect semantic incongruity. *Science, 207,* 203–205.

Liljestrom, M., Kujala, J., Jensen, O., & Salmelin, R (2005). Neuromagnetic localization of rhythmic activity in the human brain: a comparison of three methods. *Neuroimage, 25,* 734–745.

Lin, F. H., Witzel, T., Hämäläinen, M. S., Dale, A. M., Belliveau, J. W., & Stufflebeam, S. M. (2004). Spectral spatiotemporal imaging of cortical oscillations and interactions in the human brain. *Neuroimage, 23,* 582–595.

Liu, A. K., Belliveau, J. W., & Dale, A. M. (1998). Spatiotemporal imaging of human brain activity using functional MRI constrained magnetoencephalography data: Monte Carlo simulations. *Proc Natl Acad Sci USA, 95,* 8945–8950.

Lutkenhoner, B. (1992). Frequency-domain localization of intracerebral dipolar sources. *Electroencephalogr Clin Neurophysiol, 82,* 112–118.

Matsuura, K. & Okabe, Y. (1995). Selective minimum-norm solution of the biomagnetic inverse problem. *IEEE Trans Biomed Eng, 42,* 608–615.

Medendorp, W. P., Kramer, G. F., Jensen, O., Oostenveld, R., Schoffelen, J. M., & Fries, P. (2006). Oscillatory activity in human parietal and occipital cortex shows hemispheric lateralization and memory effects in a delayed double-step saccade task. *Cereb Cortex. 17,* 2364–2374.

Mitra, P. P., & Pesaran, B. (1999). Analysis of dynamic brain imaging data. *Biophys J, 76,* 691–708.

Niedermeyer, E., & Lopes da Silva, F. H. (1999). *Electroencephalography: basic principles, clinical applications, and related fields.* (4th ed.). Baltimore: Williams & Wilkins.

Nieuwenhuis, I. L., Takashima, A., Oostenveld, R., Fernandez, G., & Jensen, O. (2008). Visual areas become less engaged in associative recall following memory stabilization. *Neuroimage, 40,* 1319–1327.

Osipova, D., Takashima, A., Oostenveld, R., Fernandez, G., Maris, E., & Jensen, O. (2006). Theta and gamma oscillations predict encoding and retrieval of declarative memory. *J Neurosci, 26,* 7523–7531.

Pascual-Marqui, R. D., Michel, C. M., & Lehmann, D. (1994). Low resolution electromagnetic tomography: a new method for localizing electrical activity in the brain. *Int J Psychophysiol, 18,* 49–65.

Percival, D. B., & Walden, A. T. (1993). *Spectral analysis for physical applications: multitaper and conventional univariate techniques.* Cambridge, UK: Cambridge University Press.

Posthuma, D., Neale, M. C., Boomsma, D. I., & de Geus, E. J. (2001). Are smarter brains running faster? Heritability of alpha peak frequency, IQ, and their interrelation. *Behav Genet, 31,* 567–579.

Robinson, S. E., & Vrba, J. (1999). Functional neuroimaging by synthetic aperture magnetometry (SAM). In: *Biomag*, pp. 302–305. Sendai: Tohoku University Press.

Salmelin, R. & Hari, R. (1994). Spatiotemporal characteristics of sensorimotor neuromagnetic rhythms related to thumb movement. *Neuroscience, 60*, 537–550.

Sekihara, K., Sahani, M., & Nagarajan, S. S. (2004). Bootstrap-based statistical thresholding for MEG source reconstruction images. *Conf Proc IEEE Eng Med Biol Soc, 2*, 1018–1021.

Sekihara, K., Hild, K. E., Dalal, S. S., & Nagarajan, S. S. (2008). Performance of prewhitening beamforming in MEG dual experimental conditions. *IEEE Trans Biomed Eng, 55*, 1112–1121.

Stenbacka, L., Vanni, S., Uutela, K., & Hari, R. (2002). Comparison of minimum current estimate and dipole modeling in the analysis of simulated activity in the human visual cortices. *Neuroimage, 16*, 936–943.

Tallon-Baudry, C., & Bertrand, O. (1999). Oscillatory gamma activity in humans and its role in object representation. *Trends Cogn Sci, 3*, 151–162.

Tesche, C., & Kajola, M. (1993). A comparison of the localization of spontaneous neuromagnetic activity in the frequency and time domains. *Electroencephalogr Clin Neurophysiol, 87*, 408–416.

Uutela, K., Hämäläinen, M., & Somersalo, E. (1999). Visualization of magnetoencephalographic data using minimum current estimates. *Neuroimage, 10*, 173–180.

van Dijk, H., Schoffelen, J. M., Oostenveld, R., & Jensen, O. (2008). Prestimulus oscillatory activity in the alpha band predicts visual discrimination ability. *J Neurosci, 28*, 1816–1823.

Van Veen, B. D. (1992). *Adaptive Radar Detection and Estimation*. New York: Wiley-Interscience.

Van Veen, B.D., & Buckley, K. M. (1988). Beamforming: A versatile approach to spatial filtering. *IEEE AASP Magazine, 5*, 4–24.

Van Veen, B. D., van Drongelen, W., Yuchtman, M., & Suzuki, A. (1997). Localization of brain electrical activity via linearly constrained minimum variance spatial filtering. *IEEE Trans Biomed Eng, 44*, 867–880.

Vanni, S., & Uutela, K. (2000). Foveal attention modulates responses to peripheral stimuli. *J Neurophysiol, 83*, 2443–2452.

Welch, P. D. (1967). The use of the FFT for estimation of power spectra: a method based on averaging over short, modified periodograms. *IEEE Trans Audio and Acoustics, 15*, 70–73.

8

Anatomically and Functionally Constrained Minimum-Norm Estimates

Matti S. Hämäläinen, Fa-Hsuan Lin, and John C. Mosher

- We present a workflow of MEG source analysis which includes the steps from noise removal and sensor space analysis to source estimation
- Cortically constrained source estimates are useful for mapping the measured data to the brain space
- Depending on the source constraints applied, the results can be either focal or diffuse
- These imaging estimators make the results independent of the particular sensor array geometry
- Once the data has been transformed to the cortical space, comparison with fMRI and surface-based group analysis becomes possible

Introduction

Independently, different brain imaging methods provide compromised spatial and temporal resolutions. For example, anatomical MRI provides highly accurate images of the individual brain anatomy, but does not convey information about the dynamically changing patterns of brain activity. In functional imaging, fMRI is temporally limited by the slow time course of the hemodynamic response, but can provide a spatial sampling on a millimeter scale (Belliveau et al., 1992; Kwong et al., 1992). EEG and MEG, in turn, provide a temporal resolution of milliseconds, but the localization of sources is more complicated because of the electromagnetic inverse problem. Combining information provided by both anatomical and functional MRI with EEG and MEG data thus facilitates elucidating the spatial distribution and temporal orchestration of human brain activity (Dale et al., 2000; Daunizeau et al., 2007; Liu et al., 1998).

In order to render the solution of the electromagnetic inverse problem unique (Helmholtz, 1853), several source modeling techniques with different constraints have been proposed. In the Equivalent Current Dipole (ECD) approach, the activation is assumed to be relatively focal, and thus it can be well accounted for by a small number of current dipoles. However, the assumption of limited extent of the activity cannot always be justified. Furthermore, reliable estimation of the nonlinear dipole location parameters becomes prohibitively difficult when the number of sources increases.

Some of the limitations of the ECD model can be overcome by using a distributed source model. In this approach, the locations of a large number of dipoles are kept fixed, and their amplitudes are determined on the basis of the measured data. This problem is underdetermined; therefore, additional *a priori* constraints are required. In particular, in the l_2 minimum-norm estimate (MNE) approach (Hämäläinen & Ilmoniemi, 1984), one selects the current distribution with minimum power (l_2 norm), while maintaining the requirement that the measured data match those predicted by the model. This MNE solution was subsequently refined to incorporate cortical location and orientation constraints (Dale & Sereno, 1993). Furthermore, noise normalization has been employed to establish the statistical significance of current estimates (Dale, et al., 2000). In accordance with similar approaches employed in other functional imaging modalities (fMRI and PET), the resulting spatiotemporal estimates are often referred to as dynamic statistical parametric maps (dSPMs). Subsequently, a variation of this approach (sLORETA), with a different noise normalization factor, was introduced (Pascual-Marqui, 2002). More focal estimates than those provided by the MNE can be obtained by using an l_1-norm prior; the corresponding minimum-norm solution is often called the minimum-current estimate (MCE) (Matsuura & Okabe, 1995; Uutela et al., 1999).

It has been demonstrated that individual anatomical information, acquired with structural magnetic resonance imaging (MRI), can be incorporated into the source localization with the l_2-norm constraint. In particular, the locations of the sources can be constrained to the cortical mantle. with their orientations perpendicular to the local cortical surface (Dale & Sereno, 1993). Such a modeling constraint is motivated by the physiological information that the most significant sources of MEG and EEG signals are postsynaptic currents in the pyramidal cells on the cortex, and that the principal net direction of these currents is perpendicular to the cortical surface (Hämäläinen et al., 1993; Okada et al., 1997). Importantly, in MCE, the optimization algorithm becomes more straightforward if the orientations of the sources are known, and the scalar source amplitudes are estimated subject to l_1 constraint.

To this end, the MCE implementation described in Uutela, et al. (1999) used the current-source orientations provided by MNE.

The fusion of electromagnetic and hemodynamic data is still in its infancy. In the presently available modeling methods, a distributed current estimate confined to the cortical gray matter is usually employed, with a stronger *a priori* weighting at locations with significant fMRI activity (Dale et al., 2000; Liu et al., 1998). More elaborate methods that attempt to model the two data sets jointly under a common framework are also emerging. Furthermore, basic studies that aim at understanding the relationship between the hemodynamic and electromagnetic signals are ongoing, and will eventually result in a physiologically motivated rather than a partly heuristic model of the coupling between the hemodynamic and electromagnetic data.

In this chapter, we will first outline the overall MEG data-processing workflow, with emphasis on source estimation and incorporation of anatomical information. Thereafter, we provide an overview of analytical methods needed in the computation of the minimum-norm solutions, including application of minimum-norm solutions in the computation of time-frequency representations in the source domain. Next, we will discuss a specific workflow to compute the cortically constrained, distributed source estimates, including practical approaches to acquiring and processing the MRI and MEG data. Finally, we will discuss a few representative studies where the presented methods have been employed.

The "Workflow" of MEG Data Processing

In this section we will discuss the overall approach to processing of MEG data. One of the purposes of this section is to highlight the role of the cortically constrained minimum-norm solutions in the workflow of MEG data processing.

The General Workflow

A recommended general workflow for performing source estimation on MEG data is as follows. First, the raw sensor data need to be examined for obvious artifacts. Software provided by MEG vendors is generally quite useful for scrolling through the data, looking for dead channels, noisy channels, or channels showing jumps indicative of trapped flux, etc. Artifact-rejection software is used to automatically locate many of these defects, but it's a good idea to perform some "spot checking" as well.

The spatial pattern of the activity can also be viewed at the sensor array, by some form of interpolation from the discrete data at the sensors into a smooth color image or a contour map. These types of displays are particularly useful as "movies" of patterns over time, observing apparent sources appearing and disappearing over the epoch of interest.

With the initial observations completed, more formal noise rejection schemes should be applied. Although not always apparent to the user, noise rejection often already implies an assumption about the source, so it is indeed a first step in source estimation. With noise reduction applied, the sensor data can often be more readily observed and sources inferred directly. Some noise rejection schemes use a noise-covariance matrix estimated in the empty room, i.e., no subject present, as a basis for optimizing the noise rejection algorithm. The linear estimation approach presented in this chapter also considers "subject noise" by incorporating a noise-covariance matrix computed from the baseline signals preceding the stimuli in an evoked-response study. If ongoing background brain activity is analyzed, this separation of "brain noise" is less plausible, and we recommend using the empty room noise-covariance instead.

Next, we recommend the class of linear imaging estimators, often referred to as "minimum-norm" techniques, that are the emphasis of this chapter. These and similar techniques map the sensor data onto dense source grids. These grids are almost always based on cortical surfaces, but in the past included simple geometrical surfaces and volumes. Nonlinear imaging estimators can also be employed; see *Minimum-current Estimates* in the present chapter, and Chapters 5 and 7, for details.

Next is the class of adaptive beamformers, such as MUSIC, LCMV, and SAM, which select a source model and scan a source grid looking for agreement. The metrics generated by these scans can also be viewed as images, but they are more correctly called *pseudoimages*—since they are, more accurately, a measure of how underlying models fit, and therefore only have meaning where the measures have local maxima. The beamformer approaches are discussed in Chapter 7.

From the beamformer scans, we may often be able to discern a simpler underlying model of a few dipoles, which can be then be fully fit using maximum-likelihood or maximum-*a posteriori* methods, i.e., generalized least-squares with priors. The most widely used example is the case of fitting multiple dipoles using least-squares. This and similar techniques are discussed in Chapters 5 and 6.

The use of cortical constraints on the dipole locations can be quite useful for interpretation, but as a sanity check it is also good practice to test the data with an unconstrained dipolar model, i.e., one that does not require that the locations be on cortex. If these solutions are only shifted slightly from the cortical surface, then reasonable interpretations are that the forward model is somewhat inaccurate, or that the source is extended and is best represented by a dipole located nearby.

A gross shift, however, to a location outside the head, would be a warning that you have external contaminants not properly handled in the noise model/rejection. Similarly, a gross shift to elsewhere in the head (such as deep) is a further warning of ambiguities in the models, which are often due to edge effects of the helmet array. Another reason for using unconstrained dipole searches is that the source being modeled is not cerebral, but rather an external contaminant such as an eye movement or blink. In special cases where the signal-to-noise ratio is high, it is also possible to detect signals from deep structures outside the cortex.

In each successive step, the parameters can be tested for significance using uncertainty measures, to help simplify the model. Significance is dependent on the definition of noise, which is often defined in the first part of this process.

Imaging and Dipole Modeling

As reviewed in Baillet et al. (2001) and discussed in Chapter 5, source estimation may be broadly categorized as "imaging" or "parametric"—a somewhat artificial distinction, since the images themselves are functions of parameters, and "pseudoimages" can be generated from parametric scans. As we discussed above, a general workflow would indeed use both techniques. In the imaging techniques, we generally restrict ourselves to methods that map sensor data to the cortical surface. Typically we are mapping roughly 200 measurements onto roughly 10,000 cortical imaging points, a severely underdetermined problem. In order to solve this ambiguous problem, strong priors must be imposed to arrive at a unique solution, which can then be visualized on the cortical surface, possibly inflated to make the activity in the sulci readily visible.

This imaging-solution method goes by a variety of names and approaches, such as minimum-norm least-squares with weighting and regularization, generalized least-squares with priors, maximum *a posteriori* (MAP) or Bayesian estimation with Gaussian priors, linear minimum mean square, LORETA, or LAURA, to name a few. See Mosher, Baillet, & Leahy (2003), for a review of the mathematical approaches that all lead to the same general imaging model.

We note in passing that other imaging estimators can be derived by iterations of the priors, other norms, or other non-Gaussian priors. For instance, see the MCE discussed below and in Chapter 7.

Given that we must impose such strong priors, we might reasonably question the need to apply these techniques. One answer lies in the need to better interpret complex sensor data. For example, in the standard 10–20 EEG array, a presentation of results from the "Cz" sensor is universally understood by any researcher. But today's arrays are denser, with different gradiometric and differential designs and adaptive noise schemes. In many instances it is no longer simple to directly interpret sensor patterns. The imaging techniques incorporate the forward model directly into the transformation onto the cortex, such that many of the sensor and machine effects are suppressed in the presentation. The opportunity exists, therefore, to create cortical images that are "site independent," i.e., protocols are that are more reproducible among research instruments and sites, once the forward models have been factored out (Weisend et al., 2007).

True physical and physiological insight into neural activity is difficult, however, with such strong imaging priors on thousands of parameters. The significance tests help identify "regions of interest" (ROIs), which are "extended" sources constrained to the cortical surface. The goal is to try to simplify the number of parameters that define these ROIs. The simpler models are generally easier to interpret; for example, a single equivalent current dipole leads to a reasonable interpretation that neural activity is focused around the location.

Such low-order parametric models are difficult to generate directly when the pattern of activity is complex and extends for a long period of time. The statistical parametric maps of images and beamformer scans are intervening steps between imaging and dipole modeling. The statistical maps help identify regions of interest in the image that may be replaced with simpler patches, or even dipoles. The beamformer techniques generally require statistical assumptions about the temporal activity—e.g., linear or statistical independence—but then allow a more direct scan of the cortex for simplifying models.

Theoretical Background

This section provides technical details of the analytical methods involved in the computation of cortically constrained distributed source estimates. Our discussion includes both the l_2 minimum-norm estimates (MNE) and the more focal l_1 minimum-current estimates (MCE). We also apply the computational methods to frequency-domain analyses, in particular to the calculation of time-frequency representations and phase-locking values. While this section contains some essential mathematical details of the algorithms, it is not necessary for the reader to go into the depths of this section to understand the workflow and the section titled *Practical Implementation of Cortically Constrained Estimates*, below.

Minimum-Norm Estimates (MNE/h2)

Under the quasi-static approximation of Maxwell's equations (Hämäläinen et al., 1993), the measured MEG/EEG signals and the underlying current source strengths are related by a linear transformation:

$$\mathbf{Y} = \mathbf{AX} + \mathbf{N}, \tag{8-1}$$

where $\mathbf{Y}$ is an m-by-t matrix containing measurements from m sensors over t distinct time instants, $\mathbf{X}$ is a $3n$-by-t matrix denoting the unknown time-dependent amplitudes of the three components of n current sources, $\mathbf{A}$ is the gain matrix representing the mapping from the currents to MEG/EEG signals, i.e., the solution of the forward problem, and $\mathbf{N}$ denotes noise in the measured data.

The most feasible assumption is that $\mathbf{N}$ is Gaussian with a spatial covariance matrix $\mathbf{C}$, to be estimated from the data. If we further assume that the source amplitudes have a Gaussian *a priori* distribution with a covariance matrix $\mathbf{R}$, we obtain the Bayesian maximum *a posteriori* (MAP) estimate or l_2 minimum-norm solution, linearly related to the measurements, as (Dale & Sereno, 1993)

$$\mathbf{X}^{\mathrm{MNE}} = \mathbf{RA}^T \left(\mathbf{ARA}^T + \lambda^2 \mathbf{C}\right)^{-1} \mathbf{Y} = \lambda^{-2}\mathbf{RA}^T \left(\lambda^{-2}\mathbf{ARA}^T + \mathbf{C}\right)^{-1} \mathbf{Y} = \mathbf{WY}, \quad (8\text{--}2)$$

where λ^2 is a regularization parameter to avoid magnification of errors in data in the inversion, and the superscript T indicates the matrix transpose.

We have also implicitly assumed that $\mathbf{C}$ and $\mathbf{R}$ are time-independent, and that there are no temporal correlations. In the original unweighted minimum-norm approach, $\mathbf{R}$ is simply a multiple of the identity matrix. However, there is no direct physiological information to support this particular selection of source priors. Rather, the choice is motivated by the simple computational realization of the estimation procedure. It is also seen from Equation (8–2) that regularization corresponds to multiplying the source covariance matrix by a constant factor λ^{-2}.

Equation (8–2) can be also viewed as the analytic solution of an optimization problem where the cost function is a sum of weighted least-squares error between the measured and modeled data, and a penalty term comprising the weighted norm of the estimated currents, i.e.,

$$\mathbf{X}_{\mathrm{MNE}} = \arg\min_{\mathbf{X}} \left\{ \left\| (\mathbf{Y} - \mathbf{AX})^T \mathbf{C}^{-1} (\mathbf{Y} - \mathbf{AX}) \right\|_F^2 + \lambda^2 \left\| \mathbf{X}^T \mathbf{R}^{-1} \mathbf{X} \right\|_F^2 \right\} \quad (8\text{--}3)$$

where $\|\cdot\|_F$ indicates the Frobenius norm, a generalization of the l_2 vector norm, of the enclosed matrix.

In a later section we will consider another source prior, namely the l_1-norm prior, which corresponds to a double-exponential probability distribution function with zero mean, as discussed in Uutela et al. (1999). This prior leads to a cost function in which the penalty term is the sum of the absolute values of the source currents, while the data error term is identical to that in MNE. The optimal solution of this problem is called the minimum-current estimate (MCE). The two approaches can thus be regarded as two variants of distributed source modeling techniques with distinct prior assumptions.

In Equation (8–2), the current orientations have not been constrained. *A priori* orientation information can be easily incorporated by replacing the gain matrix by

$$\mathbf{A}_{\mathrm{fixed}} = \mathbf{A\Theta}, \quad (8\text{--}4)$$

where Θ is the $3n$-by-n matrix containing the unit vectors pointing to the directions of the currents.

If the direction cosines of the kth dipole are c_{kx}, c_{ky}, and c_{kz}, the kth column of Θ reads

$$\Theta_k = (\underbrace{0...0}_{3(k-1)} \quad c_{kx} \quad c_{ky} \quad c_{kz} \quad \underbrace{0...0}_{n-3k})^T.$$ (8–5)

Instead of applying Equation (8–2) directly, it is often convenient to use an equivalent formulation

$$\mathbf{X}^{\text{MNE}} = \mathbf{R}\tilde{\mathbf{A}}^T(\tilde{\mathbf{A}}\mathbf{R}\tilde{\mathbf{A}}^T + \lambda^2\mathbf{I})^{-1}\tilde{\mathbf{Y}} = \tilde{\mathbf{W}}\tilde{\mathbf{Y}},$$ (8–6)

where

$$\tilde{\mathbf{Y}} = \mathbf{C}^{-1/2}\mathbf{Y}$$
$$\tilde{\mathbf{A}} = \mathbf{C}^{-1/2}\mathbf{A}$$ (8–7)

are the spatially whitened data and gain matrix, respectively.

The noise-covariance matrix of the whitened data is an identity matrix, as indicated by the comparison of Equations (8–2) and (8–6). The whitening procedure also naturally leads to the choice $\lambda^2 = \zeta^2\text{tr}(\tilde{\mathbf{A}}\mathbf{R}\tilde{\mathbf{A}}^T)/m$, where ζ^2 denotes the inverse of the SNR of the whitened data, to bring the regularization parameter to the correct scale even in cases where the measurements have different units of measure—which is the case when planar gradiometer and magnetometer data, or MEG and EEG data, are combined in a single estimate.

The sensitivity of MEG sensors is not uniform across cortical locations (Hillebrand & Barnes, 2002). In fact, it follows generally from Maxwell's equations that the lead fields of both MEG sensors and EEG electrodes have a maximum at the border of the source area (Heller & van Hulsteyn, 1992). Because of the minimum-norm penalty, both MNE and MCE solutions are biased to superficial locations, to which the sensors are most sensitive. It is possible to compensate for this tendency by modifying our diagonal source-covariance matrix **R** by scaling the entries by a function increasing monotonically with source depth, e.g., a norm of the corresponding column of the gain matrix **A** (Fuchs et al., 1999; Ioannides et al., 1990; Lin, Witzel, et al., 2006).

Noise-Normalization

In the above, Equations (8–2) and (8–6) provide the best-fitting values of the current amplitudes or, in Bayesian view, the maximum *a posteriori* (MAP) estimate. To make the resulting maps conceptually similar with those calculated in other widely used functional imaging modalities (fMRI and PET), Dale et al. (2000) proposed that current values should be converted into dynamic statistical parametric maps. To this end, we need to consider the variances of the currents

$$w_k^2 = \left(\mathbf{W}\mathbf{C}\mathbf{W}^T\right)_{kk} = \left(\tilde{\mathbf{W}}\tilde{\mathbf{W}}^T\right)_{kk}.$$ (8–8)

For fixed-orientation sources, we now obtain the noise-normalized activity estimate for the kth dipole and pth time point as

$$z_{kp} = \frac{X_{k,p}^{\text{MNE}}}{w_k},$$ (8–9)

which is t-distributed under the null hypothesis of no activity at the current location k. Since the number of time samples used to calculate the noise-covariance matrix $\mathbf{C}$ is quite large (more than 100) the t distribution approaches a unit normal distribution, i.e., a z-score.

If the orientations are not constrained, the noise-normalized solution is calculated as

$$F_{kp} = \frac{\sum_{q=1}^{3}\left(X_{3(k-1)+q,p}^{MNE}\right)^2}{\sum_{q=1}^{3} w_{3(k-1)+q}^2}. \tag{8–10}$$

Note that under the null hypothesis, F_{kp} is F-distributed, with three degrees of freedom for the numerator. The degrees of freedom for the denominator is typically large, again depending on the number of time samples used to calculate the noise-covariance matrix.

As discussed in Dale et al. (2000), the noise-normalized estimates resulting from the transformations given in Equations (8–8) and (8–9) have a smaller depth bias than the MNEs obtained without applying depth weighting. Furthermore, the point-spread function, i.e., the image of a point current source, is more uniform in space in the noise-normalized estimate than in the MNE.

Another variation of the noise-normalized MNE is the sLORETA (Pascual-Marqui, 2002):

$$\bar{w}_k^2 = \left(\mathbf{W}(\mathbf{C} + \lambda^{-2}\mathbf{A}\mathbf{R}\mathbf{A}^T)\mathbf{W}^T\right)_{kk} = \left(\tilde{\mathbf{W}}(\mathbf{I} + \lambda^{-2}\tilde{\mathbf{A}}\mathbf{R}\tilde{\mathbf{A}}^T)\tilde{\mathbf{W}}^T\right)_{kk} \tag{8–11}$$

From this expression it can be clearly seen that the sLORETA noise-normalization factor differs from that given in Equation (8–8) by the addition of the term $\lambda^{-2}\mathbf{A}\mathbf{R}\mathbf{A}^T$ to the noise-covariance matrix $\mathbf{C}$. If the *a priori* information incorporated in $\lambda^{-2}\mathbf{R}$ is correct, $\mathbf{C} + \lambda^{-2}\mathbf{A}\mathbf{R}\mathbf{A}^T = \mathbf{C}_d$, the data covariance matrix. It has been shown that, in the absence of noise, sLORETA yields an unbiased estimate of the location of the activity (Pascual-Marqui, 2002). In our experience, under realistic noise conditions the difference between sLORETA and dSPM is less dramatic than claimed, as also indicated by our recent study on the depth biases of MNE and the two noise-normalized estimates (see Lin, Witzel, et al. 2006).

It is also important to realize that the roles of the MNE and the noise-normalized estimates are different. The former gives an estimate of the current amplitudes in physical units [A/m], [A/m²] while the noise-normalized distributions are test statistics to be employed as significance measures. Optimally, dSPM or sLORETA and MNE distributions should be used in combination so that the significance map is used to delineate the areas of activity with high signal-to-noise ratio and, subsequently, MNE is consulted for the true current amplitudes at that particular region.

Minimum-current Estimates (MCE)

In contrast to the MNE, the minimum-current estimate (MCE) employs the l_1-norm as constraint (Matsuura & Okabe, 1995; Uutela et al., 1999). The latter publication formulated MCE as the solution of the optimization problem:

$$\mathbf{X}_p^{MCE} = \underset{X_{i,p}}{\mathrm{argmin}} \left\{ \sum_{i=1}^{n} w_i \left| X_{i,p} \right| \right\}$$

$$\text{subject to } \tilde{\mathbf{Y}}_{rp} = \mathbf{B}_r \mathbf{X}_p^{MCE}, \tag{8–12}$$

where $\mathbf{X}_p^{MCE}$ is the solution at time point p, w_i are the weights of dipole sources, while $\tilde{\mathbf{Y}}_{rp}$ and $\mathbf{B}_r$ are derived from the measurement data and the forward solution for fixed-orientation sources to implement regularization as follows.

As before, let Θ be the n-by-3 matrix containing the source orientations and compute the singular-value decomposition

$$\tilde{\mathbf{A}}\Theta = \mathbf{U}\Pi\mathbf{V}^T. \tag{8–13}$$

Then

$$\mathbf{B}_r = \mathbf{U}_r^T \tilde{\mathbf{A}} \,\Theta,$$

$$\tilde{\mathbf{Y}}_r = \mathbf{U}_r^T \tilde{\mathbf{Y}} \tag{8–14}$$

where $\mathbf{U}_r$ is composed of the first r columns of $\mathbf{U}$.

This method of eigenvalue truncation in regularization was introduced to MCE by Uutela et al. (1999), and it is closely related to using the regularization parameter λ^2 in Equations (8–2) and (8–6). It is easy to show that the latter corresponds to weighting of the eigenvalues with a smooth transition function instead of the step function implied by Equation (8–12).

The above implementation of MCE requires the knowledge of the source orientations, to be incorporated by the matrix Θ in Equations (8–13) and (8–14). In principle, it is also possible to implement MCE without requiring Θ to be specified first. However, the solution of this minimization problem is numerically more demanding and, therefore, we prefer using the original MCE formulation proposed by Uutela, et al. (1999). The weights for currents, w_i in Equation (8–12), are usually chosen as the Euclidean norms of the columns of $\mathbf{A}\Theta$ to guard against the superficial bias mentioned above. The orientation matrix Θ can obtained either from an initial MNE using one of the orientation constraints described under *Acquisition and Processing of Anatomical MRI Data*, below. The magnitudes of the dipoles, which satisfy Equation (8–12), can be estimated using Linear Programming (Moon & Stirling, 2000).

An interesting variation of the cortically constrained MCE called VESTAL was introduced by Huang et al. (2006). The most important feature of this approach is that the usually discontinuous MCE source waveforms are projected to the subspace spanned by the most significant left singular vectors of the MEG data matrix **Y**. As a result, one obtains smooth waveforms resembling those produced by the l_2 minimum-norm approach, while preserving the focal quality of the l_1-norm solutions.

Recent work by Ou et al. (2009) addresses the same problem using a mixed $l_1 l_2$-norm approach. At each location, the source waveform is expressed as a linear combination of orthogonal basis functions, which may be determined from the SVD of the data like in VESTAL. An l_2 norm is applied among the coefficients of these basis functions to promote contributions of multiple functions at each location, while an l_1 norm among different locations encourages sparsity. This approach is computationally more efficient than VESTAL and is more principled because the regularized cost function to minimize is explicitly stated.

Computation of the Gain Matrix

In the calculation of the gain matrix **A**, a common practice is to assume dipolar sources in a dense grid covering either the entire brain or the cortical mantle. In this approach, the current estimates are dipole amplitudes, whose unit is [Am]. However, a more appropriate quantity to consider is the volume or surface dipole density given in [Am/m^3] or [Am/m^2], respectively. In case of cortically constrained currents, transformation to current density representation requires an approximation for the area of the cortical patch corresponding to each source location. We compute these patch areas using detailed cortical geometry information, as will be described below. The transformation is accomplished by multiplying each column of a 'dipolar' gain matrix by the corresponding patch area.

We have also assumed that the finite size of the pick-up coils of the MEG instrument and their configuration (magnetometers or gradiometers), as well as the effect of noise-compensation methods possibly applied to the MEG data, have been accounted for in the calculation of **A**. The size and configuration of the pick-up coils can be taken into account by approximating the sum (or difference) of the magnetic fluxes threading the elements of the pickup coil loops as a weighted sum

$$y_k = \sum_{p=1}^{N_k} w_{kp} \vec{B}(\vec{r}_{kp}) \cdot \hat{e}_{kp}, \tag{8–15}$$

where w_{kp} are weight factors specific for sensor k, $\vec{r}_{kp}$ are the integration points, $\hat{e}_{kp}$ are the unit normal vectors describing the orientation of the coil at each of the integration points, and $\vec{B}(\vec{r}_{kp})$ is the magnetic field generated by the current dipole of interest at $\vec{r}_{kp}$.

In our software packages to be discussed under *Examples of Available Software*, we have implemented Equation (8–15) for the coil geometries found in the commonly used MEG systems. We have found that depending on the coil sizes, one to eight integration points in each coil loop are necessary to ensure sufficient accuracy. If the boundary-element method (BEM) is employed in the forward solution, the calculations can be conveniently arranged so that the number of integration points (N_k) has a very modest effect on the overall computation time.

If the signal-space projection method (Tesche et al., 1995; Uusitalo & Ilmoniemi, 1997) has been employed for noise compensation, the same projection operator has to be applied to both the data and the forward solution: $\mathbf{A} = \mathbf{PA}_{orig}$, where $\mathbf{A}_{orig}$ is the unprojected gain matrix and $\mathbf{P}$ is the projection operator applied to the data. If reference sensors have been used to reject external disturbances, the measured signals $\mathbf{Y}$ are linear combinations of the data from the primary (helmet) sensors and reference sensors. Once the configurations of both sensor types and the noise compensation matrix employed are known, the effects of the noise compensation can be taken into account to compute the effective gain matrix: $\mathbf{A} = \mathbf{A}_{pri} - \mathbf{M}_{comp}\mathbf{A}_{ref}$, where $\mathbf{M}_{comp}$ is the noise compensation matrix whereas $\mathbf{A}_{pri}$ and $\mathbf{A}_{ref}$ are the gain matrices computed for the primary and reference sensors, respectively. Both of these noise compensation schemes are integrated, e.g., in the software packages presented in *Examples of Available Software*.

fMRI Constraints

The hemodynamic changes detected by fMRI are associated with changes of underlying neural activity, i.e., electrical currents flowing in and around the neurons. Therefore, it has been proposed that MEG and fMRI can be used together to obtain activity estimates with higher temporal and spatial resolution than provided by one modality alone. This joint analysis can be performed at several levels: (1) Side-by-side comparison of fMRI activity with MEG source estimates; (2) Using the fMRI information as a prior in MEG source estimation (Dale et al., 2000); (3) Joint analysis where fMRI and MEG data are handled on equal footing (Daunizeau et al., 2007); (4) Neural modeling approach where, in addition to fMRI and MEG, a plausible model of the neural ensembles and their connections is taken into account (David et al., 2006; Riera et al., 2005; 2006).

While several papers exist comparing fMRI activity with MEG source estimates using identical or similar experiments in the two modalities, combined modeling strategies are still emerging. Dale et al. (2000) describe a method to include fMRI as an additional constraint: the *a priori* variance of sources is decreased at locations with no significant fMRI activity. An optimal weighting ratio of 10:1 between active and inactive cortical locations has been suggested by simulation studies (Liu, et al., 1998).

While this approach is technically sound and can be understood in the Bayesian inference framework, it does not use a physiologically motivated, detailed model linking the electrical and hemodynamic activity. A recent comparison of hemodynamic signatures and neural activity in the soma- tosensory cortex of a rat indicates that their relationship is strongly nonlinear (Devor et al., 2003). This type of data will be eventually incorporated into joint estimation models where both fMRI and MEG are included simultane- ously, rather than employing one modality as a prior in the analysis of another; see, *e.g.*, J. Riera et al. (2005).

Time-frequency Analyses

In recent years there has been a lot of interest in frequency-domain analyses of MEG data. This includes calculation of power and coherence spectra, time-frequency representations, and phase-locking indices. These topics are covered in detail in other chapters of this book. Here, we briefly describe how time-frequency analyses can be conducted in the source domain using the linear minimum-norm solutions (Lin et al., 2004).

For localization of oscillatory neuronal activity we will first calculate the time-frequency representation (TFR) for single-trial MEG data. To this end, each single trial $s_p^{(k)}(t)$ for each sensor p is convoluted with a Morlet wavelet, which is a complex-valued sinusoidal oscillation at central frequency f weighted with a Gaussian envelope: $w(t, f) = A \exp\left(-t^2/2\sigma_t^2\right)\exp\left(2i\pi f t\right)$. In our applications we have used wavelets whose width is typically between 3 and 8 cycles. For each sensor p we thus obtain a complex TFR for trial k: $\psi_p^{(k)}(t, f) = \int w(t - \tau, f) s_p^{(k)}(\tau) d\tau$ with both amplitude and phase informa- tion. Using a minimum-norm estimate inverse operator $\mathbf{W}$, we can map the TFR from MEG sensor space onto the cortical surfaces: $\Psi^{(k)}(t, f) = \mathbf{W}\psi^{(k)}(t, f)$, where $\psi^{(k)} = \left(\psi_1^{(k)}\ldots\psi_n^{(k)}\right)^T$.

Given the TFR on cortical surfaces, the following quantities can be calcu- lated at each source location respectively: (1) averaged power, which is the modulus squared of $\psi(t, f)$ computed from the average of all trials; (2) induced power, which is the average of the squared moduli of $\psi(t, f)$ across trials; and (3) Phase-Locking Value (PLV), which is a measure of phase difference con- sistency across trials with respect to a reference signal: $\theta(t) = \left|\overline{e^{i\vartheta_k(t)}}\right|$, where $\vartheta_k(t)$ is the phase difference at time t in trial k (Lachaux et al., 1999) and $|\overline{\cdot}|$ denotes the modulus of the average over trials. The reference signal can be a waveform time-locked to the onset of the experimental stimulus during *stimulus-cortical PLV* calculation, or a waveform on the other cortical source location for *cortico-cortical PLV* calculations. As shown in Figure 8–1, fMRI information can further be utilized to improve source-localization accuracy of oscillatory activity (Lin et al., 2007; 2004).

Practical Implementation of Cortically Constrained Estimates

In this section, we will discuss the workflow of computing cortically con- strained minimum-norm solutions, including information on acquisition

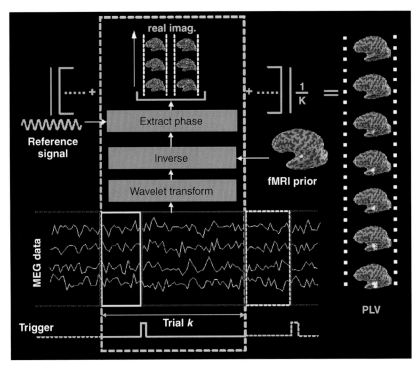

Figure 8–1. A schematic diagram illustrating the process of using raw MEG data to calculate the phase locking value (PLV) on the cortical surface The yellow and red boxes on the MEG data indicate the baseline period and the post-stimulus interval, respectively. Note that an fMRI prior can be incorporated into the calculation of the linear inverse operator. For details, see text.

of the necessary MRI and MEG data and on crucial computational steps involved.

Acquisition and Preprocessing of MEG Data

The use of cortically constrained source estimates has some implications for recommended MEG data acquisition practices. Most importantly, reliable estimation of the noise-covariance matrix requires that continuous raw data are available, as will be discussed in *Estimation of the Noise Covariance Matrix*, below. Some MEG systems provide a choice between truly continuous and epoch-based data acquisition modes. We strongly recommend that the continuous acquisition mode is employed. This approach makes off-line digital filtering straightforward, and allows the use of high-pass filters with low corner frequencies.

We also recommend that a generous bandpass is used in the actual data acquisition, since the data are invariably filtered and re-averaged off line, even if on-line averages are usually computed for quality control and initial exploratory analyses. We usually employ a highpass at 0.1 Hz or lower in the data acquisition. Depending on the system and environmental noise conditions, a DC recording may even be feasible. Since the computation of the noise-covariance matrix is a nonlinear operation, and thus does not commute with filtering, the off-line averages and noise-covariance matrix estimate should be computed with an identical bandpass. If the MEG system provides a choice of storing the data with or without noise compensation applied, we have found that it is useful to consistently save uncompensated data, and apply software noise compensation during the analysis as appropriate.

For quality control purposes, optimization of the noise-rejection algorithms, and for the computation of a noise-covariance matrix for spontaneous data analyses, about a 5-minute continuous record of empty room data without subject should be collected before each measurement session, or at least once every day.

Acquisition and Processing of Anatomical MRI Data

As described above, a feasible anatomical constraint for MEG and EEG source localization is to restrict the source locations to the cortical mantle, extracted from the individual subject's MRI. With modern segmentation methods, a representation for the geometry of the cortex can be automatically generated from high-resolution 3D MRI data sets. We routinely employ the FreeSurfer (Dale et al., 1999; Fischl et al., 2001; 1999) and BrainSuite (Shattuck & Leahy, 2002) software packages to build the triangular cortical surface mesh from T1-weighted anatomical 3D-volume MRI data. For example, on the Siemens MRI scanners, we employ the MPRAGE sequence and acquire two identical data sets to enhance the SNR by averaging. For reconstruction of the inner skull, outer skull, and scalp surfaces needed for the MEG and EEG forward solutions, and surface-based alignment of the MEG and MRI coordinate frames, we often acquire an additional 3D multi-echo FLASH sequence. However, for MEG-only modeling the MPRAGE data are usually sufficient, because the outer skull surface is not needed.

The principal surfaces generated by FreeSurfer and BrainSuite are the pial surface and the gray-white matter boundary; we use the latter to generate the cortically constrained source space. In addition to the folded surface, both FreeSurfer and BrainSuite also compute inflated and flattened representations of the cortex, which expose the parts of the cortex embedded in the sulci. These representations are thus particularly useful for visualizing MEG data, which are mainly sensitive to fissural activity. FreeSurfer also provides an automatic parcellation of the cortex, which can be useful in inquiring source waveforms in specific regions of interest. An additional benefit of the surface-based analysis is that cortical surfaces can be aligned across individuals for computation of group statistics using a morphing procedure in a spherical coordinate system (Fischl et al., 1999).

To achieve sufficient anatomical detail for visualization of the folded cortical mantle, the triangular tessellations of the cortical surface typically consist of around 130,000 – 150,000 vertices per hemisphere, corresponding to an approximate triangle size of 1 mm. For source modeling, this dense triangulation is typically subsequently decimated to a source space of 7,500 – 10,000 dipoles. The decimation is motivated by the limited spatial resolution intrinsic to the source localization using MEG/EEG, and by practical computational efficiency concerns. However, this simplified source geometry may yield inaccurate dipole orientations, which do not take into account the orientation variation over the patch belonging to each decimated current source location. Furthermore, the actual areas of the patches have to be taken into account in the calculations to estimate the current density on the cortex.

Motivated by the finite size of the cortical patches, we advocate three different approaches for handling the source orientations (Lin, Belliveau, et al., 2006): (1) Using unconstrained orientations with all three current components present; (2) Using the loose orientation constraint (LOC) whereby the orientations are constrained more or less strictly to the estimated orientation of the cortical normals, depending on the curvature of the cortex at the location of interest; (3) Using orientations which are strictly constrained by the estimated cortical normals at the source space points. In practice, the third approach often yields current estimates which contain spurious isolated spots of activation, most probably due to the fact that the normals at the relatively sparsely spaced source locations do not account for the variation of the normals within the cortical patch corresponding to the source space point. As discussed in Lin, Belliveau, et al. (2006), full implementation of the LOC approach requires computation of cortical patch statistics (CPS). This computation involves the use of the Dijkstra search (Bertsekas, 2000) to delineate the cortical patches. An analogous approach using cortical patches as elementary sources instead of current dipoles, with properties similar to our LOC procedure, also has been introduced (Wagner et al., 2000). In addition, a recent publication introduces the concept of spatial basis functions on cortical patches, to incorporate local geometrical information with a relatively small total number of unknown parameters (Limpiti et al., 2006).

Alignment of the MEG and MRI Coordinate Frames

In order to employ MRI and MEG data together, it is necessary to bring the two data sets into a common coordinate frame. For this purpose, 3 – 5 small head-position indicator (HPI) coils are usually attached on the head surface, and their locations as well as additional head surface points are digitized prior to the MEG acquisition in a coordinate frame defined by fiducial landmarks. During the MEG measurement, current is fed to the coils either intermittently (see, e.g., Fuchs et al., 1995) or continuously (Uutela et al., 2001), to compute their locations with respect to the sensor array. If a continuous head-position measurement is used, it is possible to take the head movements into account by using minimum-norm based interpolation techniques, forward model averaging, or the signal-space space separation (SSS) algorithm (Taulu et al., 2005).

One possibility to align the MRI and MEG head coordinate frames involves attaching MRI-visible markers to the fiducial locations, to be able to identify them easily from the MRI data. However, this approach has the potential of errors because the placement of the MRI markers might not be accurate and, furthermore, several investigators may share the same subject base and may prefer slightly different choices of fiducial locations. Therefore, most MEG groups have abandoned the use of markers, but instead rely on the ability to identify the fiducials from the MRI data. The correctness of the alignment can be confirmed by displaying the digitized scalp surface points overlaid with the MRI slices.

Since it is relatively straightforward to construct an accurate scalp surface triangulation from high-resolution MRI data, it is also possible to identify the fiducial locations directly from the MRI-based scalp surface reconstruction. In addition, the scalp surface points can be used to refine the fiducial-based initial alignment either manually or automatically, using the iterative closest-point algorithm (Besl & MacKay, 1992) if a MRI-based scalp surface triangulation is available.

Estimation of the Noise Covariance Matrix

The approaches introduced above employ a noise-covariance matrix estimated from the data. As indicated by the cost function in Equation (8–3), the incorporation of the noise covariance means that in noisier signal-space directions, mismatches between the measured data and those predicted by the source estimate receive a smaller weight when the optimal current distribution is determined.

Depending on the problem, different types of data can be employed to estimate the noise covariance. The most conservative choice is to employ empty-room data. The interpretation of this approach is that all brain signals are considered to be of interest, and only the environmental and instrumental noise sources are considered. Calculation of this type of covariance matrix requires that a measurement of empty-room noise without a subject is available. For the estimation of such a covariance matrix, we usually employ about five minutes of data to guarantee a reliable estimate.

Another possibility, applicable to evoked-response studies, is to consider the baseline data before stimulus presentation as noise, and to estimate the noise covariance from the baselines preceding the stimulus presentations. Since the baseline of an average typically contains no more than a few hundred samples, it is necessary to employ the individual epochs to compute a reliable estimate. We concatenate the individual baseline sections of the data after removing the DC offset from them, and use this data set to estimate noise. The DC-offset removal eliminates slow epoch-to-epoch baseline variations as a source of noise, and thus avoids overestimating the magnitude of noise. A potential confound of this approach is that the baseline periods may contain background brain activity originating in the same areas as signals of interest. Due to the combination of noise weighting, and the minimum norm constraint incorporated in Equation (8–3), the contributions of such source distributions are dampened. One possibility to address this issue is to compare solutions computed with the empty room and baseline noise covariance matrices, and investigate the source waveforms in ROIs showing significant activity in the former but not latter.

The quality of the estimated noise-covariance matrix can be evaluated by plotting its eigenvalues. Figure 8–2 compares the eigenvalue spectrum of an empty room noise covariance matrix to those of two noise estimates computed from baseline periods. It is clearly seen that if enough samples are employed in the computation of the noise covariance matrix from human data, the eigenvalue spectrum is limited from below by the empty-room estimate. If the number of data points is too small, the eigenvalues fall below the empty-room noise—which is clearly unrealistic, falsely indicating a drop in the noise level when the subject is present. If the number of data points is pathologically small, the eigenvalues may even fall below zero, which is clearly incorrect because the noise covariance matrix is theoretically positive definite.

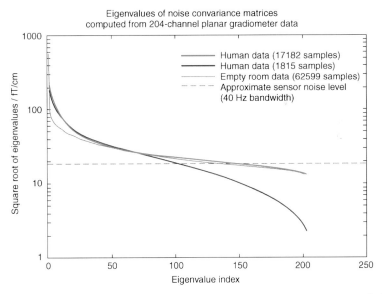

Figure 8–2. Comparison of the distribution of the square roots of the eigenvalues of three noise covariance matrix estimates: An adequate noise-covariance matrix computed from the baseline periods (green); A noise-covariance matrix computed from the baseline periods with too-small number of samples (red); A noise-covariance matrix computed from empty room data (blue). An approximate sensor noise level at the measurement bandwidth is indicated by a dashed blue line. For details, see text.

Sometimes there is not a sufficient amount of baseline-period data available to compute a reliable noise estimate. In such cases, we have used two approaches to remedy the situation: (1) Set the off-diagonal terms of the noise-covariance matrix to zero, thereby ignoring the spatial structure of the noise; (2) Regularize the noise-covariance matrix by adding a fraction of the average of its diagonal elements to each diagonal element, i.e., each sensor variance. If the latter approach is employed in a system consisting of different types of sensors, e.g., magnetometers and planar gradiometers, it is recommended that averages are calculated for each sensor type separately, and a fraction of the average corresponding to the sensor type is added to its variance for regularization.

Examples of Available Software

Our laboratories have independently developed two analysis streams, which implement the tools for MRI segmentation and geometric modeling as well as for processing MEG data to compute cortically-constrained source estimates. One of our analysis streams uses the BrainSuite software developed at the University of Southern California (Shattuck & Leahy, 2002) for MRI processing, while the other relies on the FreeSurfer package created at MGH (Dale, et al., 1999; Fischl, et al., 2001; 2004; 1999). Correspondingly, the two MEG analysis packages are called BrainStorm and MNE. BrainStorm is implemented as a Matlab toolbox and includes implementation of a wide variety of source estimation algorithms. The MNE software employs compiled C-code and includes a wealth of command-line tools as well as graphical user interfaces for visualizing the results. In addition, the MNE software includes basic signal processing tools and flexible off-line averaging capabilities. Development of new algorithms is supported by a Matlab toolbox, which gives access to all intermediate and final results of the analyses. Our groups have started a collaborative project to enhance interoperability of the two sets of software, and to verify and validate the implementations. A comparison of the BrainStorm and MNE software features is presented in Table 8–1. Both BrainSuite/BrainStorm and FreeSurfer/MNE software packages are freely downloadable from the web (see http://neuroimage.usc.edu/brainstorm/, http://brainsuite.usc.edu/, and http://www.nmr.mgh.harvard.edu/martinos/userInfo/data/index.php).

Examples

This section contains a few examples of experiments analyzed with the methods and software described above.

Consistency of Source Estimates Across Different MEG Systems

Pooling of magnetoencephalography (MEG) data across laboratories is not straightforward because of differences in hardware, software, and different

Table 8–1. Comparison of the features of BrainStorm and MNE.

Feature	BrainStorm	MNE
Implementation	Matlab	Compiled C programs, Matlab toolbox for accessing files and end-user development
MRI segmentation and reconstruction	BrainSuite recommended Other choices possible	FreeSurfer
Forward models	Sphere model, Overlapping spheres, BEM, FEM	Sphere model, BEM
BEM surface triangulations	BrainSuite, Anatomist, or other software. Program has algorithms for re-registering tessellations with MRIs. Downsampling of tessellations.	FreeSurfer or other software providing the data in the same coordinate system as FreeSurfer MRI data
Preprocessing	Filtering, data viewer, SSP, noise cancellation with reference sensors	Filtering, downsampling, raw data viewer, estimation of noise covariance matrices, SSP, noise cancellation with reference sensors. Software is also aware of the SSS method employed in Neuromag software for noise cancellation.
Input data files	Native Neuromag fif data, converters from VSM, 4D; native VSM data; native EGI data; ASCII formatted and "raw" binary data	Native Neuromag fif data, converters from VSM, 4D, and KIT data to the fif format
File formats	Matlab "mat-files"	fif files for most intermediate results, w and stc files for FreeSurfer compatible surface-based data
Graphics output	Full suite of Matlab-generated output formats	Static images: jpeg, tiff, png, PostScript, PDF; Movie files: QuickTime
Source estimation methods	LS, MNE, dSPM, MUSIC, LCMV	MNE, dSPM, sLORETA, dipole fitting.
Simulation	Simulation of data using the forward model	Simulation of data using the forward model, simulate spatially correlated noise with help of a noise-covariance matrix

environmental noise levels. To investigate these issues, we recently conducted a study with the same five subjects and stimulus-presentation equipment at three different sites with different MEG arrays: Elekta-Neuromag Vectorview (Boston), VSM MedTech Omega275 (Albuquerque), and 4D Neuroimaging Magnes 3600 WH (Minneapolis). Subjects were run twice at each site, in simple somatosensory, visual, and auditory paradigms (Weisend et al., 2007).

To assess the consistency of MEG source estimates across systems and software implementations, dynamical statistical parametric mapping (dSPM) was conducted with both the MNE and BrainStorm software packages discussed above. A high-resolution cortical surface was extracted using either FreeSurfer or BrainSuite, representing the gray-white matter boundary with approximately 300,000 vertices. The surface was downsampled to about 40,000 (BrainStorm) or 5,000 (MNE) vertices. In both MNE and BrainStorm the MEG and MRI coregistration was implemented by manual identification of three fiducial landmarks and, in MNE, this initial alignment was refined with the Iterative Closest Point (ICP) algorithm. The forward solution was computed for each of the three MEG systems using an overlapping spheres model (BrainStorm), or a single compartment BEM with linear collocation approach (MNE).

For the computation of the dSPM distributions in Brainstorm, an estimate for the diagonal noise-covariance matrix was computed from a 200-ms baseline period preceding the stimuli. In MNE, the individual epochs were used to compute the estimate; the result was divided by the number of averaged epochs in the analysis of the averages, to account for the signal-to-noise improvement. Regularization consistent with the signal-to-noise ratio of whitened data was applied in the computation of the minimum-norm estimates. The dSPM distributions were subjectively thresholded to indicate the maximum activity on the cortex.

As shown in Figure 8–3, our analyses of somatosensory data using the cortically constrained source estimates showed excellent test/retest results across instruments. This result is in line with our finding that the localization of data from the Neuromag current dipole data using a single-dipole model was accurate within less than 2 mm. Our analyses demonstrate that (1) instruments from different manufacturers yield similar results for somatosensory data, and that (2) multiple software packages produce very consistent estimates for simple source configurations.

What and Where Pathways in the Auditory Cortex

Human neuroimaging studies suggest that localization and identification of relevant auditory objects is accomplished via parallel parietal-to-lateral-prefrontal *"where"* and anterior-temporal-to-inferior-frontal *"what"* pathways, respectively. Using combined hemodynamic (fMRI) and electromagnetic (MEG) measurements, Ahveninen et al. (2006) investigated whether such dual pathways exist already in the human nonprimary auditory cortex, as

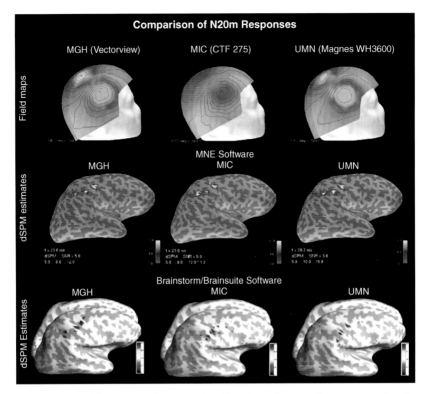

Figure 8–3. Field maps and source localizations for median nerve stimulation at 20 ms after the onset of the stimulus. The top row shows field maps for data collected on the same subject using MEG machines from three different manufacturers, after projection into a common reference frame. The second and third rows show comparisons of dSPM estimates, obtained using two different software packages (MNE/FreeSurfer and BrainStorm/BrainSuite). The estimates of activity across MEG systems and software packages within the same subject are remarkably consistent.

suggested by animal models (Rauschecker & Tian, 2000; Tian et al., 2001). This example demonstrates the potential of using anatomically and functionally constrained source estimates to study the fine details of cortical processing of sensory signals; see Figure 8–4.

During the experiments in Ahveninen et al. (2006), subjects were presented with pairs of Finnish vowels /æ/ and /ø/. Each vowel was simulated from either straight ahead or 45 degrees to the right. The sound pairs were identical, phonetically discordant (but spatially identical), or spatially discordant (but phonetically identical). Cortically constrained MEG/fMRI minimum-norm estimates of responses to "probes" preceded by identical, phonetically different, or spatially different "adaptors" were compared. The result suggested a double dissociation in response adaptation to sound pairs with phonetic vs.

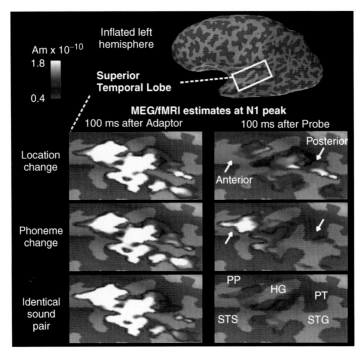

Figure 8–4. Differential adaptation to phonemes vs. sound locations in nonprimary auditory cortex. Cortical fMRI-weighted MEG minimum-norm estimates are shown in a representative subject at the N1 peak latency. The data are visualized on the inflated cortical surface, showing the convex and concave parts of the cortex in light and dark grey, respectively. The source estimate is shown with a colored overlay showing that the auditory cortex areas activated by the Adaptor (the first stimulus of the pair) are identical across the conditions, but specific adaptation-induced differences in activity patterns elicited by Probes (the second stimulus of the pair) are observed: The posterior activity is strongest (i.e., least adapted) when Adaptor and Probe differ spatially, and the anterior activity is strongest when Adaptor and Probe differ phonetically. (Abbreviations: STS, superior temporal sulcus; HG, Heschl's gyrus; PT, planum temporale; PP, planum polare; STG, superior temporal gyrus.)

spatial sound changes—demonstrating that the human nonprimary auditory cortex indeed processes speech-sound identity and location in parallel anterior "*what*" (in anterolateral Heschl's gyrus, anterior superior temporal gyrus (STG), and posterior planum polare) and posterior "*where*" (in planum temporale and posterior STG) pathways as early as ~70–150 ms from stimulus onset. These data further showed that the "*where*" pathway is activated ~30 ms earlier than the "*what*" pathway, possibly enabling the brain to utilize top-down spatial information in auditory object perception. Notably, selectively attending to phonetic content modulated the response adaptation in the *"what"* pathway, whereas attending to sound location produced analogous effects in the *"where"* pathway.

Analysis of Oscillatory Activity in VisuoMotor Coordination

The spiking activity of single neurons in the primate motor cortex is correlated with various limb movement parameters, including velocity. Recent findings obtained using local field potentials suggest that hand speed may also be encoded in the summed activity of neuronal populations. At this macroscopic level, the motor cortex has also been shown to display synchronized rhythmic activity modulated by motor behavior. Yet, whether and how neural oscillations might be related to limb speed control is still poorly understood.

Using BrainStorm, we applied MEG source imaging to the ongoing brain activity in subjects performing a continuous visuomotor (VM) task (Jerbi et al., 2007). We used coherence and phase synchronization to investigate the coupling between the estimated activity throughout the brain, and the simultaneously recorded instantaneous hand speed. We found significant phase locking between slow (2- to 5-Hz) oscillatory activity in the contralateral primary motor cortex, and time-varying hand speed (see Figure 8–5). In addition, we reported long-range task-related coupling between primary motor cortex and multiple brain regions in the same frequency band. The detected large-scale VM network spans several cortical and subcortical areas, including structures of the frontoparietal circuit and the cerebello–thalamo–cortical pathway. These findings suggest a role for slow coherent oscillations in mediating neural representations of hand kinematics in humans, and provide further support for the putative role of long-range neural synchronization in large-scale VM integration.

Dynamics of Epileptic Activity

The most important clinical application of MEG is currently the localization of epileptic foci. If clinicians are able to precisely locate where in the brain an epileptic seizure begins, then patients may be treated by surgical removal of the abnormal brain tissue, and only the abnormal brain tissue. Currently, the standard clinical approach is to find the location of the largest activation that occurs during a burst in brain activity: the epileptic spike. This is accomplished by estimating the locations and dynamics of one or more current dipoles from the MEG or EEG data. Locating the largest area of abnormal activity is often helpful, but may be misleading in many epileptic patients. For example, if the brain activity that leads to a seizure begins as a very small spike, but quickly spreads to another brain area, it is important to locate the origin of the small spike, which may be missed with the traditional analysis.

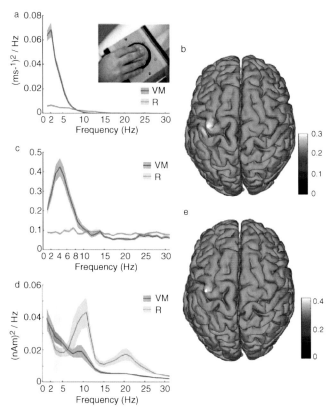

Figure 8–5. Coherence between brain activity and hand speed. (a) Trackball speed (TBS) power spectrum during visuomotor (VM – blue) and rest (R – green) conditions. (b) Cortical map of task-related Z-transformed coherence with TBS (VM vs. R) in the 2–5Hz range (P < 0.001, corrected). The white dot indicates the location of maximum coherence difference (Montreal Neurological Institute coordinates: (–42, –17, 67 mm), hand area M1). (c) M1–TBS coherence spectrum during VM and R, with a peak at 4 Hz. (d) M1 power spectrum. Compared with R (green), VM (blue) has more power in 3–5 Hz (P < 0.05, corrected), followed by the well known power suppression of 10–20-Hz oscillations. (e) Cortical map of difference in brain–TBS phase-locking at 4 Hz (+/–1Hz) between VM and R (P < 0.001, corrected). The white dot indicates the location of maximum phase-locking difference.

Using the MNE software, the Martinos Center Clinical MEG Service at MGH has begun to evaluate the utility of cortically constrained distributed-current estimates in the analysis of MEG and EEG data acquired from epileptic patients (Knake et al., 2006; Shiraishi et al., 2005). With this technique, a 'movie' is generated that shows estimates of the brain activity over the entire time course of an interictal event (see Figure 8–6). This allows a physician to determine precisely were in the brain the epileptic spike originates, and focus the treatment more specifically on the diseased tissue.

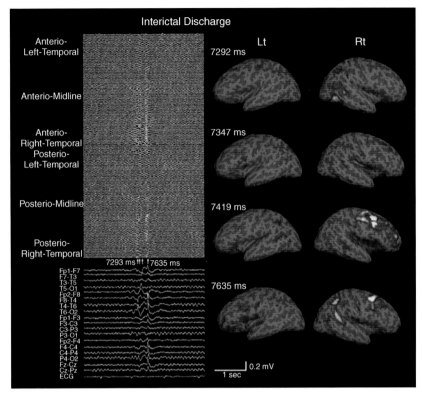

Figure 8–6. Interictal epileptiform discharges in MEG and EEG, with sources estimated using equivalent current dipoles (ECDs) and dynamic statistical parametric mapping (dSPM). *Top left:* Interictal epileptiform discharges on magnetoencephalography were observed over the right temporal and frontal regions widely. *Bottom left:* Right temporal dominant but right hemispheric spikes or polyspikes could be detected frequently on EEG. *First row, middle and right*: The equivalent current dipoles calculated by the beginning of the polyspike burst located at the right temporal operculum, some also in the lower operculum in the right frontal lobe. *Second to fifth row, middle and right:* A dynamic statistical parametric mapping showed the wide activity over the whole temporal lobe propagated to the ipsilateral frontal and parietal lobes. The threshold of displayed activity is $p < 10^{-4}$, and the full yellow area indicates $p < 10^{-9}$.

Concluding Remarks

Within the last decade, anatomical MRI has become an integral and indispensable component of MEG source analysis. MRI data are used not only as an anatomical map in the visualization of results, but also as a source of geometrical information for both forward and inverse modeling. In distributed source-modeling approaches, the cortical geometry information is particularly useful as a spatial constraint and as a vehicle of visualizing the data in a comprehensive and easily understandable way.

In contrast, only the first few steps have been taken towards joint use of fMRI with the electrophysiological measurements. Further developments in this area will clearly benefit from new experiments elucidating the exact nature of hemodynamic coupling, which leads to the development of physiologically sound models to estimate neural activity jointly from MEG, EEG, and fMRI measurements.

Acknowledgments

This work was supported by The Center for Functional Neuromaging Technologies (NIH grant P41 RR14075), grants R01-EB002010 and 1R01-EB009048-01 from the National Institute of Biomedical Imaging and BioEngineering, Department of Energy Award Number DE-FG02-99ER62764 to The MIND Institute in Albuquerque, New Mexico, and by Los Alamos National Security, LLC, for the National Nuclear Security Administration of the U.S. Department of Energy under contract DE-AC52-06NA25396.

References

Ahveninen, J., Jaaskelainen, I. P., Raij, T., Bonmassar, G., Devore, S., Hämäläinen, M., et al. (2006). Task-modulated "what" and "where" pathways in human auditory cortex. *Proc Natl Acad Sci U S A*, *103*(39), 14608–14613.

Baillet, S., Mosher, J. C., & Leahy, R. M. (2001). Electromagnetic Brain Mapping. *IEEE Signal Processing Magazine*, *18*(6), 14 – 30.

Belliveau, J. W., Kwong, K. K., Kennedy, D. N., Baker, J. R., Stern, C. E., Benson, R., et al. (1992). Magnetic resonance imaging mapping of brain function. Human visual cortex. *Invest Radiol*, *27*(2), S59–65.

Bertsekas, D. P. (2000). *Dynamic programming and optimal control* (2nd ed.). Belmont, Mass: Athena Scientific.

Besl, P., & MacKay, N. (1992). A Method for Registration of 3-D Shapes. *IEEE Trans. Pat. Anal. and Mach. Intel.*, *14*(2), 239–256.

Dale, A., & Sereno, M. (1993). Improved localization of cortical activity by combining EEG and MEG with MRI cortical surface reconstruction: A linear approach. *J. Cog. Neurosci*, *5*, 162–176.

Dale, A. M., Fischl, B., & Sereno, M. I. (1999). Cortical surface-based analysis. I. Segmentation and surface reconstruction. *Neuroimage*, *9*(2), 179–194.

Dale, A. M., Liu, A. K., Fischl, B. R., Buckner, R. L., Belliveau, J. W., Lewine, J. D., et al. (2000). Dynamic statistical parametric mapping: combining fMRI and MEG for high-resolution imaging of cortical activity. *Neuron*, *26*(1), 55–67.

Daunizeau, J., Grova, C., Marrelec, G., Mattout, J., Jbabdi, S., Pélégrini-Issac, M., et al. (2007). Symmetrical event-related EEG/fMRI information fusion in a variational Bayesian framework. *Neuroimage*, *36*(1), 69–87.

David, O., Kiebel, S. J., Harrison, L. M., Mattout, J., Kilner, J. M., & Friston, K. J. (2006). Dynamic causal modeling of evoked responses in EEG and MEG. *Neuroimage, 30*(4), 1255–1272.

Devor, A., Dunn, A. K., Andermann, M. L., Ulbert, I., Boas, D. A., & Dale, A. M. (2003). Coupling of total hemoglobin concentration, oxygenation, and neural activity in rat somatosensory cortex. *Neuron, 39*(2), 353–359.

Fischl, B., Liu, A., & Dale, A. M. (2001). Automated manifold surgery: constructing geometrically accurate and topologically correct models of the human cerebral cortex. *IEEE Trans Med Imaging, 20*(1), 70–80.

Fischl, B., Salat, D. H., van der Kouwe, A. J., Makris, N., Segonne, F., Quinn, B. T., et al. (2004). Sequence-independent segmentation of magnetic resonance images. *Neuroimage, 23, 1,* S69–84.

Fischl, B., Sereno, M. I., & Dale, A. M. (1999). Cortical surface-based analysis. II: Inflation, flattening, and a surface-based coordinate system. *Neuroimage, 9*(2), 195–207.

Fischl, B., Sereno, M. I., Tootell, R. B., & Dale, A. M. (1999). High-resolution intersubject averaging and a coordinate system for the cortical surface. *Hum Brain Mapp, 8*(4), 272–284.

Fuchs, M., Wagner, M., Kohler, T., & Wischmann, H. A. (1999). Linear and nonlinear current density reconstructions. *J Clin Neurophysiol, 16*(3), 267–295.

Fuchs, M., Wischmann, H. A., Wagner, M., & Kruger, J. (1995). Coordinate system matching for neuromagnetic and morphological reconstruction overlay. *IEEE Trans Biomed Eng, 42*(4), 416–420.

Hämäläinen, M., Hari, R., Ilmoniemi, R., Knuutila, J., & Lounasmaa, O. (1993). Magnetoencephalography-theory, instrumentation, and application to noninvasive studies of the working human brain. *Review of Modern Physics, 65,* 413–497.

Hämäläinen, M., & Ilmoniemi, R. (1984). *Interpreting measured magnetic fields of the brain: estimates of curent distributions.* Helsinki, Finland: Helsinki University of Technology.

Heller, L., & van Hulsteyn, D. B. (1992). Brain stimulation using electromagnetic sources: theoretical aspects. *Biophys J, 63*(1), 129–138.

Helmholtz, H. (1853). Ueber einige Gesetze der Vertheilung elektrischer Strome in korperlichen Leitern, mit Anwendung auf die thierisch-elektrischen Versuche. *Ann. Phys. Chem., 89,* 211–233, 353–377.

Hillebrand, A., & Barnes, G. R. (2002). A quantitative assessment of the sensitivity of whole-head MEG to activity in the adult human cortex. *Neuroimage, 16*(3 Pt 1), 638–650.

Huang, M. X., Dale, A. M., Song, T., Halgren, E., Harrington, D. L., Podgorny, I., et al. (2006). Vector-based spatial-temporal minimum L1-norm solution for MEG. *Neuroimage, 31*(3), 1025–1037.

Ioannides, A. A., Bolton, J. P., & Clarke, C. J. S. (1990). Continuous probabilistic solutions to the biomagnetic inverse problem. *Inverse Problem, 6*(4), 523–542.

Jerbi, K., Lachaux, J. P., N'Diaye, K., Pantazis, D., Leahy, R. M., Garnero, L., et al. (2007). Coherent neural representation of hand speed in humans revealed by MEG imaging. *Proc Natl Acad Sci U S A, 104*(18), 7676–7681.

Knake, S., Halgren, E., Shiraishi, H., Hara, K., Hamer, H. M., Grant, P. E., et al. (2006). The value of multichannel MEG and EEG in the presurgical evaluation of 70 epilepsy patients. *Epilepsy Res, 69*(1), 80–86.

Kwong, K. K., Belliveau, J. W., Chesler, D. A., Goldberg, I. E., Weisskoff, R. M., Poncelet, B. P., et al. (1992). Dynamic magnetic resonance imaging of human brain activity during primary sensory stimulation. *Proc Natl Acad Sci U S A, 89*(12), 5675–5679.

Lachaux, J. P., Rodriguez, E., Martinerie, J., & Varela, F. J. (1999). Measuring phase synchrony in brain signals. *Hum Brain Mapp, 8*(4), 194–208.

Limpiti, T., Van Veen, B. D., & Wakai, R. T. (2006). Cortical patch basis model for spatially extended neural activity. *IEEE Trans Biomed Eng, 53*(9), 1740–1754.

Lin, F.-H., Raij, T., Ahveninen, J., Ahlfors, S., Leuthold, A. C., Pantazis, D., et al. (2007). Imaging of oscillatory cortical activity using combined MEG and fMRI. *Elsevier Internation Congress Series, 1300*, 19–22.

Lin, F. H., Belliveau, J. W., Dale, A. M., & Hämäläinen, M. S. (2006). Distributed current estimates using cortical orientation constraints. *Hum Brain Mapp, 27*(1), 1–13.

Lin, F. H., Witzel, T., Ahlfors, S. P., Stufflebeam, S. M., Belliveau, J. W., & Hämäläinen, M. S. (2006). Assessing and improving the spatial accuracy in MEG source localization by depth-weighted minimum-norm estimates. *Neuroimage, 31*(1), 160–171.

Lin, F. H., Witzel, T., Hämäläinen, M. S., Dale, A. M., Belliveau, J. W., & Stufflebeam, S. M. (2004). Spectral spatiotemporal imaging of cortical oscillations and interactions in the human brain. *Neuroimage, 23*(2), 582–595.

Liu, A. K., Belliveau, J. W., & Dale, A. M. (1998). Spatiotemporal imaging of human brain activity using functional MRI constrained magnetoencephalography data: Monte Carlo simulations. *Proc Natl Acad Sci U S A, 95*(15), 8945–8950.

Matsuura, K., & Okabe, Y. (1995). Selective minimum-norm solution of the biomagnetic inverse problem. *IEEE Trans Biomed Eng, 42*(6), 608–615.

Moon, T. K., & Stirling, W. C. (2000). Mathematical methods and algorithms for signal processing [xxxvi, 937] Upper Saddle River, NJ: Prentice Hall.

Mosher, J. C., Baillet, S., & Leahy, R. M. (2003). *Equivalence of Linear Approaches in Bioelectromagnetic Inverse Solutions*, 2003 IEEE Workshop on Statistical Signal Processing, St. Louis, Missouri, Sep 28 – Oct 1, 2003.

Okada, Y. C., Wu, J., & Kyuhou, S. (1997). Genesis of MEG signals in a mammalian CNS structure. *Electroencephalogr Clin Neurophysiol, 103*(4), 474–485.

Ou, W., Hamalainen, M. S., & Golland, P. (2009). A distributed spatio-temporal EEG/MEG inverse solver. *Neuroimage, 44*(3), 932-946.

Pascual-Marqui, R. D. (2002). Standardized low-resolution brain electromagnetic tomography (sLORETA): technical details. *Methods Find Exp Clin Pharmacol, 24 Suppl D*, 5–12.

Rauschecker, J. P., & Tian, B. (2000). Mechanisms and streams for processing of "what" and "where" in auditory cortex. *Proc Natl Acad Sci U S A, 97*(22), 11800–11806.

Riera, J., Aubert, E., Iwata, K., Kawashima, R., Wan, X., & Ozaki, T. (2005). Fusing EEG and fMRI based on a bottom-up model: inferring activation and effective connectivity in neural masses. *Philos Trans R Soc Lond B Biol Sci, 360*(1457), 1025–1041.

Riera, J. J., Wan, X., Jimenez, J. C., & Kawashima, R. (2006). Nonlinear local electrovascular coupling. I: A theoretical model. *Hum Brain Mapp, 27*(11), 896–914.

Shattuck, D. W., & Leahy, R. M. (2002). BrainSuite: an automated cortical surface identification tool. *Med Image Anal, 6*(2), 129–142.

Shiraishi, H., Stufflebeam, S. M., Knake, S., Ahlfors, S. P., Sudo, A., Asahina, N., et al. (2005). Dynamic statistical parametric mapping for analyzing the magnetoence-phalographic epileptiform activity in patients with epilepsy. *J Child Neurol, 20*(4), 363–369.

Taulu, S., Simola, J., & Kajola, M. (2005). Applications of the Signal Space Separation Method. *IEEE Trans. Biomed. Eng., 53*(9), 3359–3372.

Tesche, C. D., Uusitalo, M. A., Ilmoniemi, R. J., Huotilainen, M., Kajola, M., & Salonen, O. (1995). Signal-space projections of MEG data characterize both distributed and well-localized neuronal sources. *Electroencephalogr Clin Neurophysiol, 95*(3), 189–200.

Tian, B., Reser, D., Durham, A., Kustov, A., & Rauschecker, J. P. (2001). Functional specialization in rhesus monkey auditory cortex. *Science, 292*(5515), 290–293.

Uusitalo, M. A., & Ilmoniemi, R. J. (1997). Signal-space projection method for separating MEG or EEG into components. *Med Biol Eng Comput, 35*(2), 135–140.

Uutela, K., Hämäläinen, M., & Somersalo, E. (1999). Visualization of magnetoence-phalographic data using minimum current estimates. *Neuroimage, 10*(2), 173–180.

Uutela, K., Taulu, S., & Hämäläinen, M. (2001). Detecting and correcting for head movements in neuromagnetic measurements. *Neuroimage, 14*(6), 1424–1431.

Wagner, M., Köhler, T., Fuchs, M., & Kastner, J. (2000). *An extended source model for current density reconstructions.* Paper presented at the Proceedings of the 12th International Conference on Biomagnetism.

Weisend, M. P., Hanlon, F. M., Montano, R., Ahlfors, S. P., Leuthold, A. C., Mosher, J. C., et al. (2007). Paving the way for cross-site pooling of magnetoencephalography (MEG) data. *Elsevier International Congress Series, 1300*, 615–618.

9

Noninvasive Functional Tomographic Connectivity Analysis with Magnetoencephalography

Joachim Gross, Jan Kujala, Riitta Salmelin, and Alfons Schnitzler

- The excellent temporal resolution of MEG can be used for the non-invasive investigation of long-range interactions between brain areas. This analysis requires statistically validated interaction measures and localization techniques
- We describe several measures for the quantification of neural interactions, their implementation and limitations
- Localization techniques are introduced and discussed with respect to their applicability for MEG connectivity studies
- We describe the identification of significant connectivity effects by using surrogate data and permutation techniques
- As an example, we present in detail the different analysis steps of one particular connectivity study

Introduction

One possible mechanism for neural communication has attracted considerable interest in recent years. Neural synchronization, i.e., temporally precise interactions between neural assemblies, may indicate functionally relevant interactions between these assemblies (Singer, 1999; Bressler & Kelso, 2001; Engel, Fries et al., 2001; Varela, Lachaux et al., 2001; Fries, 2005; Schnitzler & Gross, 2005). Investigating long-range interactions requires simultaneous measurements of neural activity in the entire brain, with high temporal resolution. Connectivity studies using fMRI have successfully been performed (e.g., Buchel & Friston, 1997; Logothetis, 2003; Mechelli, Price et al., 2003), but they are inherently restricted to investigating neuronal interactions on the rather coarse time scale of hemodynamics, which is well beyond the millisecond time range of neural signals.

In contrast, magnetoencephalography (MEG) offers whole-scalp coverage and excellent temporal resolution in the range of milliseconds and below. MEG can not only track rapid changes in the activity of neural populations, but it can also reveal changes in oscillatory activity or oscillatory interactions. Techniques for analyzing and characterizing oscillatory activity and oscillatory interactions have been used at the level of sensor recordings, both in magnetoencephalography and electroencephalography (EEG). Unfortunately, in most cases it is difficult to relate effects observed at different sensors (or EEG electrodes) to brain areas. Nevertheless, the localization is important for the interpretation of results, and adds relevant information.

The noninvasive recording of magnetic fields (associated with neural activity) outside the head leads to limitations in the localization of neural activity (see Chapter 5). Thus, performing MEG functional connectivity analysis at the level of macroscopic brain areas instead of sensor recordings requires caution and a thorough understanding of the localization procedure.

In the following paragraphs we will describe methods that allow the investigation of long-range dynamic interactions between brain areas based on MEG recordings. The aim of this chapter is not a complete review of available methods, but rather an introduction to concepts, methods and approaches that currently play a role in the rapidly evolving field of functional connectivity analysis with MEG.

Measures of Interactions

A large number of methods exist for the characterization of interdependencies between two or more time series. The aim of the characterization is a detailed description of the connection in terms of the time course and frequency of interaction, the type of interaction (e.g., linear or nonlinear) and possibly the direction of interaction. In this section we describe some dependency measures that are most frequently used in the analysis of functional interactions based on electrophysiological recordings. We focus on measures in the frequency domain.

One way to classify functional connectivity measures is the distinction between parametric and nonparametric, and between linear and nonlinear measures. Nonparametric techniques estimate dependency measures directly from the data. They usually employ the fast Fourier transform (FFT), the wavelet transform, or the Hilbert transform. In contrast, parametric techniques fit a model to the data. The estimation of interactions between two time series uses the parameters of the model, and thus relies on the accuracy of the estimated model parameters.

Linear dependency measures assume that the output of the system under investigation is linearly related to the input (scaling the input by a factor A leads to an output scaled by the same factor). Although nonlinear interactions have been demonstrated in electrophysiological recordings (e.g., Breakspear, 2002; Breakspear & Terry, 2002; Stam, Breakspear et al., 2003) linear measures are still widely used. Their advantage is a robust implementation and fast computation, but they suffer from their insensitivity to nonlinear dependencies in the data. In contrast, nonlinear measures can reveal some nonlinear dependencies, but often rely on additional parameters that must be specified by the user.

Nonparametric Dependency Measures

Coherence

Coherence is the most common measure to describe the relationship between two time series. It is defined as the magnitude squared cross spectrum, divided by the power spectra of both time series: $Cxy(f)=|Pxy(f)|^2/(Pxx(f)Pyy(f))$ and ranges between 0 and 1. The cross spectrum is defined as $Pxy(f)=X(f)Y'(f)$ (where Y' denotes the complex conjugate of Y and a capital letter represents the Fourier transform). $Cxy(f1)=1$ indicates a perfect linear relation at frequency f1. The coherence spectrum is usually computed using Welch's method, that is illustrated in Figure 9–1.

The classic coherence measures suffer from several limitations that have led to the development of related measures. First, stationarity of the data is required. Second, if coherences between a number of signals are computed, it is unclear to what extent the coherence between two signals is due to a common input from a third signal. Third, coherence is sensitive to both amplitude and phase dynamics.

Event-related coherence has been used to obtain a time-varying estimate of coherence (Andrew & Pfurtscheller, 1996; Pfurtscheller & Andrew, 1999; Pfurtscheller & Lopes da Silva, 1999) to account for instationarity in the data. Here, averaging of individual segments is not performed over time, but across trials. The FFT window is shifted relative to trial onset, and allows investigation of temporal changes of coherence.

In the second problem, one would like to distinguish the case that area A interacts with area B from the case that both areas interact with a third area C. Both cases could yield the same coherence spectrum between A and B. Partial coherence is an extension to the classical coherence measure that allows one to distinguish between the two cases (Dahlhaus, 2000; Dahlhaus, Eichler et al., 1997; Eichler, Dahlhaus et al., 2003; Halliday, Rosenberg et al., 1995). It allows the computation of coherence between A and B, taking into account the common effect of C. For the characterization of a network of areas, partial

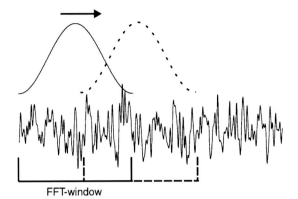

Figure 9–1. Welch's method for spectral computation. A Hanning window is applied to segments of a signal. The FFT-transform is applied to each segment. Finally, the FFT-transform is averaged over successive data segments, which overlap by half their segment length. Coherence and power estimates may be improved by replacing the Hanning window with several orthogonal functions – termed "tapers" – that are based on discrete prolate spheroidal sequences (multitaper spectra). (Thomson, 1982; Mitra & Pesaran, 1999).

coherence can be computed efficiently based on the inverse cross-spectral density matrix of the time courses of all areas (Dahlhaus, 2000).

A third problem of the classical coherence measure—its dependence on amplitude and phase dynamics—may be addressed by complementing a coherence analysis with an analysis of phase synchronization.

Phase Synchronization

It is important to separately characterize phase and amplitude dynamics and their contributions to interactions of time series, since phase dynamics, in particular, may play an important role for the interaction of neuronal processes (Rodriguez, George et al., 1999; Varela, Lachaux et al., 2001). Phase synchronization has been extensively studied for weakly coupled, self-sustained oscillators (Rosenblum & Kurths, 1998). The computation is illustrated in Figure 9–2. Coherence between an electromyographic signal (EMG) reflecting muscle activity and MEG signal is computed (Figure 9–2A) and shows strong coherence in the range 25–31 Hz.

A bandpass filter in this frequency band is applied to both signals (Figure 9–2B). One should be careful to avoid phase delays due to the filtering (e.g., by applying the filter forward and backward).

The temporal evolution of phase and amplitude is computed via the Hilbert transform (Figure 9–2C) (Rosenblum & Kurths, 1998, Le Van Quyen, Foucher et al., 2001), thus accounting for instationarity in the data.

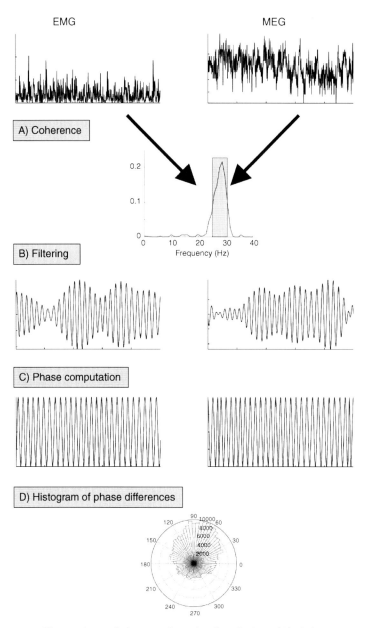

Figure 9–2. Illustration of the synchronization index. (A) Coherence spectrum of electromyographic signal (EMG) and magnetoencephalographic signal (MEG) shows a peak between 25 and 31 Hz. Computation of the synchronization index starts by applying a 25–31 Hz bandpass filter (B). The instantaneous phase is computed by means of Hilbert (or wavelet) transform (C) and phase signals are subtracted from each other. Here, the histogram of phase differences (D) shows a preferred value, i.e., the distribution of phase differences shows a strong deviation from a uniform distribution. The synchronization index quantifies this deviation, and thus the amount of phase-locking between the two signals in this particular frequency range.

To obtain a quantitative measure of synchronization, the phase difference between two time series, and the deviation of the phase difference distribution from a random distribution, can be calculated (Figure 9–2D) and tested for significance against surrogate data (Tass, Rosenblum et al., 1998; Lachaux, Rodriguez et al., 1999). (Surrogate data are artificially generated data that share almost all statistical properties with the original data except the property that is studied.)

Direction of Information Flow

Whereas the above measures are used to identify significant dependencies between time series, the interpretation of functional connectivity results would greatly benefit from further information mainly about the directionality of information flow. The information flow may be unidirectional (sending or receiving) or bidirectional. Due to the wide use of classical spectral analysis, directionality between two signals has often been inferred from a delay estimation based on the phase spectrum $PHIxy(f)=arctan(Im(Pxy(f))/Re(Pxy(f)))$. The rationale behind this idea is that oscillatory information between two areas (or a brain area and motoneuron pool) will be transmitted with a certain delay that depends on the conduction times along the pathway.

A constant delay between two stationary time series x,y would appear in the phase spectrum as a linear relationship between phase and frequency in the frequency range of significant coherence. However, it should be noted that FFT-based methods rely on the assumption of stationarity of the time series, which is usually not the case for human MEG/EEG data. In addition, fitting a line to a noisy phase spectrum requires a broad frequency range of significant coherence (the line can only be fitted in the frequency band of significant coherence). In real data this frequency range is often not broad enough for a stable fit.

Another technique has been used to estimate the time delay between primary motor cortex (M1) and muscle (Gross, Tass et al., 2000). Here, the phase difference (computed from the Hilbert transform of the signal) in the range of significant coherence was computed between the M1 oscillations and the electromyographic signal recorded with surface electrodes. The times of strongest oscillatory activity (yielding the highest signal-to-noise ratio) were selected based on the amplitude of the Hilbert transform. At these times, the phase differences were converted to delays and displayed in a histogram. Deviations from a uniform distribution (evident as peaks in the histogram) indicated a preferred delay that corresponded to known conduction times measured with TMS.

Within the framework of phase synchronization, the directionality index (DI) has been developed (Bezruchko, Ponomarenko et al., 2003; Rosenblum, Cimponeriu et al., 2002; Rosenblum & Pikovsky, 2001) to quantify the dependencies between two self-sustained, weakly coupled oscillators. It is based on the phase dynamics of two signals. The DI quantifies to what degree the phase dynamics of one signal is influenced by the phase dynamics of the other signal. The DI is normalized such that -1 and 1 represent an unidirectional effect (to and from the first time series, respectively) and 0 indicates a symmetric bidirectional effect.

Parametric Dependency Measures

Parametric dependency measures often rely on autoregressive (AR) models (Brovelli, Ding et al., 2004; Chen, Bressler et al., 2006; Ding, Bressler et al., 2000; Kaminski, Ding et al., 2001; Moller, Schack et al., 2001; Schack, Rappelsberger et al., 1999). The AR model represents a mathematical model for time series based on the assumption that values of the time series are weighted sums of the p previous values (p is called "the order of the AR model") and additive noise. A number of methods are available for computing the weights (coefficients) of a model once the order has been specified. Interestingly, power spectra are easily computed from the model coefficients. AR models can be extended to multivariate autoregressive models (MVAR) that allow not only the computation of power spectra, but also of coherence. In addition, the directed transfer function can be computed for MVAR models, and quantifies the frequency-dependent causality of time series A and B (Brovelli, Ding et al., 2004; Kaminski & Liang, 2005; Sameshima & Baccala, 1999). Here, causality is understood in the sense of Granger causality meaning that the prediction of the future of timeseries A can be improved by using the past values of time series B. Similar to the concept of partial coherence, partial directed coherence has been introduced to identify direct interactions between time series (Baccala & Sameshima, 2001).

One can account for instationarities in the data by computing model coefficients in a time window moving across the signals (Ding, Bressler et al., 2000; Moller, Schack et al., 2001).

In addition, methods based on autoregressive models have been introduced to characterize directionality between two signals. These techniques compute a frequency-domain analogue of Granger causality.

Finally, we want to point the interested reader to other (nonlinear) measures that have been applied to MEG/EEG data, particularly generalized synchronization and mutual information (Breakspear & Terry, 2002; Stam, Breakspear et al., 2003; David, Cosmelli et al., 2004; Ioannides, Poghosyan et al., 2004).

Statistical Considerations

Surrogate data offer another, very flexible possibility to identify statistically significant effects in dependency measures (David, Cosmelli et al., 2003; David, Garnero et al., 2002; Hurtado, Rubchinsky et al., 2004; Palus & Hoyer, 1998; Schreiber & Schmitz, 2000). In general, surrogate data are artificially generated data that share almost all statistical properties with the original data, except the property that is studied. We can illustrate the flexible use of surrogate data for coherence spectra. Artificial peaks in coherence spectra due to stable oscillatory signals (e.g., line noise) can be identified by shifting one time series relative to the other, e.g., by 1–2 seconds (Figure 9–3A,B). Coherences from physiological processes are most likely destroyed by the time-shift operation, whereas the artificial coherence peak should not change if the underlying oscillation is stable (Figure 9–3B). To destroy synchronization and oscillations in the time series, both time series can be independently permuted (i.e., the order of the data points is randomly changed; see Figure 9–3C). Applying the same permutation to both time series destroys oscillations but preserves non-oscillatory dependencies between the time series (Figure 9–3D). This particular approach is interesting for the validation of cerebro-cerebral coherence spectra. Depending on the quality of the data, the signal-to-noise ratio (SNR), and the possible presence of artifacts, the coherence spectrum may show a substantial offset (an artificial shift of the spectrum across all frequencies to higher coherence values). The offset is accounted for by the surrogate data, and allows the identification of significant coherence despite the offset. Another relevant type of surrogate data is computed by randomly changing the phase of a signal (for each frequency) without changing the amplitude (Figure 9–3E). The surrogate data has the same power spectrum as the original data (Figure 9–3F) but any coherence between the data is destroyed.

How can we use the methods introduced above to identify a network of interacting brain areas? Three strategies may be employed. First, selection of individual anatomical brain areas based on *a priori* information (e.g., from other studies). Further analysis is needed to establish interactions between these areas. Second, areas are selected based on their activity and subsequently tested for interactions. Third, areas may be selected directly, based on their functional connectivity to other areas. As the first strategy does not require any computation, we describe the second and third strategies in the following paragraphs.

Activation Maps for Network Analysis

In principle, any localization technique that can be applied to unaveraged data may be used for the second strategy (see Chapter 5). In the following, we refer to functional connectivity studies classified according to the localization technique—namely, minimum-norm solutions, magnetic field tomography, spatial filter, or dipole models. In addition to the localization technique, the studies differ in other analysis aspects: First, localization can be performed in the time, frequency, or time-frequency domain. Second, regions of interest can be selected anatomically, by using local maxima in activation maps or significant local maxima according to a statistical procedure. Third, the employed measures that quantify dependencies between the selected regions of interest are different. Some interesting methods are briefly described in the following paragraphs, together with their main features.

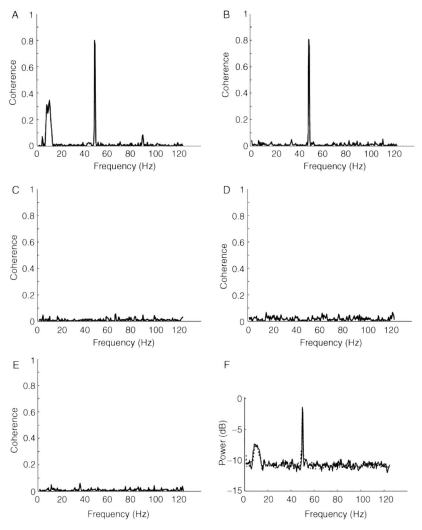

Figure 9–3. Surrogate data for coherence. Two time signals were simulated with a broadband component around 10 Hz and a 50-Hz sinusoid, representing line noise. (A) The original coherence spectrum. (B) Coherence computed with one time series shifted by 1 s. The broadband nonstationary component (representing physiological coherence) has vanished, while the 50-Hz component is not affected. (C) Coherence between the two time series, after the order of data points has been randomly changed independently for each time series (independent permutation). Physiological and artificial coherence is destroyed. (D) Coherence between the time series after the order of data points has been changed in exactly the same way for both time series (same permutation). Again, physiological and artificial coherence is destroyed. (E) Coherence spectrum after random phases have been added to one time series. (F) Power spectrum of the original time series (solid line) and the same time series after phase randomization (dashed line) indicating that the phase randomization does not affect the power spectrum.

Minimum-norm Techniques

In dSPM (dynamic statistical parametric mapping; Lin, Witzel et al., 2004) the source estimation is performed for each single trial after filtering the MEG signals with a complex Morlet wavelet. Power estimates normalized by baseline power are displayed on a cortical map without selecting regions of interest. In addition, cortical maps of phase synchronization to a reference signal can be computed and displayed.

In contrast, the method by David and coworkers (David, Cosmelli et al., 2003; David, Garnero et al., 2002) identifies significantly activated areas in relation to surrogate data. Localization is based on nonaveraged data. An iterative procedure is employed to reduce the number of active volume elements (voxels) leading to sparse and focal source representations. During the iteration, surrogate data (created from random permutation of the measured data) are used to identify significantly activated areas. The final selection of significantly activated voxels is subsequently subjected to a synchronization analysis. The method has been validated with simulated data, and has been applied to an example data set. The use of the iterative sparsening of the source representation is of particular interest in this method. Although the iteration introduces extra *a priori* parameters, it allows for the identification of *significantly* activated areas.

An interesting application of minimum norm source reconstructions has been proposed by Amor, Rudrauf et al. (2005), using the frequency flow measure introduced by Rudrauf and colleagues (Rudrauf, Douiri et al., 2006). The frequency flow analysis is based on an estimation of the instantaneous frequency, and identifies cortical areas with possibly transient common instantaneous frequencies in the time-frequency plane.

Another technique for functional connectivity analysis using the minimum norm inverse solution has been suggested by Astolfi (Astolfi, Cincotti et al., 2005). Regions of interest were identified anatomically, and the directed transfer function (DTF) was evaluated for all combinations of regions of interest. The DTF describes frequency-specific directed interactions between areas, and is computed from a multivariate autoregressive model (see previous section, Measures of Interactions).

Magnetic Field Tomography

Another example, synchronization tomography (Tass, Fieseler et al., 2003), uses a nonlinear localization algorithm—magnetic field tomography (MFT) (Ioannides, Bolton et al. 1990)—to compute current densities within the brain for each recorded data sample. Phase synchronization is subsequently computed on the current density maps for all pairs of voxels. Since MFT is a nonlinear, iterative localization procedure, synchronization tomography requires long computation times on standard workstations. MFT has also been applied to nonaveraged data to localize activated brain areas and to extract their time courses for a subsequent connectivity analysis based on mutual information (Ioannides, Liu et al., 2000; Ioannides, Poghosyan et al., 2004).

Spatial Filter

Spatial filtering is a different method that provides tomographic maps of activated brain areas (Hadjipapas, Hillebrand et al., 2005). Again, synchronization analysis was then applied on the time course of activation in the regions of interest (see the following DICS section for more information on spatial filtering).

Dipole Models

In contrast to the distributed localization techniques described above, source coherence (Hoechstetter, Bornfleth et al., 2004) uses a multidipole model to explain the measured data (see Grasman, Huizenga et al., 2004 for another example). Single-trial dipole waveforms (the time course of activation of dipoles) are subjected to a time-frequency analysis and a subsequent computation of coherence.

A different approach based on dipoles has been described by Makeig (Makeig, Debener et al., 2004; Makeig, Delorme et al., 2004). Here, independent component analysis (ICA) is applied to the nonaveraged data. Synchronization analysis of the time courses of individual components (e.g., by means of phase synchronization) shows frequency-specific interactions between components.

DICS: Activation and Connectivity Maps

Dynamic Imaging of Coherent Sources (Gross, Kujala et al., 2001) allows the tomographic mapping of both power and coherence in the entire brain, using spatial filtering (Robinson & Vrba 1997; Sekihara, Nagarajan et al. 2001a; Sekihara, Nagarajan et al., 2002a; Van Veen, van Drongelen et al., 1997) in the frequency domain (Figure 9–4).

The output of the spatial filter is a linear combination of the adequately weighted channels of the data matrix. Spatial filters can be designed according to very different objectives depending on the aim of the analysis. For source localization, the LCMV (linearly constrained minimum variance) beamformer is often used. Here, the set of coefficients or weights is computed as the solution of a constraint-minimization problem: the minimization of output power subject to the constraint that activity from the region of interest is passed with unit gain. The coefficients depend on the solution of the forward problem for the region of interest, and the covariance matrix of the data. The linear combination of the weighted channels acts like a spatial filter that leaves

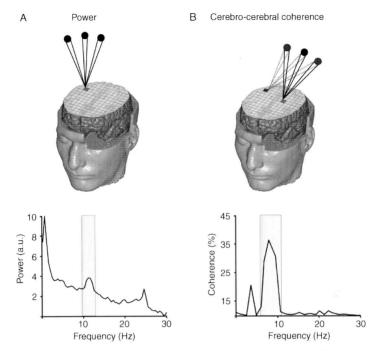

A   Power   B   Cerebro-cerebral coherence

Figure 9–4. Power and coherence mapping with DICS. Uniformly sized volume elements (voxels) are defined to cover the entire brain based on magnetic resonance images (MRI). The sensor information is used to compute the spatial distribution of power (A) or coherence (B) in a predefined frequency band (bottom row).

the signal from the region of interest unchanged and attenuates, as much as possible, signals originating elsewhere.

The filter has to be computed for each region of interest. Indeed, to create a tomographic map of power, the spatial filter must be computed for each voxel on a regular 3-dimensional grid covering the entire brain. Since synchronization is often frequency-dependent, DICS has been developed as a frequency-domain implementation of a spatial filter that allows the tomographic mapping of power and coherence in a predefined frequency band.

We employ the cross-spectral density matrix as the basic representation of the oscillatory components and their dependencies between MEG and possibly additional signals. For continuous data, the complex cross-spectral density P for signals $x(t)$, $y(t)$ is computed using Welch's method of spectral density estimation (Welch, 1967; see also Figure 9–1). For trial-based data, P should be computed using wavelets or a moving FFT window. One element $P_{i,j}$ of the cross-spectral matrix consists of the cross-spectral densities of signals i and j. Therefore, P contains the cross-spectral densities of all combinations of signals.

Two measures are derived from this matrix. First, the power spectrum of the signal i is represented by the diagonal element $P_{i,i}$. It allows identification of frequency bands containing most of the power, or those showing task-dependent changes. Second, coherence is the magnitude-squared cross spectrum divided by the power spectra of both time series.

To obtain a tomographic map of power or coherence, the spatial filter coefficients are computed sequentially for each voxel. Based on the matrix P and the coefficients, the cross spectrum can be computed between any two voxels. If the same two voxels are chosen, the resulting map will show the spatial distribution of power. Alternatively, coherence between a reference voxel and all other voxels in the brain can be mapped based on the cross spectrum of the reference voxel and all other voxels, and power of both voxels.

Except DICS, all the methods introduced in the previous section identify regions of interest based on their activation (maybe in a particular frequency band). DICS also supports the computation of maps representing oscillatory power—but, in addition, it can directly map coherence to a reference area (i.e., the third strategy listed in the section on statistical considerations).

The functioning of a spatial filter can be illustrated in a simplified scenario (Gross, Timmermann et al., 2003). We assume that a single brain area is active. The frequency-dependent power estimate at any given point can be computed as follows:

$$P(\mathbf{r},\mathrm{f})=\left[L_T(\mathbf{r})C(\mathrm{f})^{-1}L(\mathbf{r})\right]^{-1} \tag{9-1}$$

$\mathbf{r}$ denotes the position at which power is estimated, f is the frequency, L is the solution of the forward problem for position $\mathbf{r}$ and two tangential orientations (i.e., the leadfield) and C represents the cross spectrum of all MEG channels. The matrix C can be decomposed using singular value decomposition. The decomposition leads to a projection matrix M_s. M_s projects vectors onto the signal space. The power estimate can then be described (Gross, Timmermann et al., 2003) as

$$P(\mathbf{r},f)=\left[S_1^{-1}L_T(\mathbf{r})M_sL(\mathbf{r})+S_2^{-1}L_T(\mathbf{r})(I-M_s)L(\mathbf{r})\right] \tag{9-2}$$

where S_1 represents the first singular value of C and S_2 the second singular value. $(I-M_s)$ acts as a projection to the noise space.

Now the mechanism of the spatial filter becomes apparent (see Figure 9–5). For this illustration we arbitrarily assume $S_1 = 10$ and $S_2 = 1$. At the true source location (marked by +) the corresponding leadfield is in the signal space. For the first addend in equation 9–2 we get 1/10 (reciprocal value of S_1). In the second addend the projection to the noise space is zero (since $L(\mathbf{r})$ is entirely in the signal space). Consequently, we obtain a value of P=10. For a point close to the true source location (marked by *) the corresponding leadfield is not entirely in the source space but has a component in the noise space. Thus, the first addend becomes smaller (e.g., 0.9/10) and the second addend takes a

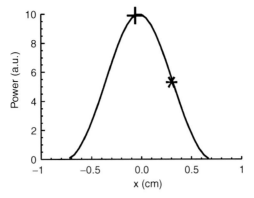

Figure 9–5. Illustration of spatial filter. At each location along the x–axis the power of a point source located at 0 is displayed as computed from a spatial filter directed to this position. The + sign marks the true location for which the solution of the forward problem is entirely in the signal space. The * marks a point for which the solution of the forward problem has a component in noise-space leading to a reduced power estimate.

nonzero value (e.g., 0.1). The resulting value is P=5.3 (Figure 9–5). As we move away from the true source location, the estimated power decreases. The steepness of the decrease depends on the signal-to-noise ratio (SNR, here the ratio S_1/S_2) and the change of the leadfields. This underlines the importance of the SNR for the spatial resolution of beamformer tomographic maps. Efforts to increase the SNR during measurement and analysis (e.g., by using an optimal signal representation) would be rewarded by an increased spatial resolution.

Starting from Activation Maps: Choice of a Localization Method

The choice of the localization procedure should be governed by several considerations. In general, one should be aware of the particular advantages and limitations of the different methods. In addition to considerations that are relevant also for source localizations, functional connectivity analysis imposes further requirements on localization techniques. The method should be robust in the presence of sources with a physiologically plausible degree of correlation (or coherence). In addition, methods yielding sparse source representations should be preferred. Otherwise it is difficult to separate two interacting areas that are close to each other.

Dipole models are well suited for data that show a small number of dipolar field patterns in the topographical maps (e.g., signals recorded from primary sensory areas). For more complex data it is difficult to estimate the correct number of sources, and the assumption of point-like generators may not be valid.

Distributed inverse solutions based on the minimum-norm technique can be efficiently computed, and they are robust in the presence of even highly correlated sources. In their standard implementation they result in rather smooth source representations that have a bias towards superficial generators. More complex, iterative techniques like MFT are also insensitive to high correlations between sources. They provide focal sources but need long computation times. Spatial filtering techniques are computationally very efficient but they are affected by high correlations between areas (Gross, Kujala et al., 2001; Van Veen, van Drongelen et al., 1997). This is due to their adaptive, data-dependent formulation that also leads to a possibly high spatial resolution (see DICS section). Simulations have demonstrated that under physiological conditions (i.e., no correlations or coherence of 1), spatial filtering techniques provide an acurate localization of correlated sources (Gross, Kujala et al., 2001; Hadjipapas, Hillebrand et al., 2005; Sekihara, Nagarajan et al., 2002b). The adaptive, data-dependent nature of spatial filtering techniques can be exploited by optimizing the filter design (e.g., for a particular frequency range of interest), thus improving the spatial resolution of the tomographic maps.

Several software packages are available that implement some of the above-mentioned methods.[1] The source coherence technique is implemented in the commercial software Besa 5 (www.besa.de). LORETA is a free software package that implements low-resolution brain electromagnetic tomography (see http://www.uzh.ch/keyinst/loreta.htm). Several methods are implemented in freely available Matlab toolboxes. Fieldtrip implements spatial filtering techniques and a number of spectral analysis methods (http://fieldtrip. fcdonders.nl/). Another implementation of spatial filters is provided in Nutmeg (www.nutmeg.edu/). Brainstorm implements dipole models and minimum norm solutions (neuroimage.usc.edu/brainstorm). EEGlab contains an algorithm for independent component analysis (ICA) and a plugin for dipole fitting (sccn.ucsd.edu/eeglab/).

Selecting Regions of Interest: Significance Tests

The identification of regions of interest (either from activation maps or functional connectivity maps) should be based on statistical methods. This requirement is not specific to functional connectivity analysis, but holds true for any localization study. As described above, regions of interest may be selected *a priori*, based on their activity or based on their interaction with some reference signal (e.g., muscle activity or activity of a cerebral reference area). DICS allows the direct mapping of either power or coherence. The other methods first generate distributed source representations and subsequently create maps of coherence to a given reference signal. In most cases, tomographic functional maps representing either oscillatory activity, or coupling with a reference area, are obtained.

In principle, regions of interest can be selected from activation maps after normalization to pseudo-T maps using noise estimates (Dale, Halgren et al., 2000; Van Veen, van Drongelen et al., 1997; Vrba & Robinson, 2001). Preferably, methods should be used that account for the multiple-comparison problem. Performing a statistical test for each voxel (or surface node) results in an increase of the possible numbers of false positive results. Consequently, the statistical procedure should account for the number of tests. The simplest method is the Bonferroni correction that can be performed by multiplying the resulting p-values by the number of tests. For spatially correlated maps (as in our case) with many elements, this method is not effective and too conservative. Two approaches may be used that are more efficient.

First, random field theory has successfully been applied for the corresponding problem of statistically analyzing fMRI (functional magnetic resonance imaging) or PET (positron emission tomography) data (Worsley & Friston, 1995). It has recently been adapted for distributed source representations from MEG/EEG recordings (e.g., Barnes & Hillebrand, 2003; Carbonell, Galan et al., 2004; Pantazis, Nichols et al., 2005); see also Kiebel, Tallon-Baudry et al. (2005). The approach from Carbonell, Galan et al. (2004) offers a unified statistical framework for the identification of significant components in topographic and tomographic representations of the data. Thus, the method can be applied to the data recorded by the sensors, and the data linearly mapped into the brain to create maps of brain activity. Barnes and coworkers (Barnes & Hillebrand, 2003) employed random field theory to specifically address the multiple-comparison problem on tomographic maps created by spatial filtering. A limitation of random field theory for MEG is dependence on the assumptions of sufficient smoothness, gaussianity, and stationarity of the underlying data.

Second, permutation methods may be used to extract significant regions of interest while correcting for multiple tests. Similarly to random field theory, permutation tests have been applied to functional magnetic resonance data (Nichols & Holmes, 2002). Permutation methods rely on very few assumptions, which are illustrated in the following example. Let us assume that MEG data was continuously recorded during two experimental conditions, A (e.g., rest) and B (e.g., continuous finger movements). We want to know which areas in the brain show a significantly different activation between the two conditions. Specifically, the null hypothesis is that a change of the experimental condition has no effect on the activation of brain areas. Any of the described localization procedures can be used to compute a distributed source representation for condition A and B. Statistics can then be computed that characterize the difference between A and B. As preparation for the permutation approach, each data set is split into a number of segments of equal length.[2] Before carrying out the localization, the data segments from A and B are randomly exchanged. Thus, the first and the second localization is now performed on a random set of data segments from both conditions. Subsequently, the same test statistics (e.g., relative difference) is evaluated on both functional maps. The random exchange of segments, localization, and evaluation of the test statistics, is repeated a large number of times. For each repetition the maximum of the test statistics is identified. This results in the distribution of the maximum statistics. The critical threshold corresponding to a given significance level α (e.g., 0.05) can be identified as the $(\alpha^{\star}N)+1$ largest element of the distribution where N is the number of repetitions. It can be shown that the use of the maximum statistics provides a strong protection against Type 1 error, i.e., rejecting the null hypothesis when it is true (Nichols & Holmes, 2002).

Permutation methods make no assumptions on the distribution of the data (and can thus be applied to activation or connectivity maps) but they require the exchangeability of the segments.

Using permutation methods with the maximum statistics on real data may lead to problems if the null distribution is too variable across voxels. If the simple difference between two conditions is used, the maximum statistics may be dominated by some voxels with a large variability in the mean difference. This leads to a reduced sensitivity for other voxels. When that is the case, other statistics (such as t-statistics) that lead to more homogeneous distributions across voxels should be used (Nichols & Holmes, 2002; Pantazis, Nichols et al., 2005).

Pantazis and coworkers performed a comparison of random field theory and permutation methods for functional maps obtained from MEG data (Pantazis, Nichols et al., 2005). For simulated data both methods showed valid results, although the method based on random field theory demonstrated conservative performance and a dependence on the smoothness of the data. Differences in real data that were observed between the methods may have been caused by violations of the distribution assumption of random field theory.

Permutation statistics for MEG data have been used by several groups in various ways (e.g., Chau, McIntosh et al., 2004; Greenblatt & Pflieger, 2004; Gross, Schmitz et al., 2004; Singh, Barnes et al., 2003) that demonstrate the flexibility of permutation methods. They can be applied to test for significant differences between two conditions for single subjects or for a group of subjects, or to test for significant differences between two groups of subjects for one condition.

Permutation methods are implemented in SnPM (www.sph.umich.edu/ ni-stat/SnPM/; Nichols & Holmes, 2002). This particular implementation has been used for the analysis of MEG tomographic maps (Gross, Schmitz et al. 2004; Singh, Barnes et al., 2003). Another noncommercial Matlab toolbox that implements permutation methods is Fieldtrip (for web page, see above).

An interesting approach that should be mentioned in this context is the application of partial least squares (PLS) analysis on tomographic maps (www. rotman-baycrest.on.ca/index.php?section=84) (McIntosh & Lobaugh, 2004). PLS is a multivariate method that performs a singular value decomposition of the covariance of sets of variables. The method is very flexible, since the variables may contain MEG signals, spectra, behavioral results like reaction times, tomographic maps, or other data from different conditions and subjects.

A simple application may be the singular value decomposition of the covariance of the experimental design matrix, and the tomographic maps of the different conditions. The results are singular values and latent variables. The singular values represent the covariance explained by the latent variables. The latent variables optimally capture the effect of the experimental conditions on the data—i.e., they reveal which parts of the data have the strongest covariance with the experimental design matrix. Significance of latent variables is assessed by means of permutation test.

Analysis Strategies and Practical Considerations

A critical step in tomographic functional connectivity studies using MEG is network identification. If regional activation (the second strategy described in the section on statistical considerations) is used for network identification, one should carefully choose the signal representation that is used for localization. The optimal signal representation ultimately determines the quality of the network identification. The choice of the signal representation should be made based on the maximization of the signal-to-noise ratio of the effect of interest (after careful artifact rejection). For example, frequency spectra are the optimal signal representation for oscillatory signal components. If one aims at localizing continuous oscillations, Welch's method can be applied on the continuous recordings to obtain the cross spectra (after carefully choosing the length of the FFT window). Peaks in the power spectra can then be localized. For transient oscillations, wavelet transforms are more appropriate.

If little *a priori* information is available about the effect of interest (e.g., its time or frequency) one should start at the sensor level. A computation of spectra (for continuous data) or time-frequency maps (for epoch data) for each sensor is a reasonable first step. In order to account for the stronger power of low-frequency components, a frequency-specific normalization is advisable (e.g., (A-mean(B))/mean(B) or (A-mean(B))/std(B) where A is the post-stimulus data, B is the baseline data, and std represents the standard deviation). These signal representations can then be tested for significant differences between experimental conditions. Parameters of the frequency or time-frequency computation can be optimized to increase the signal-to-noise ratio (e.g., the use of multi-taper spectra can be particularly beneficial for effects in the gamma frequency range [Mitra & Pesaran, 1999]).

The second approach usually requires the choice of a reference signal. In some studies, muscle activity was used as the reference signal to identify the brain area to which it showed strongest coupling (e.g., Pollok, Gross et al., 2004; Sudmeyer, Pollok et al., 2004; Timmermann, Gross et al., 2003). This area can then be used as a reference region for a cerebro-cerebral coherence analysis. Often, this extra information is not available. Using modern computers, a matrix can be computed that represents coherence (or any other dependency measure) between all voxel combinations at a particular frequency. The diagonal of the matrix could contain power for each voxel at this frequency.

Permutation tests could reveal significant differences between conditions. Thus, an entire network can be identified from this matrix.

Several problems may arise if broad-band activation time courses are computed for regions of interest that were identified in tomographic maps. If localization is performed in the frequency domain (e.g., on the cross-spectral matrix), the properties (e.g., the spatial resolution) of the spatial filters are different compared to a filter based on the covariance matrix (including all frequency components).

Another relevant point for the computation of activation time courses is the choice of the exact coordinates of the spatial filter. Tomographic maps can only be computed with a limited spatial resolution (usually a few millimeters), which may not allow optimal identification of the center of the region of interest. The maximum obtained from the tomographic map can be used as an initial estimate for a nonlinear bounded optimization (e.g., using the Nelder-Mead algorithm implemented in Matlab). Within the optimization procedure, activation time courses are computed for various positions and orientations. The criteria for optimization depend on the data (e.g., to maximize the ratio of mean post-stimulus power to mean baseline power). This optimization may significantly improve the time-course estimation.

Example: Slow Finger Movements

In the following paragraphs we describe a particular MEG functional connectivity study (Gross, Timmermann et al., 2002) and guide the reader through the different steps of the analysis.

Paradigm

This study employed a mapping of cerebro-cerebral coherence without the intermediate step of localizing activated brain areas. The study used DICS to map cerebro-cerebral coherence during slow finger movements (Gross, Timmermann et al., 2002). Subjects were asked to perform slow flexion and extension movements of the right index finger, sinusoidally, at a frequency of 0.5 Hz (Figure 9–6). Subjects were trained with a visual target signal and feedback of their finger position. Subjects were recorded during three 2-minute periods of self-paced movements. Neural activity was measured with 122 sensors at a temporal resolution of 1 millisecond. Simultaneously, muscle activity from three hand and finger muscles was recorded with surface electrodes (EMG), together with the position of the tip of the right index finger using an ultrasound device. In the analysis presented here, the EMG signal from the right *extensor digitorum communis* (EDC) muscle and the velocity of the finger tip is used.

The slow movements are known to be associated with rhythmic changes at 6–9 Hz in the velocity of the finger (Vallbo & Wessberg, 1993; Wessberg & Vallbo, 1995; Wessberg & Vallbo, 1996; Wessberg & Kakuda, 1999).

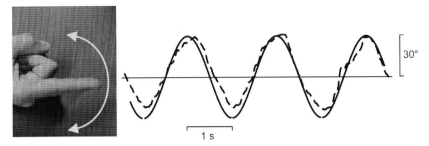

Figure 9–6. Study of slow finger movements. The subjects were asked to perform smooth and slow (0.5 Hz) flexions and extensions of the right index finger. The solid line shows the visually presented target signal used for training. The dashed line corresponds to the actual movement of the subject measured with an ultrasound device.

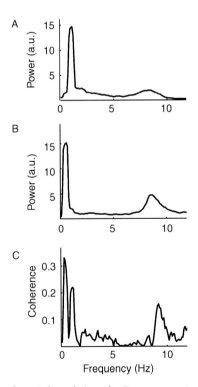

Figure 9–7. Spectra of peripheral signals. Power spectra of velocity of right finger tip (A) and muscle activity (EMG signal, B) show maxima at the movement frequency (or harmonics) and at about 8 Hz. (C). Coherence of both signals shows interdependencies at the movement frequency (and first harmonics) and at about 8 Hz.

235

After excluding peripheral mechanisms as causes of the discontinuities, the authors suggested a central origin.

Peripheral Signals

First, power and coherence spectra were computed for muscle activity and finger velocity for all subjects. As expected from the previous studies, regular changes in finger movements were seen at about 8 Hz in power spectra of muscle activity and finger velocity, and also in coherence between those signals (Figure 9–7). The frequency of these regular changes varied across subjects in the range 6–9 Hz. For each individual subject, the exact frequency of maximum power in the finger velocity was determined for the subsequent analysis. The findings from this analysis step confirmed the previously published results (e.g., Vallbo & Wessberg, 1993).

Cerebro-muscular Coherence

The aim of the next analysis step was the identification of possible cerebro-muscular coherence. To this end, coherence between all MEG signals and the muscle activity was computed for each subject. Figure 9–8 shows the results

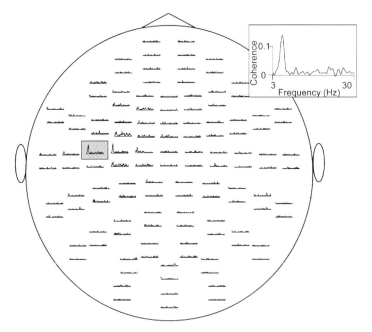

Figure 9–8. Topography of cortico-muscular coherence. Coherence spectra of EMG signal and all MEG signals are shown in a flattened view of the sensor layout. Strongest coherence to muscle signal can be seen at about 8 Hz in a sensor overlying the left sensorimotor cortex.

from an individual subject. Coherence at about 8 Hz can be seen between sensors above the left sensorimotor area and muscle activity from the right EDC muscle. This result was confirmed in the other subjects and indicated the existence of cerebro-muscular coherence at the frequency of the regular velocity changes of finger movements.

In the next step DICS was applied to localize cerebro-muscular coherence in each subject. The frequency of maximum cerebro-muscular coherence was determined for each individual subject from the sensor plots (Figure 9–8). A 2-Hz frequency range around these individual frequencies was used to perform the localization with DICS. Figure 9–9A shows the thresholded map of coherence to the right EDC muscle for one subject. All 9 subjects showed the strongest cerebro-muscular coherence to muscle in the contralateral sensorimotor cortex.

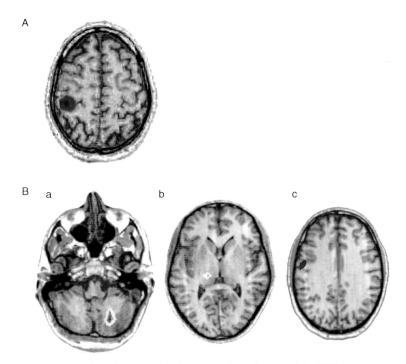

Figure 9–9. Localization results for a single subject. (A). DICS was used to compute a functional map of cerebro-muscular coherence. For each voxel in the brain, coherence of activity in this voxel to muscle activity is computed, and coherence at 8 Hz is used for color coding. Maximum coherence is evident in the contralateral sensorimotor cortex. (B). Coherence between the contralateral primary motor cortex and all other voxels in the brain was computed with DICS. Local maxima in the coherence map were found in ipsilateral cerebellum (a), contralateral thalamus (b) and contralateral premotor cortex (c).

Cerebro-cerebral Coherence

The computation of cerebro-cerebral coherence requires the selection of a reference point. Our previous localization of cerebro-muscular coherence leads to a natural selection of a reference point: the individual maximum of cerebro-muscular coherence at 6–9 Hz, which is located in the primary motor cortex. Using this approach, we track the peripherally observed effect to the cortex and further on to other areas in the brain. If this approach is not possible (e.g., because the effect can not be observed in peripheral signals) one has to resort to an *a priori* selection of a reference area, to select it from the set of significantly activated areas, or to compute the coherence between all combinations of voxels.

The cerebro-cerebral coherence analysis with DICS resulted in tomographic maps of coherence to primary motor cortex. Again, the individual frequency band (from the cerebro-muscular coherence analysis) was used for localization. Visual inspection of local maxima in the coherence maps revealed a number of areas. Figure 9–9B displays local maxima in the coherence maps in ipsilateral cerebellum (a), thalamus (b), and premotor cortex (c). To identify the areas that are consistently involved across subjects, the individual tomographic maps were spatially normalized in SPM99, and subjected to a statistical group analysis (one sample t-test). This procedure resulted in the identification of a network consisting of contralateral primary motor cortex, premotor cortex, thalamus, and ipsilateral cerebellum (Figure 9–10).

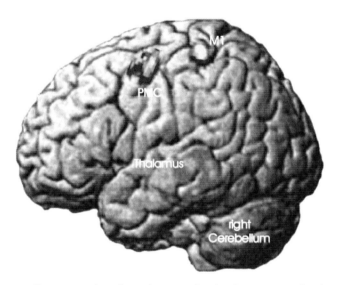

Figure 9–10. Group results of cerebro-cerebral coherence. Individual maps of coherence to left motor cortex in the 6–9 Hz band were spatially normalized and subjected to a one-sample t-test in SPM99. Significant areas are shown (p<0.05, corrected, modified from Gross, Timmermann et al., 2002).

The significance of these results does not lie in the identification of the cerebello-thalamo-cortical loop (which has been described before) but in the functional characterization of the loop in the current paradigm. The study showed for the first time an oscillatory interaction at 6–9 Hz within this loop, and its relation to finger velocity changes at the same frequency. The oscillatory interplay within the network may well implement discrete movement control (Gross, Timmermann et al., 2002).

In this particular study, network identification as a critical part of the functional connectivity analysis was performed using group statistics of coherence maps. A similar approach has been used in other studies (Pollok, Gross et al., 2004; Sudmeyer, Pollok et al.,. 2004; Timmermann, Gross et al., 2003).

Discussion and Perspectives

Noninvasive functional connectivity analysis with MEG is a new field that opens up exciting possibilities to significantly enhance our understanding about basic principles governing efficient information processing in the brain. Neural activity is recorded with high temporal resolution that allows to analyze the transient neural dynamics. In conjunction with localization techniques, time courses of activity in selected regions of interest can be computed and subjected to further analysis, characterizing the temporal evolution of dependencies between the regions. Due to its high temporal resolution and whole-scalp coverage, MEG offers unique information about long-range interactions in the human brain. With further methodological developments that are currently underway, we can expect to reliably observe neural communication processes under physiological and pathological conditions.

Nevertheless, one should keep in mind the limitations of functional tomographic connectivity analysis with MEG, particularly when interpreting the results. For example, it is important to realize that most localization techniques cannot reliably estimate the extent of an activated brain area. Even if statistical criteria are used for the computation of a threshold, the size of a distributed source representation is often more related to particular properties of the data (e.g., signal-to-noise ratio) than to the extent of an activated area. One should also be cautious in the interpretation of interactions between areas. Even if sophisticated measures (like partial coherence, or the directed transfer function) are used on a carefully selected network, there is no way to assure the completeness of the network. Thus, interactions that have been identified as direct may be due to the influence of an "invisible" area. In addition, the existence of significant dependency during a specific experimental condition does not necessarily mean that this dependency is functionally relevant. Significant differences in dependency measures are more reliable for the identification of task-relevant interactions.

In this rapidly evolving field, methodological developments take place in several directions. Statistical methods primarily based on permutation techniques and surrogate data are developed, adapted and validated for high-dimensional data. Similarly, algorithms for data mining and dimensionality reduction become increasingly important. These methods often rely on principal component analysis (see, e.g., PLS), independent component analysis, hierarchical clustering, or multidimensional scaling. An interesting approach that has recently been developed is dynamic causal modeling (DCM). DCM is specifically designed to allow the investigation of effective connectivity. In DCM the brain is described as a deterministic dynamical system that is perturbed by external stimuli. The stimuli cause changes in modeled areas. The measurement is predicted based on a forward model, and the parameters describing the areas and their interactions are fitted to minimize the deviation from the measured signals (Friston, Harrison et al., 2003). In addition, neural mass models are used to understand the relation between certain physiologically meaningful parameters and phenomena observable in EEG/MEG recordings, such as particular spectral peaks or event-related components. (David, Cosmelli et al., 2004; David, Harrison et al., 2005; Rennie, Robinson et al., 2002). Furthermore, functional connectivity analysis will very likely benefit from the incorporation of anatomical connectivity information (e.g., Passingham, Stephan et al., 2002; Sporns, Tononi et al., 2005).

Notes

1 Please note that this list is not complete.
2 For localizations in the frequency domain, Fourier-transformed data segments can be used.

References

Amor, F., Rudrauf, D., et al. (2005). Imaging brain synchrony at high spatio-temporal resolution: application to MEG signals during absence seizures. *Signal Processing 85*, 2101–2111.

Andrew, C., & Pfurtscheller, G. (1996). Event-related coherence as a tool for studying dynamic interaction of brain regions. *Electroencephalogr Clin Neurophysiol 98*(2), 144–148.

Astolfi, L., & Cincotti, F., et al. (2005). Assessing cortical functional connectivity by linear inverse estimation and directed transfer function: simulations and application to real data. *Clin Neurophysiol 116*(4), 920–932.

Baccala, L. A., & Sameshima, K. (2001). Partial directed coherence: a new concept in neural structure determination. *Biol Cybern, 84*(6), 463–474.

Barnes, G. R., & Hillebrand, A. (2003). Statistical flattening of MEG beamformer images. *Hum Brain Mapp 18*(1), 1–12.

Bezruchko, B., Ponomarenko, V., et al. (2003). Characterizing direction of coupling from experimental observations. *Chaos, 13*(1), 179–184.

Breakspear, M. (2002). Nonlinear phase desynchronization in human electroencephalographic data. *Hum Brain Mapp, 15*(3), 175–198.

Breakspear, M., & Terry, J. R. (2002). Nonlinear interdependence in neural systems: motivation, theory, and relevance. *Int J Neurosci 112*(10), 1263–1284.

Bressler, S. L., & Kelso, J. A. (2001). Cortical coordination dynamics and cognition. *Trends Cogn Sci 5*(1), 26–36.

Brovelli, A., & Ding, M., et al. (2004). Beta oscillations in a large-scale sensorimotor cortical network: directional influences revealed by Granger causality. *Proc Natl Acad Sci USA 101*(26), 9849–9854.

Buchel, C., & Friston, K. J. (1997). Modulation of connectivity in visual pathways by attention: cortical interactions evaluated with structural equation modelling and fMRI. *Cereb Cortex 7*(8), 768–778.

Carbonell, F., Galan, L., et al. (2004). Random field-union intersection tests for EEG/MEG imaging. *Neuroimage, 22*(1), 268–276.

Chau, W., McIntosh, A. R., et al. (2004). Improving permutation test power for group analysis of spatially filtered MEG data. *Neuroimage, 23*(3), 983–996.

Chen, Y., Bressler, S. L., et al. (2006). Frequency decomposition of conditional Granger causality and application to multivariate neural field potential data. *J Neurosci Methods 150*(2), 228–237.

Dahlhaus, R. (2000). Graphical interaction models for multivariate time series. *Metrika, 51*, 157–172.

Dahlhaus, R., Eichler, M., et al. (1997). Identification of synaptic connections in neural ensembles by graphical models. *J Neurosci Methods, 77*(1), 93–107.

Dale, A., Halgren, E., et al. (2000). Spatiotemporal cortical activation patterns during semantic processing of novel and repeated words as revealed by combined fMRI and MEG. *Neuron, 26*, 55–67.

David, O., Cosmelli, D., et al. (2004). Evaluation of different measures of functional connectivity using a neural mass model. *Neuroimage, 21*(2), 659–673.

David, O., Cosmelli, D., et al. (2003). A multitrial analysis for revealing significant corticocortical networks in magnetoencephalography and electroencephalography. *Neuroimage, 20*(1), 186–201.

David, O., Garnero, L., et al. (2002). Estimation of neural dynamics from MEG/EEG cortical current density maps: application to the reconstruction of large-scale cortical synchrony. *IEEE Trans Biomed Eng, 49*(9), 975–987.

David, O., Harrison, L., et al. (2005). Modelling event-related responses in the brain. *Neuroimage, 25*(3), 756–770.

Ding, M., Bressler, S. L., et al. (2000). Short-window spectral analysis of cortical event–related potentials by adaptive multivariate autoregressive modeling: data preprocessing, model validation, and variability assessment. *Biol Cybern 83*(1), 35–45.

Eichler, M., Dahlhaus, R., et al. (2003). Partial correlation analysis for the identification of synaptic connections. *Biol Cybern 89*(4), 289–302.

Engel, A. K., Fries, P., et al. (2001). Dynamic predictions: oscillations and synchrony in top-down processing. *Nat Rev Neurosci 2*(10), 704–716.

Fries, P. (2005). A mechanism for cognitive dynamics: neuronal communication through neuronal coherence. *Trends Cogn Sci, 9*(10), 474–480.

Friston, K. J., Harrison, L., et al. (2003). Dynamic causal modelling. *Neuroimage, 19*(4), 1273–1302.

Grasman, R. P., Huizenga, H. M., et al. (2004). Frequency domain simultaneous source and source coherence estimation with an application to MEG. *IEEE Trans Biomed Eng 51*(1), 45–55.

Greenblatt, R. E. & Pflieger, M. E. (2004). Randomization-based hypothesis testing from event-related data. *Brain Topogr, 16*(4), 225–232.

Gross, J., Kujala, J., et al. (2001). Dynamic imaging of coherent sources: Studying neural interactions in the human brain. *Proc Natl Acad Sci U S A 98*(2), 694–699.

Gross, J., Schmitz, F., et al. (2004). Modulation of long-range neural synchrony reflects temporal limitations of visual attention in humans. *Proc Natl Acad Sci U S A, 101*(35), 13050–13055.

Gross, J., Tass, P., et al. (2000). Cortico-muscular synchronization during isometric muscle contraction in humans as revealed by magnetoencephalography. *J Physiol (Lond) 527*(3), 623–631.

Gross, J., L. Timmermann, et al. (2002). "The neural basis of intermittent motor control in humans." *Proc Natl Acad Sci U S A 99*(4): 2299–2302.

Gross, J., Timmermann, L., et al. (2003). Properties of MEG tomographic maps obtained with spatial filtering. *Neuroimage 19*(4), 1329–1336.

Hadjipapas, A., Hillebrand, A., et al. (2005). Assessing interactions of linear and nonlinear neuronal sources using MEG beamformers: a proof of concept. *Clin Neurophysiol 116*(6), 1300–1313.

Halliday, D. M., Rosenberg, J. R., et al. (1995). A framework for the analysis of mixed time series/point process data–theory and application to the study of physiological tremor, single motor unit discharges and electromyograms. *Prog Biophys Mol Biol 64*(2–3), 237–278.

Hoechstetter, K., Bornfleth, H., et al. (2004). BESA source coherence: a new method to study cortical oscillatory coupling. *Brain Topogr, 16*(4), 233–238.

Hurtado, J. M., Rubchinsky, L. L., et al. (2004). Statistical method for detection of phase-locking episodes in neural oscillations. *J Neurophysiol, 91*(4), 1883–1898.

Ioannides, A. A., Bolton, J. P. R., et al. (1990). Continous probabilistic solutions to the biomagnetic inverse problem. *Inverse Problems, 6*, 523–542.

Ioannides, A. A., Liu, L. C., et al. (2000). Coupling of regional activations in a human brain during an object and face affect recognition task. *Hum Brain Mapp 11*(2), 77–92.

Ioannides, A. A., Poghosyan, V., et al. (2004). Real-time neural activity and connectivity in healthy individuals and schizophrenia patients. *Neuroimage, 23*(2), 473–482.

Kaminski, M., Ding, M., et al. (2001). Evaluating causal relations in neural systems: granger causality, directed transfer function and statistical assessment of significance. *Biol Cybern, 85*(2), 145–157.

Kaminski, M. & Liang, H. (2005). Causal influence: advances in neurosignal analysis. *Crit Rev Biomed Eng, 33*(4), 347–430.

Kiebel, S. J., Tallon-Baudry, C., et al. (2005). Parametric analysis of oscillatory activity as measured with EEG/MEG. *Hum Brain Mapp, 26*(3), 170–177.

Lachaux, J. P., Rodriguez, E., et al. (1999). Measuring phase synchrony in brain signals. *Hum Brain Mapp 8*(4), 194–208.

Le Van Quyen, M., Foucher, J., et al. (2001). Comparison of Hilbert transform and wavelet methods for the analysis of neuronal synchrony. *J Neurosci Methods 111*(2), 83–98.

Lin, F. H., Witzel, T., et al. (2004). Spectral spatiotemporal imaging of cortical oscillations and interactions in the human brain. *Neuroimage, 23*(2), 582–595.

Logothetis, N. K. (2003). MR imaging in the non-human primate: studies of function and of dynamic connectivity. *Curr Opin Neurobiol, 13*(5), 630–642.

Makeig, S., Debener, S., et al. (2004). Mining event-related brain dynamics. *Trends Cogn Sci, 8*(5), 204–210.

Makeig, S., Delorme, A., et al. (2004). Electroencephalographic brain dynamics following manually responded visual targets. *PLoS Biol, 2*(6), e176.

McIntosh, A. R. & Lobaugh, N. J. (2004). Partial least squares analysis of neuroimaging data: applications and advances. *Neuroimage, 23* Suppl 1, S250–63.

Mechelli, A., Price, C. J., et al. (2003). A dynamic causal modeling study on category effects: bottom-up or top-down mediation? *J Cogn Neurosci*, *15*(7), 925–934.

Mitra, P. P. & Pesaran, B. (1999). Analysis of dynamic brain imaging data. *Biophys J*, *76*(2), 691–708.

Moller, E., Schack, B., et al. (2001). Instantaneous multivariate EEG coherence analysis by means of adaptive high-dimensional autoregressive models. *J Neurosci Methods*, *105*(2), 143–158.

Nichols, T. E. & Holmes, A. P. (2002). Nonparametric permutation tests for functional neuroimaging: a primer with examples. *Human Brain Mapping 15*(1), 1–25.

Palus, M. & Hoyer, D. (1998). Detecting nonlinearity and phase synchronization with surrogate data. *IEEE Eng Med Biol Mag*, *17*(6), 40–45.

Pantazis, D., Nichols, T. E., et al. (2005). A comparison of random field theory and permutation methods for the statistical analysis of MEG data. *Neuroimage*, *25*(2), 383–394.

Passingham, R. E., Stephan, K. E., et al. (2002). The anatomical basis of functional localization in the cortex. *Nat Rev Neurosci*, *3*(8), 606–616.

Pfurtscheller, G. & Andrew, C. (1999). Event-related changes of band power and coherence: Methodology and interpretation. *J Clin Neurophysiol*, *16*(6), 512–519.

Pfurtscheller, G. & Lopes da Silva, F. H. (1999). Event-related EEG/MEG synchronization and desynchronization: basic principles. *Clin Neurophysiol*, *110*(11), 1842–1857.

Pollok, B., Gross, J., et al. (2004). The Cerebral Oscillatory Network of Voluntary Tremor. *J Physiol*, *554*, 871–878.

Rennie, C. J., Robinson, P. A., et al. (2002). Unified neurophysical model of EEG spectra and evoked potentials. *Biol Cybern 86*(6), 457–471.

Robinson, S. E. & Vrba, J. (1997). Functional neuroimaging by synthetic aperture magnetometry (SAM). In: T. Yoshimoto, M. Kotani, S. Kuriki, H. Karibe & B. Nakasato. *Recent Advances in Biomagnetism*. Sendai: Tohoku University Press, pp. 302–305.

Rodriguez, E., George, N., et al. (1999). Perception's shadow: long-distance synchronization of human brain activity. *Nature*, *397*(6718), 430–433.

Rosenblum, M. G., Cimponeriu, L., et al. (2002). Identification of coupling direction: application to cardiorespiratory interaction. *Phys Rev E Stat Nonlin Soft Matter Phys*, *65*(4 Pt 1), 041909.

Rosenblum, M. G. & Kurths, J. (1998). Analysing Synchronization Phenomena from Bivariate Data by Means of the Hilbert Transform. In: Kantz, H., Kurths, J. & Mayer-Kress, G. (pp. 91–99). *Nonlinear Analysis of Physiological Data*. Berlin: Springer.

Rosenblum, M. G. & Pikovsky, A. S. (2001). Detecting direction of coupling in interacting oscillators. *Phys Rev E Stat Phys Plasmas Fluids Relat Interdisc Topics*, *64*(4-2), 1–4.

Rudrauf, D., Douiri, A., et al. (2006). Frequency flows and the time-frequency dynamics of multivariate phase synchronization in brain signals. *Neuroimage*, *31*(1), 209–227.

Sameshima, K. & Baccala, L. A. (1999). Using partial directed coherence to describe neuronal ensemble interactions. *J Neurosci Methods*, *94*(1), 93–103.

Schack, B., Rappelsberger, P., et al. (1999). Adaptive phase estimation and its application in EEG analysis of word processing. *Journal of Neuroscience Methods 93*(1), 49–59.

Schnitzler, A. & Gross, J. (2005). Normal and pathological oscillatory communication in the brain. *Nat Rev Neurosci*, *6*(4), 285–296.

Schreiber, T. & Schmitz, A. (2000). Surrogate time series. *Physica D, 142*, 346–382.

Sekihara, K., Nagarajan, S. S., et al. (2001). Reconstructing spatio-temporal activities of neural sources using an MEG vector beamformer technique. *IEEE Trans Biomed Eng 48*(7), 760–771.

Sekihara, K., Nagarajan, S. S., et al. (2002a). Application of an MEG eigenspace beamformer to reconstructing spatio-temporal activities of neural sources. *Hum Brain Mapp 15*(4), 199–215.

Sekihara, K., Nagarajan, S. S., et al. (2002b). Performance of an MEG adaptive-beamformer technique in the presence of correlated neural activities: effects on signal intensity and time-course estimates. *IEEE Trans Biomed Eng 49*(12 Pt 2), 1534–46.

Singer, W. (1999). Neuronal synchrony: a versatile code for the definition of relations? *Neuron 24*(1), 49–65, 111–125.

Singh, K. D., Barnes, G. R., et al. (2003). Group imaging of task-related changes in cortical synchronisation using nonparametric permutation testing. *Neuroimage 19*(4), 1589–1601.

Sporns, O., Tononi, G., et al. (2005). The human connectome: a structural description of the human brain. *PLoS Comput Biol 1*(4), e42.

Stam, C. J., Breakspear, M., et al. (2003). Nonlinear synchronization in EEG and whole-head MEG recordings of healthy subjects. *Hum Brain Mapp, 19*(2), 63–78.

Sudmeyer, M., Pollok, B., et al. (2004). Postural tremor in Wilson's disease: A magnetoencephalographic study. *Mov Disord, 19*(12), 1476–1482.

Tass, P., Rosenblum, M. G., et al. (1998). Detection of n:m Phase Locking from Noisy Data: Application to Magnetoencephalography. *Phys Rev Lett 81*(15), 3291–3294.

Tass, P. A., Fieseler, T., et al. (2003). Synchronization tomography: a method for three-dimensional localization of phase synchronized neuronal populations in the human brain using magnetoencephalography. *Phys Rev Lett, 90*(8), 088101.

Thomson, D. J. (1982). Spectrum estimation and harmonic analysis. *Proc IEEE 70*(9), 1055–1096.

Timmermann, L., Gross, J., et al. (2003). The cerebral oscillatory network of parkinsonian resting tremor. *Brain 126*(Pt 1), 199–212.

Vallbo, A. B., & Wessberg, J. (1993). Organization of motor output in slow finger movements in man. *J Physiol (Lond), 469*, 673–691.

Van Veen, B. D., van Drongelen,W., et al. (1997). Localization of brain electrical activity via linearly constrained minimum variance spatial filtering. *IEEE Trans Biomed Eng 44*(9), 867–880.

Varela, F., Lachaux, J. P., et al. (2001). The brainweb: phase synchronization and large-scale integration. *Nat Rev Neurosci 2*(4), 229–239.

Vrba, J. & Robinson, S. E. (2001). Signal processing in magnetoencephalography. *Methods 25*(2), 249–271.

Welch, P. D. (1967). The use of Fast Fourier Transform for the estimation of power spectra: A method based on time averaging over short, modified periodograms. *IEEE Trans Audio Electroacout, AU-15*, 70–73.

Wessberg, J., & Kakuda, N. (1999). Single motor unit activity in relation to pulsatile motor output in human finger movements. *J Physiol (Lond) 517*(Pt 1), 273–285.

Wessberg, J., & Vallbo, A. B. (1995). Coding of pulsatile motor output by human muscle afferents during slow finger movements. *J Physiol (Lond) 485*(Pt 1), 271–282.

Wessberg, J., & Vallbo, A. B. (1996). Pulsatile motor output in human finger movements is not dependent on the stretch reflex. *J Physiol (Lond), 493*(Pt 3), 895–908.

Worsley, K. J., & Friston, K. J. (1995). Analysis of fMRI time-series revisited–again. *Neuroimage 2*(3), 173–181.

10

Statistical Inference in MEG Distributed Source Imaging

Dimitrios Pantazis and Richard M. Leahy

- This chapter reviews the statistical tools available for MEG analysis
- We describe how statistical maps of brain activation are created on the cortex using the General Linear Modeling approach
- We review methods to threshold these maps and establish statistical significance while controlling for multiple comparisons

Introduction

As more whole-head systems become available, magnetoencephalography (MEG) is increasingly being used in clinical and cognitive neuroscience to image human brain function. With the use of novel experimental paradigms, researchers are using MEG to explore many aspects of the workings of the human brain. To assure an objective scientific interpretation of these studies, it is important that experimental findings be accompanied by appropriate statistical analysis that effectively controls for false positives.

This chapter reviews the statistical tools available for the analysis of dis tributed activation maps, defined either on the 2D cortical surface or throughout the 3D brain volume. Statistical analysis of MEG data bears a great resemblance to the analysis of fMRI or PET activation maps; therefore much of the methodology can be borrowed or adapted from the functional neuroimaging literature. In particular, we describe the General Linear Modeling (GLM) approach, where the MEG data are first mapped into brain space, and then fit to a univariate or multivariate model at each surface or volume element. A desired contrast of the estimated parameters produces a statistical map, which is then thresholded for evidence of an experimental effect.

Statistical thresholding at each surface or volume element introduces the multiple hypothesis testing problem, where thousands of elements or voxels are tested against the null hypothesis of no experimental effect. Uncorrected thresholding of the brain activation maps could introduce an unacceptably large number of false positives. For example, naive thresholding of 10,000 independent voxels at $\alpha = 5\%$ threshold is inappropriate, since this could produce approximately 500 false positives in data in which there is no experimental effect (the null condition). In practice, MEG maps exhibit a high degree of spatial correlation, which further confounds their interpretation. Therefore, a means of controlling for multiple hypothesis testing is essential for meaningful interpretation of statistical maps. In this chapter we describe several approaches that can produce corrected thresholds and control for false positives: Bonferroni, Random Field Theory (RFT), permutation tests, and False Discovery error Rate (FDR).

Why MEG Statistical Inference is Different than that for Other Neuroimaging Modalities

Statistical inference in MEG distributed-activation maps uses the GLM framework (Kiebel, 2003), which has been widely successful and is considered a standard in fMRI and PET neuroimaging studies. However, there are important differences from the other neuroimaging modalities related to how observations are created and fitted in GLM models, as well as how subsequent statistical inference is performed.

The temporal resolution of MEG is on the order of milliseconds, much higher than fMRI and PET. Standard analysis of MEG data involves the use of stimulus-locked averaging over epochs to produce the evoked response. Recently there has also been a great deal of interest in analysis of the induced response, which corresponds to stimulus-related variations in power in different oscillatory bands as a function of time. This allows us to detect experimental oscillatory effects corresponding to modulations in power in specific frequency bands, even though the oscillations themselves are not phase-locked to the stimulus or response. Induced effects are typically investigated using a time-frequency decomposition such as the Morlet wavelet transform (Teolis, 1998). Averaging over epochs of the power in the time-frequency maps gives us an estimate of induced components, which can then be tested for experimental effects. These two forms of processing, stimulus-locked averaging and averaging of time-frequency power maps, are the two basic approaches that are used for analyzing, respectively, evoked and induced components in the MEG data (Figure 10–1).

The fact that we often want to identify and localize experimental effects—not only over space, as traditionally done in fMRI with the notion of voxels, but also in time and possibly frequency—introduces challenges that differentiate MEG analysis from that of PET and fMRI. The high dimensionality of the data (space × time × frequency × experimental design) presents challenges in terms of high computational costs, but also possibilities in terms of greater flexibility in the design of the linear models.

Another important difference relative to fMRI is that MEG offers only limited spatial resolution. Distributed cortical imaging involves the reconstruction of thousands of elemental current sources from a few hundred measurements. The problem is highly underdetermined and requires regularization to produce a stable solution. The resulting images are typically of low resolution, so that reconstructions of focal sources are blurred with extended point-spread functions (PSF). The shape of the PSF will depend on the reconstruction space, cortical or volumetric, and whether the orientations of the sources are constrained to be normal to the cortical surface. Unlike in fMRI, the PSFs for MEG are highly asymmetric and can extend over multiple gyri or sulci. As a result, even after thresholding to control for false positives, one can still observe false positives at locations within the point spread of truly active regions and, therefore, care must be taken in interpreting these results. Figure 10–8, shown later in this chapter, illustrates this issue; the reconstructed statistical map has much greater spatial extent than the single simulated cortical patch, and subsequent thresholding procedures identify significant activity in broad cortical areas.

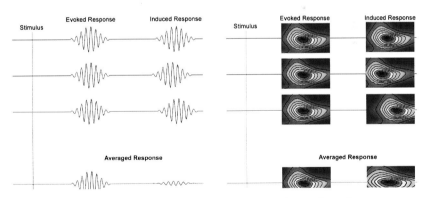

Figure 10–1. MEG brain activity in response to a task consists of two components: evoked responses that are phase locked to the stimuli, and induced responses that are not. Averaging the MEG time-series over epochs preserves the evoked components, but suppresses the induced components (left). Averaging the power time-frequency decompositions of the time-series preserves both evoked and induced components (right).

This issue is closely related to the MEG resolution kernel and the actual hypothesis being tested. In MEG, the channel measurements m are linearly related with the brain activation s as: $m = Gs + n$, where G is the lead field matrix that depends on the shape and conductivity of the head as well as the position of the sensors, and n is the channel noise. We obtain an estimate of the MEG sources $\hat{s}$ with some linear inverse method: $\hat{s} = Wm = WGs + Wn$, where W is the inverse operator and $R = WG$ is the resolution kernel. In distributed cortical imaging, where we estimate more sources than the available channel measurements, R is not the identity matrix and our solution is biased. For a particular cortical location i, when we test the hypothesis $\hat{s}_i = 0$, we are effectively testing $(WG)_i s = 0$, where $(.)_i$ represents the ith row of a matrix. Our true null hypothesis is, therefore, not that the cortical activity at location i is zero, but rather that the whole brain activity, linearly weighted by the resolution kernel at location i, is zero. Waldorp et al. (2006) therefore suggests performing hypothesis testing on multivariate models where spatially smooth regions of interest lead to more interpretable hypotheses than univariate models.

Analysis in fMRI is typically performed in the 3D volumetric space, while in MEG the 2D cortical surface is often chosen as the source space. Cortically constrained maps can complicate the analysis in several ways. For example, isotropic smoothing on the cortical surface when applying random field methods requires the use of the Laplace-Beltrami operator (Chung, 2001). In group analysis the data should be brought into a common coordinate system, which requires cortical surface alignment rather than volumetric registration (Joshi et al., 2007b; Fischl et al., 1999), and the resulting areas of activation should be reported with respect to cortical anatomy rather than the standard Talairach coordinates. Orientation-free MEG reconstructions produce vector rather than scalar fields (3 elemental dipoles at each location), which can also complicate analysis.

In addition to producing a nonuniform PSF, the MEG inverse operator also introduces a highly non-stationary spatial covariance structure in reconstructed images. Contributions to the covariance can include trial-to-trial variations in induced and evoked responses, as well as physiological and environmental noise. Furthermore, the covariance can also vary substantially over the course of an experiment so that we can often not assume temporal stationarity. In comparison, variations in fMRI data can often reasonably be approximated as spatially and temporally stationary. As a result, statistical inference for MEG with random field theory requires the use of special formulas that correct for non-stationarity (Worsley et al., 1999).

Creation of Statistical Maps

In this section we review several methods for generating statistical maps of brain activation based on distributed source imaging. They all consist of three steps: process the MEG measurements to create a collection of observations, use a general linear model to fit the observations at each location, and finally, generate a contrast of the estimated parameters and normalize with its variance to create a map of pivotal statistics (t-maps, F-maps etc). This methodology is a standard approach in fMRI and PET data analysis, and together with subsequent statistical inference, is generally referred to as Statistical Parametric Mapping (SPM) (Friston et al., 1995).

Observations

Typically, the MEG channel measurements are converted into 2D cortical or 3D volumetric maps of brain activation using a source imaging method (Figure 10–2a). Inverse methods include the regularized minimum-norm (Hämäläinen & Ilmoniemi, 1984) and its variants (depth-weighted (Fuchs et al., 1999); Tikhonov-regularized (Tikhonov & Arsenin, 1977), and noise-normalized (Dale et al., 2000); beam-formers (Veen et al., 1997); MUSIC

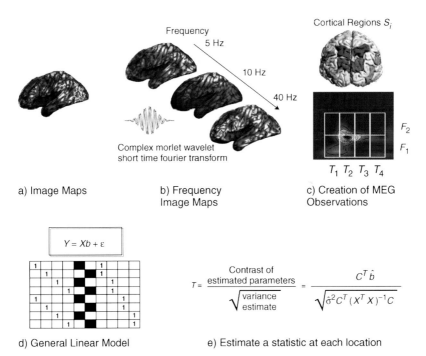

a) Image Maps   b) Frequency Image Maps   c) Creation of MEG Observations

$$Y = Xb + \varepsilon$$

$$T = \frac{\text{Contrast of estimated parameters}}{\sqrt{\text{variance estimate}}} = \frac{c^T \hat{b}}{\sqrt{\hat{\sigma}^2 c^T (X^T X)^{-1} c}}$$

d) General Linear Model   e) Estimate a statistic at each location

Figure 10–2. Creation of statistical maps of brain activation: (a) Inverse methods produce distributed cortical activation maps; (b) Time-frequency decompositions expand the data in the frequency domain; (c) MEG data observations are created over several spatial-temporal-spectral bands. Alternative data reduction techniques can be used, such as singular value decomposition; (d) The observations are fitted into a general linear model following a mass-univariate approach, a multivariate approach, or a general univariate formulation; (e) A contrast of interest is defined and the statistic is normalized by its standard deviation.

maps (Mosher & Leahy, 1998); and sLORETA (Pascual-Marqui, 2002). Different source assumptions underlie each of these methods, e.g., the dipole model in MUSIC and beamforming vs. the distributed source model in the minimum norm methods. However, in each case a statistic can be computed at each voxel in the 2D or 3D space.

To explore the spectral components of induced brain activation, it is also common to perform time-frequency decompositions of the image maps, using for example the complex Morlet wavelet transform, or the short-time Fourier transform (Bruns, 2004) (Figure 10–2b). As described before, the resulting inverse solutions are of high dimension: (2D or 3D) space, time, frequency and experimental condition for each subject. There is, therefore, tremendous flexibility in processing the MEG data; we can create observations using any of these dimensions, treat them as univariate or multivariate observations, and fit them to different general linear models.

Some form of data reduction is desirable. For example, we can summarize information by forming discrete regions or "bands" with respect to the time, frequency and/or spatial dimensions and integrating brain activity over these bands (Figure 10–2c). Even though this reduces resolution, as we have no discrimination power within each band, it can benefit the analysis in multiple ways: reduce data storage requirements, improve the signal-to-noise ratio, and ameliorate the multiple comparison problem by reducing the number of concurrent hypothesis tests. Data reduction in the spatial, temporal, and frequency dimension, is a common practice in MEG studies. For example, Pantazis et al. (2007) defined 10 temporal bands (100ms each), a single α-frequency band (8–14Hz), and 6 spatial bands (or equivalently, cortical regions of interest) and integrated power over these bands in each trial. Brooks et al. (2004) analyzed the data only in a couple of frequency bands. Kilner et al. (2005) completely collapsed the spatial information by performing time-frequency analysis on a single channel, or equivalently, a single source. Finally, Singh et al. (2003) filtered the data into four frequency bands and averaged out the temporal dimension using a spatial power map computed from an LCMV beamformer output.

If oscillatory analysis is not required, a time-frequency decomposition is not necessary and the frequency dimension is ignored (Barnes & Hillbrand, 2003; Sekihara et al., 2005; Carbonell et al., 2004; Pantazis et al., 2005b). An alternative form of data reduction is the application of singular value decomposition (SVD) or independent component analysis (ICA) to the MEG data. For example, Friston et al. (1996) used SVD in the spatiotemporal dimension to reduce the set of components for each multivariate observation.

General Linear Modeling

After the construction of observations, a GLM approach is used to model the data at each location (Figure 10–2d). The MEG observations, as described before, can be current density estimates, time-frequency power maps, or others. GLM theory assumes normal distributions, which is reasonable for averaged evoked responses due to the central limit theorem. However, power time-frequency decompositions of single trial data have a χ^2-distribution. Fortunately, Kiebel et al. (2005) has shown that, under most circumstances, one can appeal to the central limit theorem, or transform the MEG power estimates with a log or square-root transform, to make the error terms normal, and thus GLM theory is still appropriate.

Under the GLM framework, the MEG observations Y are predicted from the parameters b:

$$Y = Xb + \varepsilon \qquad (10\text{--}1)$$

where ε is the modeling error. X is the design matrix whose elements model an experimental paradigm and consist of qualitative (0s or 1s) and/or quantitative variables.

To provide intuition on using the GLM theory for MEG data modeling, consider the following example. In a MEG visual attention study, we acquire multi-trial data for two conditions: subject attends to the right (condition 1), or to the left (condition 2). By combining an inverse method with time-frequency analysis of individual trials, we produce dynamic images of brain activity in the α-frequency band. The α-power observations for a single voxel, $y_{11}, \ldots, y_{1N}$ for condition 1 and $y_{21}, \ldots, y_{2M}$ for condition 2, are fitted into a one-way ANOVA GLM model with two predictor variables, b_1 and b_2, for the two conditions:

$$y_{ij} = b_i + \varepsilon_{ij} \qquad (10\text{--}2)$$

where $i = \{0, 1\}$ denotes the condition, j the trial repetition for each condition, and ε_{ij} is the model error.

The same ANOVA model can be written in matrix notation. If the observations y_{ij} are arranged on a single observation vector Y, and the rows of the design matrix X have 0s and 1s to indicate the condition for each MEG observation, the ANOVA model becomes $Y = Xb + \varepsilon$, explicitly written as:

$$
\begin{bmatrix} y_{11} \\ y_{12} \\ \vdots \\ y_{1N} \\ y_{21} \\ y_{22} \\ \vdots \\ y_{2M} \end{bmatrix}
=
\begin{bmatrix} 1 & 0 \\ 1 & 0 \\ & \vdots \\ 1 & 0 \\ 0 & 1 \\ 0 & 1 \\ & \vdots \\ 0 & 1 \end{bmatrix}
\begin{bmatrix} b_1 \\ b_2 \end{bmatrix}
+
\begin{bmatrix} \varepsilon_{11} \\ \varepsilon_{12} \\ \vdots \\ \varepsilon_{1N} \\ \varepsilon_{21} \\ \varepsilon_{22} \\ \vdots \\ \varepsilon_{2M} \end{bmatrix}
\qquad (10\text{--}3)
$$

By assuming independent Gaussian error distributions with equal variance for both conditions, $N(0, \sigma^2)$, we can solve the GLM using an ordinary least squares solution:

$$\hat{b} = (X^T X)^{-1} X^T Y = \begin{bmatrix} \overline{y}_{1.} \\ \overline{y}_{2.} \end{bmatrix} \qquad (10\text{–}4)$$

where the bar denotes the mean over the dotted subscript. The estimated error variance $\hat{\sigma}^2$ has $N + M - 2$ degrees of freedom, because two of them where used to estimate the model predictors. The error and error variance are estimated as:

$$\hat{\varepsilon} = Y - X\hat{b} = (I - X(X^T X)^{-1} X^T)Y = PY \qquad (10\text{–}5)$$

$$\sigma^2 = \frac{\hat{\varepsilon}^T \hat{\varepsilon}}{\text{trace}\{P\}} = \frac{\Sigma_i (y_{1i} - \overline{y}_{1.})^2 + \Sigma_i (y_{2i} - \overline{y}_{2.})^2}{N + M - 2} \qquad (10\text{–}6)$$

where P is a projection operator onto the left null space of X. We want to test whether there is a difference between the two conditions, or equivalently whether the difference $b_1 - b_2$ is significantly different from zero. The statistic of interest is therefore the contrast of the two parameters, $c^T \hat{b} = \begin{bmatrix} 1 \\ -1 \end{bmatrix}^T \hat{b} = b_1 - b_2$,

which is then normalized with an estimate of its standard deviation. The resulting statistic T is a two-sample t-test between the two conditions.

$$T = \frac{c^T \hat{b}}{\sqrt{\hat{\sigma}^2 c^T (X^T X)^{-1} c}} = \frac{\overline{y}_{1.} - \overline{y}_{2.}}{\sqrt{\hat{\sigma}^2 (1/N + 1/M)}} \qquad (10\text{–}7)$$

Even though we could have derived the T statistic directly, it is useful to see how it is estimated in the GLM framework and get intuition for more complex designs where the theory becomes really important. The design matrix X can have multiple columns with indicator variables, as above, but also quantitative variables that correspond to covariates. The observations can be arranged in multiple ways and several contrasts can capture the experimental effect of interest.

Types of GLMs

There are three ways to organize the MEG data into GLM observations Y: a mass-univariate approach, a multivariate approach, and a general univariate formulation (Kiebel and Friston, 2004). The mass-univariate approach considers the data at each location in isolation. Therefore, a separate but identical GLM is fitted at each spatial-temporal-spectral location and analyzed using an ANOVA or ANCOVA approach. The data correlations in the respective dimensions are ignored at this stage, and accommodated at the inference stage through adjusting the P-values associated with the statistical maps. For example, even though the activation of nearby voxels is correlated, the mass-univariate approach ignores the spatial correlation, but corrects for it when random field theory or permutation tests define a threshold for significant activation. The mass-univariate approach can identify regionally specific effects, since it can test for rejection of the null hypothesis independently at each location. This property, together with its ease of implementation, has made it the most popular approach in functional neuroimaging. Examples in MEG/EEG include mass-univariate models in the spatial dimension (Park et al., 2002; Barnes & Hillbrand, 2003; Brooks et al., 2004); spatial-temporal dimensions (Pantazis et al., 2003, 2005b; Sekihara et al., 2005); spatial-spectral dimensions (Singh et al., 2003); and spatial-temporal-spectral dimensions (Pantazis et al., 2005c, 2007).

In the multivariate approach, we use the Multivariate Analysis of Variance (MANOVA) or Multivariate Analysis of Covariance (MANCOVA) framework. In this case, the MEG observations are organized into vectors and stacked as rows in an observation matrix Y. Classical analysis of this model proceeds by computing sample covariance matrices of the data and the residuals, and then estimating test statistics such as Roy's maximum root, Wilk's lambda, Pillai's trace, or Hotelling's trace (Seber, 2004).

An important difference between the multivariate model and the univariate model is that the former makes inferences on distributed models, whereas the latter makes inferences on regionally specific effects. For example, if the observation vector represents a group of neighboring voxels, then rejection of the null hypothesis allows one to infer there is an experimental effect, but it does not indicate a subset of these voxels at which this has occurred. Because of this limitation, and the requirement to fully specify the covariance structure, MANOVA models are rarely used in the spatial dimension. Interestingly, Waldorp et al. (2006) argues that mass-univariate approaches are inappropriate for hypothesis testing in MEG, and multivariate models are more suitable, because of the limited spatial resolution and bias of MEG inverse methods (see also earlier in this chapter). Friston et al. (1996) used a multivariate model with MEG data where whole trials (spatial and temporal dimension) were formed into single observation vectors. Even though MANOVA models are generally not convenient for the spatial dimension, they can be useful when applied in the temporal or spectral dimension, because of their potential to improve statistical power. (Soto et al., 2009) Therefore, we expect mass-multivariate analysis, where MANOVA models with temporal-spectral observations are fitted separately in each spatial voxel, to be useful in practice.

In the general univariate formulation, the observations from multiple locations are stacked together into a long vector and fitted into a univariate GLM. The parameter and error variables are similarly vectorized. Therefore, a dimension of the observation variables (either space, time, frequency, or combinations of these) is used as an experimental factor with the same number of levels as there are bands in this dimension. This model is the most general case of GLM; if the error covariance terms are unconstrained, then it is equivalent to the MANOVA model (where the corresponding dimension is used to build multivariate observations); if the between-location covariance terms are forced to zero, it is equivalent to the mass-univariate approach (where a GLM is fitted independently in each location). We can also force different constraints that will allow us to estimate fewer variance parameters. For example, we could assume that in the spatial dimension the covariances depend only on the spatial distance between voxels. Kiebel and Friston (2004) propose the use of a mass-univariate formulation where a different GLM is fitted in each spatial location and the temporal dimension is included as a factor. The advantage of this approach is that we can make inferences about the temporal extent of evoked responses, which would have not been possible if the temporal dimension was modeled with a mass-univariate approach. With the general univariate formulation, in this case we can make inferences about differential latencies among trial types or groups.

Contrast Statistic and Normalization

After selection of a GLM approach, the MEG observations are fitted to the models and a contrast (or linear combination) of the parameters is computed (Figure 10–2e). This contrast statistic captures the effect of interest—for example, the difference between two experimental conditions—or the correlation of a response variable with brain activation. It is then preferable to normalize the statistics into known parametric distributions (pivotal statistics). This allows the application of random field theory, which, as we will see, requires a Gaussian distribution or one derived from Gaussian data (e.g., a t or F statistic). The normalization also helps when using nonparametric permutation methods, because it makes the variance at all voxels homogeneous under the null hypothesis, which should produce approximately uniform specificity; i.e. false positives are equally likely at all locations.

We conclude by showing that the GLM framework is parsimonious in MEG analysis. Consider, for example, the simple case where the MEG data are used to create dSPM maps (Dale et al., 2000), i.e. minimum-norm inverse maps normalized with an estimate of the noise standard deviation at each location. This corresponds to the simplest case of GLM analysis following a mass-univariate approach: the one-way ANOVA model $y_j^{it} = b^{it} + \varepsilon_j^{it}$ is fitted to the data separately at each spatial location i and temporal location t, where j is the trial repetition index and b^{it} is the main effect (brain response) (Pantazis et al., 2005b). We use superscripts for i and t to denote that the same model is fit separately in each spatial-temporal location. The estimated contrast of interest is the parameter itself, which is equal to the trial average according to the minimum-norm solution: $c^T \hat{b}^{it} = [1]\hat{b}^{it} = \hat{b}^{it} = \bar{y}_\cdot^{it}$, where the bar indicates an average over the dotted subscript. Since the error terms ε_j^{it} are assumed to be Gaussian, the estimated contrast is also a Gaussian statistic. Finally, to create a map of t-distribution statistics, we normalize with the standard deviation at each location $T^{it} = \dfrac{\hat{b}^{it}}{\hat{\sigma}^{it}/\sqrt{J}}$ where $\hat{\sigma}^{it}$ is the estimated standard deviation and J is the total number of trials. This is equivalent to the noise normalization performed in dSPM for orientation-constrained linear inverses. For the unconstrained case, the dSPM output is an F-map. The sLORETA solution (Pascual-Marqui, 2002) is similar to dSPM, but with a different normalization coefficient. In this case we normalize by the standard deviation computed from the data covariance, rather than the noise-only covariance. Under the null hypothesis of noise-only (or equivalently, a zero experimental effect), sLORETA and dSPM are identical. Similarly, the beam-former neural activity index (Veen et al., 1997) corresponds to a t-map for the orientation-constrained case, or an F-map for the orientation-free case, which can be again cast in a GLM framework.

Multisubject Studies

In multisubject studies, the measurement variance has two sources, the within-subject variance and the between-subject variance. Depending on how we model the error variance, two types of statistical analysis can be used: fixed-effect and mixed (or random) effect. Fixed-effect analysis considers only the within-subject variance, and therefore all measurements are fitted to the same GLM in the same manner as they would be for a single subject. Statistical inferences apply only to the particular subjects participating in the experiment. To generalize to the whole population, mixed-effect analysis is required, where both within- and between-subject variances are considered in making statistical inferences.

Mixed-effect analysis typically involves fitting hierarchical models (Friston et al., 2002; Mumford & Nichols, 2006), where we specify the complete model in stages, a first or lower level model fits the data for each subject separately, and a second level combines the different subjects. The estimation of the parameters in the two-stage analysis is a challenge, since it involves iterative optimization and is generally not practical unless we follow the summary statistics approach. This approach is computationally efficient because it dissociates estimation of the parameters of the two-stage models, and can be implemented with algorithms such as Markov chain Monte Carlo (Beckmann et al., 2003), or Restricted Maximum Likelihood (Verbeke & Molenberghs, 2000).

Under specific assumptions, the summary statistics approach simplifies and the parameters can be estimated without the need for an iterative procedure (Mumford & Nichols, 2006; Holmes & Friston, 1998). We describe this method here, because it has become the most popular approach for multisubject analysis in MEG. The first-stage model fits the data from each subject $k = 1 \cdots K$ separately (To ease notation, we now use subscripts for indices where we follow a mass-univariate approach):

$$Y_k = X_k b_k + \varepsilon_k \tag{10-8}$$

where Y_k are the MEG observations and b_k are the model parameters of subject k. While each design matrix X_k can have a different number of rows (for example, different number of MEG trials per subject), all the design matrices must have the same number of columns, with each column expressing the same effect among subjects. The subject parameters are estimated using a generalized least-squares solution, which normally requires the estimation of the error covariance matrix C_k:

$$\hat{b}_k = (X_k^T C_k^{-1} X_k)^{-1} X_k^T C_k^{-1} \qquad (10\text{–}9)$$

The second stage model takes only one contrast $c^T \hat{b}_k$ from each subject and fits it to the group GLM:

$$\begin{bmatrix} c^T \hat{b}_1 \\ c^T \hat{b}_2 \\ \vdots \\ c^T \hat{b}_K \end{bmatrix} = X_g b_g + \varepsilon_g \qquad (10\text{–}10)$$

where X_g and b_g are the group design matrix and group level parameters respectively. The summary statistics model error ε_g has two variance components, the intrasubject and intersubject variance. Under the assumption of homogeneous intrasubject variance (i.e. $c^T \hat{b}_k$, has the same variance for all subjects), the intrasubject variance is a scaled identity matrix. Similarly, under the assumption of independent subjects, the intersubject variance is a scaled identity matrix. Therefore, the covariance of ε_g is also a scaled identity matrix, and the generalized least-squares solution of the second stage model (which normally requires estimation of the error covariance matrix) becomes equivalent to an ordinary least-squares solution that does not require the covariance matrix:

$$\hat{b}_g = (X_g^T X_g)^{-1} X_g \hat{b} \qquad (10\text{–}11)$$

The key assumption here is the homogeneity of the intrasubject variances; without it, the ordinary least-squares solution could not have been used, iterations would be necessary to estimate both the intrasubject and the intersubject components of the variance.

With multisubject studies, we first coregister all subjects to a common coordinate system, using either volumetric brain coregistration (Christensen & Johnson, 2001; Shen & Davatzikos, 2002; Hellier et al., 2002) or cortical surface alignment methods (Fischl et al., 1999; Thompson et al., 2001; Joshi et al., 2007a). Then the first-stage model, which can be a mass-univariate approach, a multivariate approach, or a general univariate framework, estimates subject-specific parameters. These parameters are then fitted to a second-stage model, and finally a statistic map is computed on the common coordinate system using a contrast of the group parameters b_g at each voxel.

This statistic map can then be thresholded for significant activity at the group level, using any of the methods described later in this chapter.

Consider the following example. In Pantazis et al. (2007), the first-stage model consisted of fitting a univariate model for each subject in the alpha band, for each of several cortically defined regions of interest and time bands. A contrast statistic was then estimated that captured an attention effect: ipsilateral minus contralateral alpha power in each spatiotemporal band. The contrast for all subjects was then fitted to a second-stage GLM (Equation 10–10), whose design matrix X_g is a column of 1s. This simply leads to averaging the responses from all subjects (Equation 10–11), since the assumption of homogeneous intrasubject variance allows application of the simple summary statistics approach described above. Finally, the FDR approach, as described below, was used to threshold the resulting statistic map. Other examples of multisubject MEG studies can be found in Singh et al. (2003), and Kiebel and Friston (2004).

Thresholding Statistical Maps and Establishing Statistical Significance

The first half of this chapter reviewed several approaches to creating statistical maps of brain activation in MEG distributed cortical imaging using the GLM methodology. Arbitrary thresholding of these maps can lead to different interpretations of brain activation (Figure 10–3) and undermine the validity of a functional neuroimaging study. Objective assessment of the statistic maps requires a principled approach to identifying regions of activation. This involves testing thousands of hypotheses (one for each spatial/temporal/frequency band or region of interest) for statistically significant experimental effects (Figure 10–4), and raises the possibility of large numbers of false positives simply as a result of multiple hypothesis testing.

In the following, we first define measures of false positives and show the important role that the maximum statistic plays in statistical inference. We then describe the Bonferroni correction, Random Field Theory (RFT), permutation methods, and False Discovery error Rate (FDR), which provide corrected thresholds for statistical maps.

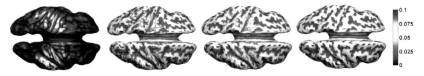

Figure 10–3. A statistic map thresholded at several arbitrary levels. Do both hemispheres show experimental effects, or just the right one? Interpretation of these activation results clearly depends on principled selection of the threshold for significance.

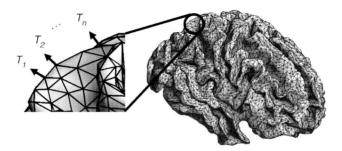

Figure 10–4. A statistical map typically consists of activation measures at thousands of voxels T_i on the brain surface. In the case of multidimensional statistical maps, we acquire activation measures for multiple timepoints and frequencies at each voxel.

False Positive Measures

Thresholding statistical maps should control some measure of the false-positive rate that takes into account the multiple-hypothesis tests. Several measures of false positives have been proposed, the most popular of which is the familywise error rate (FWER), i.e., the probability of making at least one false positive under the null hypothesis that there is no experimental effect. The Bonferroni method, and two approaches based on the maximum statistic distribution—RFT, and permutation test—control the FWER. Another measure that is becoming increasingly popular is FDR, which controls the expected proportion of errors among the rejected hypotheses. Other measures of false positives exist, such as positive false-discovery rate, false discovery-rate confidence, and per-family error-rate confidence (Nichols & Hayasaka, 2003), but they are not as common, and not covered in this chapter.

There are two types of FWER control: weak and strong. In *weak FWER control*, false positives are controlled only when the complete null hypothesis holds, i.e., when there is no experimental effect at any location in the brain. If a cortical site (or a temporal/spectral band) is truly active, control of false positives is not guaranteed anywhere in the brain. Effectively, this implies that with weak FWER control we cannot achieve any localization of an experimental effect, but rather only reject the complete null hypothesis. Conversely, in *strong FWER control*, the false positives are controlled for any subset where the null hypothesis holds. So, even if there is true brain activation at some locations, false positives are still controlled at the other locations, and therefore we can localize experimental effects. Fortunately, the Bonferroni, RFT, and permutation methods achieve strong control of FWER, and therefore have localization power. On the other hand, the FDR method only has weak control of FWER.

FWER methods control the false positives at an α level, typically 5%. This means that with 100 repetitions of the entire experiment only 5 of them will have one or more false positives, or type I errors, at any location in the brain. We now investigate how the FWER is related to the maximum statistic.

Maximum Statistic

The FWER is directly related to the maximum value in the statistical image; one or more voxels T_i will exceed the threshold u_α under the null hypothesis H_0 only if the maximum exceeds that threshold:

$$
\begin{aligned}
P(\text{FWER}) &= P(\cup_i \{T_i \geq u_\alpha\} \mid H_o) && (\text{Prob. any voxel exceeds the threshold}) \\
&= P(\max_i T_i \geq u_\alpha \mid H_o) && (\text{Prob. max voxel exceeds the threshold}) \\
&= 1 - F_{\max T \mid H_o}(u_\alpha) && (\text{1-cum. density function of max voxel}) \\
&= 1 - (1 - \alpha) = \alpha && (10\text{--}12)
\end{aligned}
$$

where $F_{\max T \mid Ho}$ is the cumulative density function of the maximum statistic under the null. Therefore, we can control the FWER if we choose the threshold u_α to be in the $(1 - \alpha)100^{th}$ percentile of the maximum distribution (Figure 10–5).

To control FWER, random field theory estimates the right tail of the maximum statistic distribution using a topological measure called the Euler Characteristic. Permutation tests, on the other hand, resample the data to estimate the empirical distribution of the maximum statistic. The Bonferroni method relies on the Bonferroni inequality and makes no use of the maximum distribution described here.

Rather than use the statistic values directly, these can first be converted to P-values by either assuming a parametric distribution, or by estimating an empirical distribution at each location (Pantazis et al., 2005b). P-values can improve control of FWER in cases where the distribution of the statistic is spatially variant. In this case we use the distribution of the minimum P-value

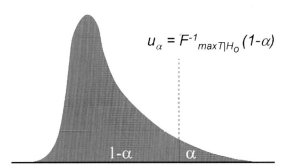

$$u_\alpha = F^{-1}_{\max T \mid H_0}(1 - \alpha)$$

$1 - \alpha$ α

Figure 10–5. Probability density function of the maximum statistic. By choosing a threshold u_α which leaves only α (typically 5%) of the distribution to the right of u_α, we control the FWER at level α.

for control of FWER. As we see below, P-values are also used when controlling the FDR.

Bonferroni Correction

The simplest approach to controlling the FWER is the Bonferroni correction method (Hochberg & Tamhane, 1987; Nichols & Hayasaka, 2003). It is based on the Bonferroni inequality, and assumes independence of each of the multiple hypothesis tests; under dependency, Bonferroni is still valid but can be very conservative. To control false positives at an α level, we threshold each voxel separately at the $\alpha_b = \alpha/V$ level, where V is the total number of voxels.

$$
\begin{aligned}
P(\text{FWER}) &= P(\cup_i \{T_i \geq u_{\alpha_b}\} \,|\, H_o) \\
&\leq \sum_i P(T_i \geq u_{\alpha_b}\} \,|\, H_o) \quad \text{(Bonferroni inequality)} \\
&= \sum_i \alpha_b \\
&= \sum_i \alpha/V = \alpha
\end{aligned}
\tag{10–13}
$$

The Bonferroni method requires the estimation of the marginal distribution at each location in the statistical map, or equivalently, its conversion into a P-value map. We can do this either parametrically—by assuming for example a Gaussian, t, or F distribution at each voxel—or non-parametrically, by resampling the data using a permutation scheme and estimating the empirical distribution separately at each voxel. In Figure 10–8, we estimated the distributions using the latter approach. Since the cortical surface was defined using 7501 nodes, the Bonferroni-adjusted 5% level threshold was $\alpha_b = 0.05/7501 = 6.66 \cdot 10^{-6}$ and no voxel exceeded this very small threshold.

This is not suprising, as the Bonferroni method produces very conservative thresholds unless the tests are independent or have weak dependency (Nichols & Hayasaka, 2003). This is rarely, if ever, the case in MEG, since the number of MEG sensors rarely exceeds a few hundred, while the number of voxels in a statistical map may number several thousand. The inverse procedure that maps from sensors into brain space will inevitably introduce correlation among voxels. Many Bonferroni variants have been proposed, such as the Kounias inequality, and step-up or step-down procedures (Hochberg & Tamhane, 1987). However, they offer little improvement over the original Bonferroni method.

Random Field Methods

As shown in Equation (10–12), the FWER can be determined directly from the probability distribution of the maximum statistic. Adler (1981) demonstrated that the expected value of the Euler Characteristic (EC), a topological measure of the suprathreshold region of a statistical map, is a good approximation of this probability when the threshold is large. Therefore, Random Field Theory (RFT) approximates the upper tail of the maximum distribution F_{maxT} using the expected value of the EC of the thresholded image (Worsley et al., 1996). Computational procedures for calculating this value are implemented in several software packages for analysis of functional imaging data (SPM - http://www.fil.ion.ucl.ac.uk; VoxBo - http://www.voxbo.org; and FSL - http://www.fmrib.ox.ac.uk/fsl among others), and are widely used in fMRI and PET functional neuroimaging studies.

Worsley et al. (1996) provides a formula for the expected value of the EC that unifies the results for all types of random fields:

$$P(\text{FWER}) = P(\cup_i \{T_i \geq u\} \mid H_o)$$

$$\approx \sum_{d=0}^{D} R_d(S)\rho_d(u) \qquad (10\text{–}14)$$

This equation gives the probability of a FWER for threshold u in a D-dimensional random field T_i in a search region S, which can be the cortical surface ($D = 2$) or the brain volume ($D = 3$). The term $R_d(S)$ is the d-dimensional RESEL (RESolution Element) count, a unitless quantity that depends only on topological features of the statistical map in the search region S (Figure 10–6) and is a measure of smoothness of the field under the null hypothesis. The term $\rho_d(u)$ is the EC density that depends only on the threshold u and the type of statistical field (such as z, t, X^2, and Hotelling's T^2). In Equation 10–14 the lower dimensional terms ($d < D$) compensate for the case when the excursion set, i.e., the regions of voxels in a field above a threshold u, touches the boundary. They can usually be omitted because they have only a small impact on the RESEL count.

While in fMRI and PET the random fields can be assumed to be statistically stationary, in MEG we need to compensate for nonstationarity in the spatial, temporal, and spectral dimensions (Worsley et al., 1999), both for maximum statistic inference and for cluster size tests (Hayasaka et al., 2004).

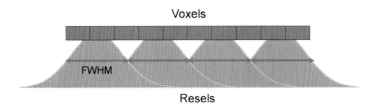

Figure 10–6. Random field theory uses the topological features of a statistical map to convert the voxels into RESELS, a dimensionless quantity that represents the image with interpretable units of smoothness. Under the null hypothesis of no experimental effects, it is the degree of spatial correlation in the noise in the statistical maps that determines the RESEL count.

Such corrections in the spatial dimension were applied by Pantazis et al. (2005b), and Barnes and Hillbrand (2003), to threshold 2D cortical maps and 3D volumetric maps, respectively. Singh et al. (2003) and Park et al. (2002) used RFT as implemented in the SPM software to threshold beamformer and LORETA (Pascual-Marqui et al., 1994) volumetric maps from a multisubject MEG/EEG study. Kilner et al. (2005) used single channel EEG data to create time-frequency maps that were thresholded with SPM under the assumption of stationarity. Finally, Carbonell et al. (2004) applied RFT on a 1D Hotelling T^2 statistical map created from multichannel EEG data in the temporal dimension.

To derive corrected thresholds for statistical maps, RFT relies on several assumptions, including the following: the image has the same parametric distribution at each spatial location; the point spread function has two derivatives at the origin; the field has sufficient smoothness to justify application of continuous RFT; and the threshold is sufficiently high for the asymptotic results to be accurate. When these assumptions hold, RFT is a very powerful method; when this is not possible—for example, with statistical maps of nonstandard distribution—nonparametric alternatives should be considered.

To apply RFT in Figure 10–8, the statistical map was first smoothed with the Laplace-Beltrami operator (Chung, 2001), a generalization of Gaussian smoothing on an arbitrary Riemannian manifold. The spatial filtering corresponded to a 16.7mm Full-Width Half-Maximum (FWHM). Since the mean distance between the vertices in the tessellated cortical surface was 5.7mm, the spatial filtering was equivalent to 2.93 vertices FWHM, which is considered sufficient when smoothing 3D Gaussian images (Hayasaka & Nichols, 2003). On the smoothed statistical map, RFT produced 334.91 RESELS from 7501 cortical vertices or voxels. Using Equation 10–14, the adjusted 5% level threshold was 4.12.

RFT results are available not only for the maximum statistic (peak statistic height), but also for the size of a cluster, the number of clusters, and joint inference on peak height and cluster size (Poline et al., 1997; Hayasaka et al., 2004; Hayasaka & Nichols, 2004). Furthermore, the theory is applicable to the multivariate analog of the F-statistic, Roy's maximum root, and therefore multivariate GLM modeling can also be used in conjunction with RFT (Worsley et al., 2004).

Permutation Methods

The standard approach to permutation tests is to find units exchangeable under the null hypothesis. Units are exchangeable if, by randomly rearranging these units, we can create permutation samples that are statistically equivalent under the null hypothesis to the original data. The simplest example involves a study in which we want to detect differences between two experimental conditions. Under the null hypothesis that there is no difference, epochs from the two conditions can be exchanged.

A test statistic is computed from each permutation sample and, together with the statistic representing the original data, constitute the reference set for determining significance. The proportion of data permutations in the reference set that have test statistic values greater than or equal to the value for the experimentally obtained results, is the P-value (significance or probability value). An excellent treatment of permutation tests can be found in Edgington (1995) and in; Nichols and Holmes (2001).

For FWER control, the test statistic is the maximum in the statistical map. Therefore, unlike the RFT approach, which estimates the upper tail of the maximum distribution based on geometrical features of a parametric statistical map, permutation methods resample the data and create an empirical maximum distribution. By setting a threshold at the α100th percentile of the upper tail of the empirical distribution, we have exact control of the FWER.

Since the permutation samples must be statistically equivalent to the original data, permutations that destroy the inherent correlation structure of the MEG data are not allowed. For example, we cannot exchange channel labels or randomize time-series because the spatial or temporal structure would be altered. Therefore, it is important to apply valid permutation schemes for both single-subject and multi-subject studies.

In single-subject studies, permutations are feasible between experimental conditions (Maris & Oostenveld, 2007). The MEG data are assigned to conditions either beforehand, with respect to the baseline and types of stimuli provided, or on the fly based on the subject's responses, such as fast/slow button presses. In between-trials design, every trial is assigned to one experimental condition; in within-trials design, every trial is assigned to multiple experimental conditions in different time segments. The latter is far more common, as a baseline is typically included before the presentation of a stimulus, and therefore a single trial has two conditions. Most researchers are willing to assume statistical independence between MEG trials, or between non-overlapping time segments within trials, especially if they are separated by some minimum time interval, and thus satisfy the exchangability requirement. Figure 10–7 shows an example permutation scheme used in Pantazis et al. (2005b) to threshold minimum-norm cortical maps while controlling for false positives.

In multi-subject studies, permutations are only performed on the second-level GLM for random-effect statistical inference (see description of multi-subject studies earlier in the chapter). In the simple summary statistics approach in Equation 10–10, each subject's estimated contrast $c^T \hat{b}_k$ is assumed to have a symmetric distribution around zero under the null hypothesis. Therefore, randomly multiplying it by 1 or -1 does not change its distribution under the null hypothesis. With K subjects (and thus K contrasts), a total of 2^K permutation samples can be created, which can then each be fitted to the second level GLM, to estimate permuted group parameters that are used in turn to estimate the empirical distribution of the group-averaged map. Such an approach was followed, for example, by Singh et al. (2003) and

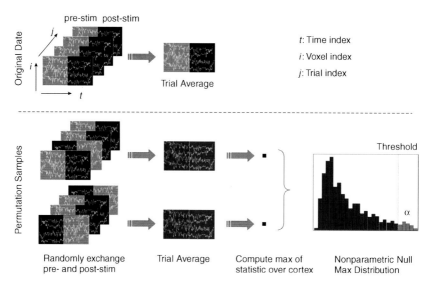

Figure 10–7. Permutation scheme on a single-subject multi-trial MEG study. Top: averaging of original statistical maps, Bottom: generation of permutation samples by randomly exchanging pre- and post-stimulus conditions within each trial. An empirical distribution of the maximum statistic is generated by averaging the permuted trials and computing the max over the cortex. The α level threshold at the upper tail of the empirical distribution is applied to the original averaged data to control the FWER.

Pantazis et al. (2007). Unfortunately, with small K the empirical distribution may be coarsely quantized, and more subjects may be necessary to achieve a desired FWER control.

Permutation tests have many advantages. They are exact, i.e., give precise control of FWER; they do not assume parametric distributions; they adapt to underlying correlation patterns in the data; and they are very flexible, as any test statistic can be used. The only assumptions required are those to justify permuting the labels of the conditions, such as, that the distributions under the null hypothesis have the same shape or are symmetric. Even though we are free to consider any statistic summarizing evidence for the effect of interest at each location, it is usually best to use the same statistics for a non-parametric approach as we would for a comparable parametric approach. The reason is that parametric statistics often have optimal power; for example, a t-statistic is the most powerful in detecting differences between populations in many circumstances. Further, to achieve uniform specificity, i.e., equal chances of false positives at any location in the statistical map, we should use statistics that have approximately homogeneous null permutation distributions.

Because of their flexibility, permutation tests are more commonly used in MEG than the parametric RFT. Permutation tests have been proposed to control false positives in the channel domain (Blair & Karnisky, 1993, 1994; Karnisky et al., 1994; Maris, 2004; Achim, 2001; Galan et al., 1997) and in the source domain (Park et al., 2002; Pantazis et al., 2003, 2005b; Chau et al., 2004; Singh et al., 2003; Sekihara et al., 2005). These methods have been applied in multiple MEG studies (Kaiser et al., 2000; Lutzenberger et al., 2002; Cheyne et al., 2006; Bayless et al., 2006; Itier et al., 2006; Pantazis et al., 2005a,c, 2007). Reviews on the application of permuation tests in MEG are available in Maris and Oostenveld (2007); and in Maris et al. (2007).

Various thresholding methods are illustrated in Figure 10–8. The permutation method was based on that described in Pantazis et al. (2005b) and produced a threshold of 3.99, which controls FWER over the whole cortex at a 5% level.

Control of the False Discover Rate (FDR)

In contrast to the above methods that control the FWER, FDR controls the expected proportion of errors among the rejected hypotheses (Benjamini & Hochberg, 1995; Genovese et al., 2002). For example, if we set an $\alpha = 5\%$ FDR threshold, then on average we should expect 5% of our suprathreshold voxels to be false positives.

The standard FDR method proposed by Benjamini and Hochberg (1995) is conservative, as it controls the FDR at a $\frac{V_0}{V}\alpha$ level, where V is the total number of voxels and V_0 is the number of voxels where the null hypothesis is true:

$$E(FDR) = E\left(\frac{\text{false positives}}{\text{suprathreshold voxels}}\right) \leq \frac{V_0}{V}\alpha \qquad (10\text{–}15)$$

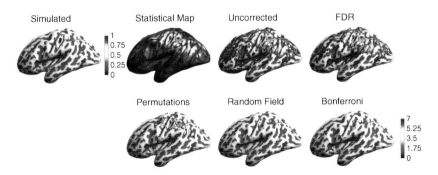

Figure 10–8. Simulated MEG source on the left hemisphere and reconstructed dSPM statistical map, thresholded using several methods to control false positives. Uncorrected thresholding (P-value = 0.05) and FDR (P-value = 0.0065) produced many false positives. Permutations and random field theory gave thresholds $t = 3.99$ and $t = 4.12$, respectively. The Bonferroni approach was very conservative (P-value 0.05/7501 = 6.6610 [6]) and did not identify the source.

When the true brain activation extends over broad areas, V_0 may become small and the FDR procedure too conservative. Thus, a number of adaptive procedures improve on the original FDR approach by first estimating V_0, and then using this estimate to tighten the threshold (Benjamini et al., 2006).

The FDR methods adapt to the properties of the data; when a large number of voxels are truly active, the threshold will adjust to allow for more false positives; when no truly activated voxels exist, FDR controls the FWER, but in a weak sense (see False Positive Measures earlier in the chapter). They are more powerful than Bonferroni, random field, and permutation control of FWER, and for this reason may become popular for thresholding MEG maps.

The FDR approach requires the estimation of the marginal distribution at each location in the statistical map, or, equivalently, conversion of the statistic value at each location into an equivalent P-value. We can do this parametrically or non-parametrically, as described for the Bonferroni approach.

Once the maps are converted to P-values, implementation of the standard FDR method is relatively straightforward (Genovese et al., 2002). If V is the total number of voxels being tested, the procedure is as follows:

(1) Order the voxel P-values from smallest to largest:

$$P_{(1)} \leq P_{(2)} \leq \cdots P_{(V)} \tag{10-16}$$

(2) Let r be the largest i for which

$$P_{(i)} \leq \frac{i}{V} \frac{\alpha}{c(V)} \tag{10-17}$$

(3) Declare all voxels corresponding to the P-values $P_{(1)}, \ldots, P_{(r)}$ active.

where $c(V) = \sum_{i=1}^{V} 1/i$ if no assumptions on the joint distribution of the P-values across voxels is made, and $c(V) = 1$ if the P-values in different voxels are independent or they have positive dependence (Benjamini & Yekutieli, 2001).

The procedure is demonstrated graphically in Figure 10–9 for the FDR procedure applied to the statistical map in Figure 10–8. The estimated threshold for 7501 cortical voxels at the 5% level was 0.065, and produced an extended region of suprathreshold voxels. Unfortunately, the large extent of the significantly active region determined using FDR, is a result of the limited spatial resolution of MEG; many voxels surrounding the true simulated source exhibit significant activity in the statistical map, and FDR is sensitive enough to identify them. Conversely, the more conservative thresholds from FWER control tend to reduce the size of activated regions, as also shown in Figure 10–8. Other examples of the application of FDR in MEG maps include Edwards et al. (2005); Jacobs et al. (2006); Pantazis et al. (2007); and Jacques and Rossion (2007).

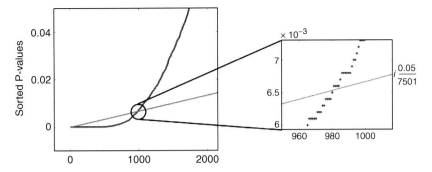

Figure 10–9. Graphical representation of the FDR procedure. The blue line represents the sorted P-values of the statistical map in Figure 10–8, and the red line is $i\frac{\alpha}{V} = i\frac{0.05}{7501}$. The largest P-value below the line is 0.0065 and corresponds to a 5% level FDR threshold.

Discussion

We have presented a GLM framework to produce statistical maps from MEG distributed cortical imaging, and subsequently threshold them while controlling for false positives. Choosing a thresholding method depends on the data available: Bonferroni is simple and efficient for a small number of tests with minimal dependence; random fields are robust when their parametric assumptions are satisfied, and strong correlation exists in the data; permutation tests are very general, adapt to the underlying data correlations, can use any statistic, and are more powerful than random fields for data with low degrees of freedom (e.g., studies with a few subjects); FDR is more powerful, works well with sparse signals, and is recommended when we can afford a few false positives. However, as we have shown in our simulations, FDR can produce large regions of significant activation as a result of the limited resolution of MEG inverses.

A number of important statistical issues are beyond the scope of this chapter, such as conjunction analysis (Nichols et al., 2005), i.e., the identification of brain areas that are simultaneously active in multiple tasks; extraction of confidence intervals for distributed solutions using the bootstrap (DiNocera and Ferlazzo, 2000; Gross et al., 2003; Darvas et al., 2005); and thresholding using cluster-size tests (Hayasaka et al., 2004). Also, the theory was developed for distributed inverse methods in MEG. However, discrete solutions are also popular in MEG, especially with well localized activation when a few equivalent current dipoles can represent most cortical activity. In this case, alternative approaches can be used to establish significance; for example, the bootstrap resampling approach, or Monte Carlo simulations to find localization accuracy and confidence intervals for current dipoles (Darvas et al., 2005; Braun et al., 1997).

A related problem in MEG data analysis is testing for the statistical significance of cortical interactions (Varela et al., 2001; Gross et al., 2001; Hui & Leahy, 2006; Jerbi et al., 2007; Maris et al., 2007). In some cases, a few cortical locations are investigated and corrections for multiple comparisons are generally not employed. In the case where tests are made for interactions between multiple pairs of locations, the theory described in this chapter can be applied. The DICS algorithm, for example, can be used to investigate cortical coherence at all locations in the cortex relative to a reference, which may be a single cortical location or an electromyograph reference signal (Gross et al., 2001). The resulting maps are a measure of coherence at each cortical location for a single frequency band, but can be easily extended to multiple frequency bands. The methods described in this chapter for analysis of time-frequency representations of brain activity can be adapted to testing for significant activation in these coherence maps.

References

Achim, A. (2001). Statistical detection of between-group differences in event-related potentials. *Clinical Neurophysiology, 112*, 1023–1034.

Adler, R. J. (ed.) (1981). *The Geometry of Random Fields.* New York: Wiley.

Barnes, G. R., & Hillbrand, A. (2003). Statistical flattening of MEG beamformer images. *Human Brain Mapping, 18*, 1–12.

Bayless, S. J., Gaetz, W. C., Cheyne, D. O., & Taylor, M. J. (2006). Spatiotemporal analysis of feedback processing during a card sorting task using spatially filtered MEG. *Neuroscience Letters, 410*, 31–36.

Beckmann, C. F., Jenkinson, M., & Smith, S. M. (2003). General multilevel linear modeling for group analysis in fMRI. *Neuroimage, 20*(2), 1052–1063.

Benjamini, Y., & Hochberg, Y. (1995). Controlling the false discovery rate: a practical and powerful approach to multiple testing. *Journal of the Royal Statistical Society, 57*, 289–300.

Benjamini, Y., Krieger, A. M., & Yekutieli, D. (2006). Adaptive linear step-up procedures that control the false discovery rate. *Biometrica, 93*(3), 491–507.

Benjamini, Y., & Yekutieli, D. (2001). The control of the false discovery rate in multiple testing under dependency. *The Annals of Statistics, 29*(4), 1165–1188.

Blair, R. C., & Karnisky, W. (1993). An alternative method for significance testing of waveform difference potentials. *Psychophysiology, 30*, 518–524.

Blair, R. C., & Karnisky, W (1994). Distribution-free statistical analyses of surface and volumetric maps. In: R. W. Thatcher, M. Hallett, T. Zeffiro, E. R. Jony, and M. Huerta, eds.)*Functional Neuroimaging* (pp. 19–28). New York: Academic Press.

Braun, C., Kaiser, S., Kinces, W., & Elbert, T. (1997). Confidence interval of single dipole locations based on EEG data. *Brain Topography, 10*(1), 31–39.

Brooks, M. J., Gibson, A. M., Hall, S. D., Furlong, P. L., Barnes, G. R., Hillebrand, A., et al. (2004). A general linear model for MEG beamformer imaging. *Neuroimage, 23*, 936–946.

Bruns, A. (2004). Fourier-, hilbert and wavelet-based signal analysis: are they really different approaches? *Journal of Neuroscience Methods, 137*, 321–332.

Carbonell, F., Galan, L., Valdes, P., Worsley, K., Biscay, R. J., Diaz-Comas, L., et al. (2004). Random field - union intersection tests for EEG/MEG imaging. *NeuroImage, 22*, 268–276.

Chau, W., McIntosh, A. R., Robinson, S. E., Schulz, M., & Pantev, C. (2004). Improving permutation test power for group analysis of spatially filtered MEG data. *NeuroImage, 23*, 983–996.

Cheyne, D., Bakhtazad, L., & Gaetz, W. (2006). Spatiotemporal mapping of cortical activity accompanying voluntary movements using an event-related beamforming approach. *Human Brain Mapping, 27*, 213–229.

Christensen, G. E., & Johnson, H. J. (2001). Consistent image registration. *IEEE Transactions on Medical Imaging, 20*(7), 568–582.

Chung, M. K. (2001). Statistical morphometry in neuroanatomy. Ph.D. thesis, McGill University, Montreal.

Dale, A. M., Liu, A. K., Fischi, R. B., Buckner, R. L., Belliveau, J. W., Lewine, J. D., et al. (2000). Dynamic statistical parametric mapping: Combining fMRI and MEG for high-resolution imaging of cortical activity. *Neuron, 26*, 55–67.

Darvas, F., Rautiainen, M., Pantazis, D., Baillet, S., Benali, H., Mosher, J. C., et al. (2005). Investigations of dipole localization accuracy in MEG using the bootstrap. *NeuroImage, 25*, 355–368.

DiNocera, F., & Ferlazzo, F. (2000). Resampling approach to statistical inference: bootstrapping from event-related potentials data. *Behavioral Research Methods, Instruments and Computers, 32*(1), 111–119.

Edgington, E. S. (ed.). (1995). *Randomization Tests* (3rd ed.). New York: Marcel Dekker.

Edwards, E., Soltani, M., Deouell, L. Y., Berger, M. S., & Knight, R. T. (2005). High gamma activity in response to deviant auditory stimuli recorded directly from human cortex. *Journal of Neurophysiology, 94*, 4269–4280.

Fischl, B., Serano, M., Tootell, R., & Dale, A. M. (1999). High-resolution intersubject averaging and a coordinate system for the cortical surface. *Human Brain Mapping, 8*(4), 272–284.

Friston, K. J., Holmes, A. P., Worsley, K. J., Poline, J. B., Frith, C., & Frackowiak, R. S. J. (1995). Statistical parametric maps in functional imaging: A general linear approach. *Human Brain Mapping, 2*, 189–210.

Friston, K. J., Penny, W., Phillips, C., Kiebel, S., Hinton, G., & Ashburner, J. (2002). Classical and bayesian inference in neuroimaging: Theory. *NeuroImage, 16*, 465–483.

Friston, K. J., Stephan, K. M., Heather, J. D., Frith, C. D., Ioannides, A. A., Liu, L. C., et al. (1996). A multivariate analysis of evoked responses in EEG and MEG data. *Neuroimage, 3*, 167–174.

Fuchs, M., Wagner, M., Kohler, T., & Wischmann, H. (1999). Linear and non-linear current density reconstructions. *Journal of Clinical Neurophysiology, 16*, 267–295.

Galan, L., Biscay, R., Rodriguez, J. L., Abalo, M. C. P., & Rodriguez, R. (1997). Testing topographic differences between event related brain potentials by using non-parametric combinations of permutation tests. *Electroencephalography and clinical Neurophysiology, 102*, 240–247.

Genovese, C., Lazar, N., & Nichols, T. (2002). Thresholding of statistical maps in functional neuroimaging using the false discovery rate. *NeuroImage, 15*, 870–878.

Gross, J., Kujala, J., Hämäläinen, M., Timmermann, L., Schnitzler, A., & Salmelin, R. (2001). Dynamic imaging of coherent sources: Studying neural interactions in the human brain. *Proceedings of National Academy of Sciences, 98*(2), 694–699.

Gross, J., & Timmermann, L., Kujala, J., Salmelin, R., & Schnitzler, A. (2003). Properties of MEG tomographic maps obtained with spatial filtering. *Neuroimage*, *19*, 1329–1336.

Hämäläinen, M. S., & Ilmoniemi, R. J. (1984). Interpreting magnetic fields of the brain: minimum norm estimates. *Medical and Biological Engineering and Computing*, *32(1)*, 35–42.

Hayasaka, S., & Nichols, T. E. (2003). Validating cluster size inference: Random field and permutation methods *20 (4)*, 2343–2356.

Hayasaka, S., & Nichols, T. E. (2004). Combining voxel intensity and cluster extent with permutation test framework. *Neuroimage*, *23(1)*, 54–63.

Hayasaka, S., Phan, K. L., Libarzon, I., Worsley, K. J., & Nichols, T. E. (2004). Nonstationary cluster-size inference with random field and permutation methods. *NeuroImage*, *22*, 676–687.

Hellier, P., Ashburner, J., Corouge, I., Barillot, C., & Friston, K. J. (2002). Inter-subject registration of functional and anatomical data using textSPM. In: *Medical Image Computing and Computer-Assisted Intervention - MICCAI 2002*, pp. 590–597.

Hochberg, Y., & Tamhane, A. C. (eds.). (1987). *Multiple Comparison Procedures.* New York: Wiley.

Holmes, A., & Friston, K. J. (1998). Generalisability, random effects and population inference. *NeuroImage*, *7*, S754.

Hui, H., Leahy, R. M. (2006). Linearly constrained MEG beamformers for MVAR modeling of cortical interactions. In: *Biomedical Imaging: From Macro to Nano, 2006. 3rd IEEE International Symposium*, pp. 237–240.

Itier, R. J., Herdman, A. T., George, N., Cheyne, D., & Taylor, M. J. (2006). Inversion and contrast-reversal effects on face processing. *Brain Research*, *1115*, 108–120.

Jacobs, J., Hwang, G., Curran, T., & Kahana, M. J. (2006). EEG oscillations and recognition memory: Theta correlates of memory retrieval and decision making. *NeuroImage*, *32*, 978–987.

Jacques, C., & Rossion, B. (2007). Early eloctrophysiological responses to multiple face orientations correlate with individual discrimination performance in humans. *NeuroImage*, *36*, 863–876.

Jerbi, K., Lachaux, J. P., N'Diaye, K., Pantazis, D., Leahy, R. M., & Garnero, L. (2007). Coherent neural representation of hand speed in humans revealed by MEG imaging. *PNAS*, *104(18)*, 7676–7681.

Joshi, A. A., Shattuck, D. W., Thompson, P. M., Leahy, R. M. (2007a). A finite element method for elastic parameterization and alignment of cortical surfaces using sulcal constraints. In: *Biomedical Imaging: From Macro to Nano, 2007. 4th IEEE International Symposium*, pp. 640–643.

Joshi, A. A., Shattuck, D. W., Thompson, P. M., & Leahy, R. M. (2007b). Surface constrained volumetric brain registration using harmonic mappings. *IEEE Transactions on Medical Imaging*, *26(12)*, 1657–1669.

Kaiser, J., Lutzenberger, W., Preissl, H., Mosshammer, D., & Birbaumer, N. (2000). Statistical probability mapping reveals high-frequency magnetoencephalographic activity in supplementary motor area during self-paced finger movements. *Neuroscience Letters*, *283(1)*, 81–84.

Karnisky, W., Blair, R. C., & Snider, A. D. (1994). An exact statistical method for comparing topographic maps with any number of subjects and electrods. *Brain Topography*, *6*, 203–210.

Kiebel, S. (2003). The general linear model. In: Frackowiak, R., Friston, K., Frith, C., Dolan, R., Friston, K., Price, C., Zeki, S., Ashburner, J., Penny, W. (eds.), Human Brain Function, (2nd ed.). San Diego: Academic Press.

Kiebel, S. J., & Friston, K. J. (2004). Statistical parametric mapping for event-related potentials: I. generic considerations. *Neuroimage, 22*, 492–502.

Kiebel, S. J., Tallon-Baudry, C., & Friston, K. J. (2005). Parametric analysis of oscillatory activity as measured with EEG/MEG. *Human Brain Mapping, 26*, 170–177.

Kilner, J. M., Kiebel, S. J., & Friston, K. J. (2005). Applications of random field theory to electrophysiology. *Neuroscience Letters, 374*, 174–178.

Lutzenberger, W., Ripper, B., Busse, L., Birbaumer, N., & Kaiser, J. (2002). Dynamics of gamma-band activity during an audiospatial working memory task in humans. *Journal of Neuroscience, 22*(*13*), 5630–5638.

Maris, E., (2004). Randomization tests for ERP topographies and whole spatiotemporal data matrices. *Psychophysiology, 41*, 142–151.

Maris, E., & Oostenveld, R. (2007). Nonparametric statistical testing of EEG- and MEG-data. *Journal of Neuroscience Methods, 164*, 177–190.

Maris, E., Schoffelen, J.-M., & Fries, P. (2007). Nonparametric statistical testing of coherence differences. *Journal of Neuroscience Methods, 163*, 161–175.

Mosher, J. C., & Leahy, R. M. (1998). Recursive MUSIC: A framework for EEG and MEG source localization. *IEEE Transactions of Biomedical Engineering, 45* (*11*), 1342–1354.

Mumford, J. A., & Nichols, T. (2006). Modeling and inference of multisubject fmri data. *IEEE Engineering in Medicine and Biology Magazine,* March/April, 42–51.

Nichols, T., Brett, M., Andersson, J., Wager, T., & Poline, J.-B. (2005). Valid conjunction inference with the minimum statistic. *NeuroImage, 25*, 653–660.

Nichols, T. E., & Hayasaka, S. (2003). Controlling the familywise error rate in functional neuroimaging: A comparative review. *Statistical Methods in Medical Research, 12* (*5*), 419–446.

Nichols, T. E., & Holmes, A. P. (2001). Nonparametric permutation tests for functional neuroimaging: A primer with examples. *Human Brain Mapping, 15*, 1–25.

Pantazis, D., Merrifield, W., Darvas, F., Sutherling, W., & Leahy, R. M. (2005a). Hemispheric language dominance using MEG cortical imaging and non-parametric statistical analysis. *WSEAS Transactions on Biology and Biomedicine, 2*(*3*), 318325.

Pantazis, D., Nichols, T. E., Baillet, S., & Leahy, R. M. (2003). Spatiotemporal localization of significant activation in MEG using permutation tests. In: Taylor, C., Noble, J. A. (eds.), *Proc. 18th Conf. Information Processing in Medical Imaging,* pp. 512–523.

Pantazis, D., Nichols, T. E., Baillet, S., & Leahy, R. M. (2005b). A comparison of random field theory and permutation methods for the statistical analysis of MEG data. *Neuroimage, 25*(*2*), 383–394.

Pantazis, D., Simpson, G., Weber, D., Dale, C., Nichols, T., & Leahy, R. (2007). Exploring human visual attention in an meg study of a spatial cueing paradigm using a novel ancova design. In: 2007 IEEE International Symposium on Biomedical Imaging: From Nano to Macro.

Pantazis, D., Weber, D., Dale, C., Nichols, T., G.V. Simpson, & Leahy, R. (2005c). Imaging of oscillatory behavior in event-related MEG studies. In: Bouman, C., Miller, E. (Eds.), *Proceedings of SPIE, Computational Imaging III.* Vol. 5674. (pp. 55–63).

Park, H., Kwon, J., Youn, T., Pae, J., Kim, J., Kim, M., & Ha, K. (2002). Statistical parametric mapping of LORETA using high density EEG and individual MRI: application to mismatch negativities in schizophrenia. *Human Brain Mapping, 17*, 168–178.

Pascual-Marqui, R. D. (2002). Standardized low resolution brain electromagnetic tomography (sLORETA): technical details. *Methods and Findings in Experimental Clinical Pharmacology, 24D*, 5–12.

Pascual-Marqui, R. D., Michel, C. M., & Lehmann, D. (1994). Low resolution electromagnetic tomography: a new method for localizing electrical activity in the brain. *International journal of Psychophysiology, 18*, 49–65.

Poline, J.-B., Holmes, A. P., Worsley, K. J., & Friston, K. J. (1997). Statistical inference and the theory of random fields. In: Friston, K., Frith, C. D., Dolan, R. J., Mazziotta, J. C., Frackowiak, R. (eds.), *Human Brain Function*, (1st edn.) San Diego: Academic Press.

Seber, G. A. F. (2004). *Multivariate Observations.* New Jersey: Wiley Series in Probability and Statistics.

Sekihara, K., Sahani, M., & Nagarajan, S. S. (2005). A simple nonparametric statistical thresholding for MEG spatial-filter source reconstruction images. *Neuroimage, 27*, 368–376.

Shen, D., & Davatzikos, C. (2002). HAMMER: hierarchical attribute matching mechanism for elastic registration. *IEEE Transactions on Medical Imaging, 21(11)*, 1421–1439.

Singh, K., Barnes, G. R., & Hillebrand, A. (2003). Group imaging of task-related changes in cortical synchronization using nonparametric permutation testing. *Neuroimage, 19*, 1589–1601.

Soto, J. L. P., Pantazis, D., Jerbi, K., Lachaux, J-P., Garnero, L., &, Leahy, R. M. (2009). Detection of event-related changes in brain activation with multivariate statistical analysis of MEG data, *Human Brain Mapping*, 30(6), 1922–1934.

Teolis, A. (ed.), (1998). *Computational Signal Processing With Wavelets (Applied and Numerical Harmonic Analysis).* Boston: Birkhauser.

Thompson, P., Mega, M., Woods, R. P., Zoumalan, C. I., Lindshield, C. J., Blanton, R. E., et al. (2001). Cortical change in alzheimer's disease detected with a disease-specific population-based brain atlas. *Cerebral Cortex, 11(1)*, 1–16.

Tikhonov, A., & Arsenin, V. (1977). *Solutions of ill-posed problems.* Winston D.C.: winston.

Varela, F., Lachaux, J.-P., Rodriguez, E., & Martinerie, J. (2001). The brainweb: phase synchronization and large-scale integration. *Nature Reviews, 2*, 229–239.

Veen, B. D. V., Drongelen, W. V., Yuchtman, M., & Suzuki, A. (1997). Localization of brain electrical activity via linearly constrained minimum variance spatial filtering. *IEEE Transactions of Biomedical Engineering, 44(9)*, 867–880.

Verbeke, G., & Molenberghs, G. (2000). *Linear mixed models for longitudinal data.* New York: Springer-Verlang.

Waldorp, L. J., Huizenga, H. M., Grasman, R. P. P. P., Bocker, K. B. E., & Molenaar, P. C. M. (2006). Hypothesis testing in distributed source models for EEG and MEG data. *Human Brain Mapping, 27*, 114–128.

Worsley, K. J., Andermann, M., Koulis, T., MacDonald, D., & Evans, A. C. (1999). Detecting changes in non-isotropic images. *Human Brain Mapping, 8*, 98–101.

Worsley, K. J., Marrett, S., Neelin, P., Vandal, A. C., Friston, K. J., & Evans, A. C. (1996). A unified statistical approach for determining significant signals in images of cerebral activation. *Human Brain Mapping, 4*, 58–73.

Worsley, K. J., Taylor, J. E., Tomaiuolo, F., & Lerch, J. (2004). Unified univariate and multivariate random field theory. *NeuroImage, 23*, s189–195.

11

Combining Neuroimaging Techniques:
The Future

Jean-Baptiste Poline, Line Garnero and
Pierre-Jean Lahaye

- Combining neuroimaging techniques is important to acquire a better understanding of brain processes, and can be characterized by three types of combination: converging evidence, quantified data with shared information, and generative models
- Much remains to be understood about the complexity of the neural mechanisms and their related biological phenomena before the combined results of different imaging techniques can be solidly interpreted
- The advantages and disadvantages of simultaneous EEG-fMRI versus MEG/EEG and fMRI are summarized
- Acquiring information about brain states using different neuroimaging techniques is likely to yield more interesting information about the brain mechanisms than just using a single methodology

Introduction

Combining Techniques: The Enticements

Since any measurement technique has its own strengths and limitations, combining different experimental approaches to better probe a scientific question is a commonplace idea. In the human brain-imaging domain, it is now common to combine two or more imaging techniques to investigate a cognitive process or a disease, in addition to using other measures such as behavioral testing.

Recently, the combination of electro- or magnetoencephalography with functional magnetic resonance imaging (fMRI) or positron emission tomography (PET) has become more and more popular among neuroscientists. Clearly, if one could obtain the temporal resolution of the electric methods while maintaining the spatial precision of true imaging techniques that can resolve activity at the level of ocular dominance columns (Kim et al., 2000), the data obtained would be immensely useful for understanding how the brain implements cognitive processes, or how it malfunctions in various pathologies. In this sense, the combination of techniques with different limitations can be seen as the construction of a "super-technique" with much greater effectiveness. This argument is extremely widespread (e.g., Stippich et al., 1998; Dale et al., 2000; and many more).

Furthermore, the results obtained by combining neuroimaging techniques may be more than the sum of the results obtained separately. This is because different techniques observe different phenomena, and the interpretation of the data obtained in one modality may depend on parameters that are only accessible with the other (as, for example, in defining vigilance state or epileptic activity). Rather than a "super-technique," we may be able to construct a technique that allows us to look at other phenomena (Laufs et al., 2003).

Combining Techniques: The Difficulties

While potentially extremely useful and sometimes necessary, combining information is a challenge at several levels—when designing the experimental paradigm, when acquiring the data and during the interpretation of the data. For instance, if the same cognitive protocol has to be conducted with MEG and fMRI on the same subjects, the effect on a subject of "having a second session" may have to be carefully considered. One may want to randomize the order of the acquisitions across imaging techniques, but the repetition effect would still have to be appropriately modeled. In other words, the constraints or additional complexity involved at the protocol design stage can be (and usually is, in our opinion) underestimated.

Multimodal acquisition of data may also prove to be a technical challenge. The simultaneous acquisition of both EEG and fMRI data is a typical example. In this case, we may find that the signal-to-noise loss on the EEG signal precludes fine studies of those signals (Benar et al., 2003), while the fMRI echo planar imaging (EPI) acquisition quality is degraded as well (Krakow et al., 2000a; 2000b). While theoretically the best idea, the technological limitations may, in fact, render multimodal data useless for the study.

Thirdly, the interpretation of the data would often be more difficult. Because current models of brain functions and diseases are likely to be only crude approximations, complex data may not easily fit into the current model interpretation (here, "model" is taken in a loose sense, as the researcher's formal or informal representation of the brain mechanism under investigation), and therefore be too big a step forward. Multimodal experiments add complexity, and are therefore even more likely to lead to large deviations from current models' predictions. This phenomenon is accentuated when theoretical models are still under construction or poorly conceptualized, which is a common situation in neuroimaging.

For those reasons, multimodal studies should probably be planned even more carefully than others, and based on a solid theoretical framework for sound interpretation.

Three Ways of Combining Information

"Fusion" and "combining" do not reflect the same operations in the literature. In their article, "How can PET/fMRI and EEG/MEG can be combined?", Horwitz and Poeppel (2002) distinguish three levels of combination. Here, we briefly summarize and comment on them.

Converging evidence. This is simply the combination of different information originating from different experiments, and possibly different fields, to permit better interpretation. A vast majority of studies use converging evidence within modalities, but also across modalities (Guy et al., 1999; Ball et al., 1999). For instance, Dehaene et al. (1998) report the location, but also the timing, of the process of masked numerical primes using both fMRI and EEG techniques. Two difficulties have been highlighted by Horwitz and Poeppel (2002). First, it is very difficult to actually decide whether measurements from different studies or modalities refer to the same process or the same brain region. Second, not all evidence is usually accounted for. The most common problem is that "null results", i.e., studies that failed to report activity, are not included as evidence. This problem is magnified by the classical hypothesis-testing framework, and by the strong publication bias towards "significant" results. Adapted meta-analysis techniques could address this issue. It should be noted that converging evidence is certainly crucial for diagnosis in a clinical environment.

Quantified data, shared information. This relies on establishing quantitative relationships between measurements of a different nature. The shared information can be inferred in the time or spatial domain, but the models used are phenomenological (correlation, registration between modalities; e.g., Singh et al., 2003). If the models are crude, or might be based on invalid assumptions, then the presence or absence of shared information is difficult to interpret. The causes for the presence or absence of a given effect can be due to numerous unknown factors. Nevertheless, this is probably a necessary first step.

Generative models. The most ambitious and possibly most fruitful direction is to establish generative models for which parameters are estimated from data of different nature or provenance. Only a few examples of this can be found in the literature. One was proposed by Horwitz et al. (1999) who considered the possibility of constructing a large-scale, biologically realistic neural network model that can perform a specific cognitive task. The model construction would allow the simulation of fMRI/PET and MEG/EEG data that could be compared to experimentally observed values. Here, different data types with different spatiotemporal properties are *not directly compared*, but are informing a *common neural model*. Note that this model should include not only current knowledge about the neurophysiology and the measurement process, but also how the full model can achieve the cognitive operation under study. Pushing the idea further, one can use the data of different imaging or non-imaging techniques to estimate the parameters of the model.

Combining Brain Imaging Techniques: On What Basis?

We briefly review the biophysics principle underlying both BOLD (blood-oxygen-level dependent) and MEG/EEG signals. For MEG/EEG, the signals are believed to originate from the synchronous postsynaptic currents in the pyramidal cells. An electric dipole is the simplest and most commonly used model to represent the electric activity. On the other hand, fMRI is based on the measure of the combination of three phenomena: the increased oxygen extraction, blood flow and blood volume following increased neural cell activity. Animal experiments using simultaneous BOLD and intracerebral electrode measures (Logothetis et al., 2001) show that both action potentials and local field potentials (LFPs) correlate with BOLD activity, the link with LFP being the strongest. Further work and references can be found in Logothetis (2003) and in Logothetis & Wandell (2004, and references 27, 29, 54, 55 and 81 therein). While the question of the effect of inhibitory signals on BOLD is still under study, negative BOLD has been convincingly reported as a consequence of decreased neural activity (Shmuel et al., 2002; Duong et al., 2000).

In human neuroimaging, a number of studies report correlation between electric and hemodynamic measures. For instance, using non-simultaneous data, Arthurs et al. (2000) showed linear coupling between fMRI and ERP (evoked related response) amplitude in four out of five subjects for the early N20-P22 amplitude (see also Sammer et al., 2005). However, a number of other studies report discrepancies between the two measurements, such as in Nunez and Silberstein (2000), that might be explained with blind sources or other non- direct links between LFP or action potential activity.

This very short summary leads to the following points:

- BOLD activity can occur without EEG or MEG activity (MEG/EEG silent sources). Specific spatial configurations of the cells or of the sources may annihilate signals at the surface of the scalp. Electric signal synchronization is needed for MEG/EEG detection, but not necessarily for BOLD detection.

- MEG/EEG activity can occur in the absence of BOLD activity (fMRI silent sources) because synchronization may not necessarily consume enough energy to be seen in BOLD.
- The two activities are not necessarily spatially congruent. Many studies have found discrepancies between EEG dipolar localization and fMRI (in Bagshaw et al., 2005, up to 60 mm, but see also the differences reported for the early SI response in Kober et al., 2001; Stippich et al., 1998). These values can be regarded as alarmingly large in the first instance. However, the discrepancy can potentially be caused not only by the variability in the cell types and neuronal activities producing each particular signal of interest, but also by the approximate modeling of dipolar activities.
- The differences in the temporal scales make the direct comparison of the process temporality difficult: BOLD cannot be resolved in time unless very strong assumptions are made both on the hemodynamic model and on the neuronal activity to allow a stable deconvolution process.

To summarize, much remains to be understood about the complexity of the neurotransmission mechanisms and their related biological phenomena before the combined results of different imaging techniques can be solidly interpreted.

Nevertheless, neural activity as seen by electric techniques should often consume enough energy to produce a measurable BOLD effect, even though the BOLD signal does not seem to correspond to the neural activity that consumes the *most* energy (Attwell & Iadecola, 2002). The spatial precision of the BOLD effect that can be observed at the cortical column level (Kim et al., 2000) is also an argument in favor of a mechanism tightly coupled with local electrical activity. At a more macroscopic level, the literature also reports that in some parts of the brain, the spatial consistency can be excellent; for example in the primary visual cortex (Moradi et al., 2003). Therefore, while keeping in mind the limitations listed above, neurophysiology provides us with a good basis for the fusion of the two types of information within a spatial and temporal range that could eventually be close to the cortical column activity.

Non-Simultaneous MEG/EEG and fMRI: The Assumptions and Constraints on Protocol Design

With MEG, only non-simultaneous acquisitions are possible since there is (yet) no apparatus able to capture MRI and MEG signals concurrently (there are, however, projects that have combined MEG and MRI scanners). Since simultaneous acquisition for EEG and fMRI has only been made available recently, the first techniques developed were for separate acquisitions. It is important to note that while MEG signals have to be acquired separately, they are better resolved in space (Leahy et al., 1998) and may therefore be an excellent choice for a multimodal experiment. For further discussion on the pros and cons of simultaneous versus nonsimultaneous acquisitions, see the section below, titled "Simultaneous EEG-fMRI."

Assumptions

Non-simultaneous functional data fusion on one subject makes the assumption that average signal over time will be a reproducible feature. Typically, a subject undergoing a MEG experiment designed to investigate working memory may have slightly different brain networks involved when scanned later with fMRI. While intrasubject reproducibility has been studied (for instance in fMRI, see Symms, 1999) and has been shown to be good in general, it is certainly not perfect, and variations are to be expected. In Schultz et al. (2004), the reproducibility of the intraindividual data was evaluated on one subject, who was scanned 10 times with MEG and 5 times with fMRI. *Intra* subject position confidence interval is shown to be often twice or three times less than the *inter*subject variability. The reproducibility of combined studies has only recently begun to be investigated (Waites et al., 2005).

These between-session variations can be different in nature. First, the networks involved are the same, but acquisition noise slightly alters the measured signals. In this case, signals are assumed to be stationary, and long sessions should reduce the estimator variability. Second, the specificities of the experimental environment lead to a variation in the networks involved. In this case, there is an unknown systematic bias that will be confounded with other factors such as the differing nature of the signals. A typical example, when comparing the MEG and fMRI environments, is the noise produced by the magnet gradient as a consequence of using a standard EPI sequence. The difference between the environment can be diminished by reproducing the EPI noise in the MEG scanner. For instance Kircher et al. (2004) implemented this idea to study mismatched negativity responses in normal and schizophrenic patients in a MEG–fMRI experiment. Third, subjects' physiological and mental states at the moment of the scan can vary and influence the results. This might be thought of as an 'intrasubject random effect factor'. This variance can be reduced by either measuring the signals with similar physiological states—for instance, avoiding scanning at different times during the day (Foucher et al., 2003)—or by measuring several times and averaging results. Finally, time (experiment repetition) can be a significant factor. In this case, and whenever possible, randomizing subjects' order of acquisition should subtract bias while increasing subject-to-subject variability, and therefore should require an increased number of subjects for detecting a given signal.

In the time domain, the issue is complicated by the different time scale of MEG/EEG and fMRI. Often, the assumption is that the time course of the electrical signals are similar between experiments (intra- and intersubject alike). However, since it is not possible to retrieve the electrical (LFP) dynamic from BOLD data—in other words, to solve for the fMRI inverse problem—this assumption will never be adequately addressed. In principle, EEG recordings could play a key role, for instance, in bridging the gap between modalities such as fMRI and MEG, using conjoint recordings in both cases. However, it is certainly not impossible that a different dynamic can be found within the same network of regions between the two acquisitions, which should permit the use of a common localization, but not of a common dynamical description.

In summary, non-simultaneous acquisitions rely on the strong assumption of stationary signals in space and in time, and this needs to be further validated.

In the following, we review the techniques used to analyze jointly non-simultaneous signals (MEG-fMRI, non-simultaneous EEG-fMRI).

Methods for Analyzing MEG and fMRI or Non-Simultaneous EEG and fMRI

As any combination or fusion (above, we distinguished these two notions) will rely on a common spatial localization, where the anatomical structure plays a fundamental role.

For group analyses, subjects can either be scanned with both modalities, or different groups may have to be chosen. The advantage of having two different groups is that there will be no repetition effect: each subject will undergo the experimental protocol only once. The disadvantage is that there is an additional variability due to subject sampling (Goncalves et al., 2005) and this may require a larger number of subjects (e.g., 25). Fusion or combination of information will require a template of the anatomical space.

If individual subjects are scanned twice, the individual cortical gray matter (and subcortical structure) is the common space shared by all functional signals, if inverse problems are solved. Nevertheless, we will see also that a number of techniques do not make use of the individual anatomical structure. The reason lies within the fundamental problem of inter-individual anatomo-functional variability. Since there is no simple mapping between the anatomy of a single subject to another or a template, group analyses have to perform approximations that blur anatomical sulcogyral details, but also individual functional details. In the rest of the chapter, we therefore distinguish between methods than can use the individual space (use of MRI for MEG/EEG source reconstruction, simultaneous EEG/fMRI acquisitions) and methods that have to rely on an average anatomy such as the MNI template. Clearly, fusion or multimodal combinations of information for intersubject analyses bring together two separate difficulties: how to combine or fuse multimodal data, and how to extract summary knowledge from the data of a group of subjects.

The Comparison of Separated Analysis Results

Dipolar Analyses

Most of the comparison data available in the literature are for the spatial domain. Early studies report the distances between fMRI or PET activations with source localization, estimated using inverse problems on MEG or EEG. Those early studies often used simple tasks (Takanashi et al., 1996; Rossini et al., 1998; Ahlfors et al., 1999) or, more recently, for interictal epileptic dipolar localization with simultaneous EEG/fMRI recordings (Lemieux et al., 2001; Bagshaw et al., 2005; Benar et al., 2006). If good concordances of localizations were occasionally observed, the mean distance between the dipoles and the hemodynamic activations has often been reported to reach 1 to 2 cm (for instance, in the somatosensory cortices; Del Gratta et al., 2002). Furthermore, in epileptic analysis many sources seen with EEG were not detected as fMRI activations and, conversely, some fMRI activations did not correspond to close ECD (Equivalent Current Dipole) localization (Benar et al., 2006). This may be explained by (1) the difference between the physiological process observed, (2) the limitations of the dipolar localization method in MEG or EEG, or (3) by the fMRI detection sensitivity difference (Bagshaw et al., 2005).

Distributed Models
If dipolar source reconstruction is the most widely used technique, some authors have employed other localization techniques, such as the distributed source model, to compare the results from different modalities. For example, Moradi et al. (2003) have compared the localization obtained in a retinotopic experiment using fMRI with those obtained using Magnetic Field Tomography (MFT). They found small discrepancies between the two experiments, on the order of 3 to 5 mm.

Beamformer (scanning) Analysis
Perhaps the best way to compare MEG/EEG and fMRI activations is to use beamformer inverse techniques. Indeed, these techniques do not require averaging of the signals across events, and are better adapted to recover evoked or induced activities in different frequency bands. Furthermore, for those reconstructed data, one can use statistical detection procedures similar to those of fMRI at the individual and group levels. Comparisons are then straightforward. Singh et al. (2002) have shown converging activated networks by comparing BOLD activations and event-related desynchronization or synchronization in different frequency bands.

Alternatively, results can be compared through the fMRI and MEG/EEG responses to different experimental conditions. The assumption is that the modulations of the electric responses can be attributed to regions showing differences in BOLD activity in the different conditions. In other words, the region responsible for the modulation of the ERP response must be the one that changes its activity under the same experimental modulation, while the timing of the change is obtained from the ERP response. This reasoning led to the localization in time and space of activity modulation without an inverse problem (Downing, 2001; Dehaene, 1998).

Finding Resemblances in MEG/EEG and fMRI Data:
Multivariate Techniques

Since the two data sets share a common spatial dimension, it is, in principle, simple to look for the instances where the spatial information is the most coherent. This necessitates the reconstruction of distributed sources at a resolution comparable to the fMRI, or degrading the fMRI spatial information to the point that it can be compared to MEG/EEG. Note that using the fMRI information to reconstruct the MEG/EEG source at this stage would bias results. Once the two data sets have exactly the same number of "voxels," it is a straightforward matter to compute their cross-correlation. The result is a matrix (fMRI_time X MEG/EEG_time) in which high values indicate the times for which both electrical and metabolic maps are most correlated. The cross-correlation can then be decomposed by standard singular-value decomposition techniques, and corresponding BOLD pattern and MEG/EEG timing extracted.

To quantify this equivalence in an experiment combining MEG and fMRI to study the sensory cortex representation of digit and lip, Schultz et al. (2004) describe the reconstruction of MEG activity with the SAM beamformer technique (SAM: Synthetic Aperture Magnetometry) and obtained an image with space-dimension equivalent to fMRI. The SAM images are constructed for different frequency bands, and a voxel-per-voxel multiplication is performed between the unthresholded fMRI and SAM images. The results are summarized through standard singular-value decomposition. The authors report some areas within SI that are not found by either fMRI nor MEG. While the idea is interesting, the interpretation of the voxel-per-voxel multiplication of SAM and fMRI images is not clear, raises intensity and spatial normalization issues, and will cancel out signals that are not present in only one of the two modalities.

A similar approach considers the space defined by the scalp as the shared common space. While this would strongly diminish the fMRI resolution, it avoids the difficult source reconstruction step. Assuming—again—that the BOLD activity will coincide with sources having significant electrical energy, a projection onto the scalp (or electrode) space would make the two data sets directly comparable. The MEG/EEG data would then be transformed to retain only the energy, and the same dimension-reduction techniques can be further used to decompose this cross-correlation and extract the conjoint time/space information.

Using fMRI Information to Constrain EEG Localization Information

As the MEG/EEG inverse problem is underdetermined, and does not offer a unique solution, it seems at first sight reasonable to use the localization information given by fMRI to constrain the inverse problem, yielding an estimate of the activity time courses in the fMRI-detected regions.

However, because of the different nature of the data (as reviewed in the introduction), this approach raises several questions: (1) What fMRI information should be used? Spatial localization, or amount of activation? Information resulting from group or individual analysis? (2) Which types of constraints should be implemented—hard constraints (assuming complete equivalence between MEG/EEG and fMRI localizations), or enabling extra sources or small displacements (soft constraints)? (3) What is the influence of those constraints in the results?

As these different concerns depend on the EEG/MEG inverse method, we will address these questions separately for dipolar and distributed-source reconstructions. Those methods are described in detail in other chapters of this book, so we will review the literature only with respect to combining multimodal information. See also the review by Halchenko et al. (2005) on this topic.

Dipole Reconstruction with fMRI Information

In this technique (Pouthas et al., 2000; Ahlfors et al., 1999; Toma et al., 2002; Torquati, 2005), the MEG/EEG signals are first modeled by a number of ECDs at or around the location of BOLD or PET peak activity. The time courses of these constrained dipoles are then obtained by simple linear minimization techniques. These time courses are most often obtained at the group level, since the evoked responses are commonly computed after averaging all subjects. Similarly, the fMRI activations often result from a group analysis, although the fMRI group of subjects is not necessarily the same as the MEG/EEG group. A critical aspect of the procedure is that the set of regions is strongly dependent on the threshold chosen to detect BOLD activity, and the results may not be robust with this threshold. Our opinion is, therefore, that the technique should be used very carefully, and its results can only give a crude view of the spatiotemporal neuronal processes under investigation. Often, the "BOLD linked dipoles" are not sufficient to account for the MEG/EEG data and the goodness-of-fit of the model can be improved by adding a number of dipoles with free locations.

The strategy can also be reversed by first finding the ECD with no constraints, then adding a number of dipoles with positions close to regions that elicit BOLD activity. The detected ECDs without fMRI information can be constrained to their positions found initially (Brunetti et al., 2005), or can be restricted to a location close to their initial position (Torquati et al., 2005).

Another approach to using fMRI information for the dipolar analysis is to help in deciding which MEG inverse solution is better among those with a reasonable goodness-of-fit. This is especially useful when the goodness-of-fit for the dipole model is similar in two solutions, in which case the solution showing the closest resemblance to the fMRI activity would be preferred. (Ahlfors et al., 1999)

Because fMRI activation can extend over several square centimeters, the activity of such a large region may not be well modeled by a single dipole placed at the maximum, or center of mass, of the suprathreshold cluster. Fujimaki et al. (2002) developed a method for constraining ECD in fMRI activation areas, but they divide large fMRI activation volumes into subvolumes, in each of which a dipole is placed.

Importantly, as many authors report distances between dipole position and BOLD localization estimated independently to be greater than the constraints put on the dipoles location, there are indications that *hard and soft constraints based on fMRI data for M/EEG reconstruction should be use cautiously.*

Distributed Reconstruction with fMRI Information

Distributed-inverse techniques reconstruct the amplitudes of a great number of dipolar sources, uniformly spaced on multiple locations in a source space (volumic or surfacic) at each timepoint. The localization of active regions is derived from the variation of amplitudes in time and space. Clearly, the problem is undetermined (see Chapter 5), as the number of unknowns is greater compared to the number of EEG or MEG data, and additional information or constraints must be introduced. The selected solution would be the only one that satisfies the constraints, and corresponds best to the *a priori* information. In this context, the information derived from fMRI can help define prior constraints for the source reconstruction process.

Different source spaces may be considered. The seminal paper of Dale and Sereno (1993) showed how the cortical surface can be used to reduce the possible set of solutions for the inverse problem, and more precisely how the grey-white matter interface enables one to constrain both source localization and source orientation. Furthermore, because BOLD should originate mainly from the capillaries irrigating the cortex layers, cortical surface is the natural space on which fMRI and MEG/EEG should be merged.

In further work, Liu and collaborators have suggested that the local fMRI response can be used to bias the electrical activity estimate toward those regions that show the greatest fMRI response (Liu et al., 1998; Dale et al., 2000; Bonmassar et al., 2001; Liu et al., 2002). The principle of the method is to take fMRI signals into account in the diagonal elements of the *a priori* source covariance matrix. Those diagonal elements represent the spatial locations of the potential sources. Liu et al. (1998) computed with large Monte Carlo simulations that a coefficient of 1 and 0.1 respectively, for locations with and without fMRI activation, gave the "best" results. This corresponds to a 90% weighting toward locations that are believed to contain fMRI activity, and "best" is used in the sense that the dipoles were found to be influenced, but not too influenced, by fMRI information. However, simulation studies from the same authors show that the solution can then be easily overconstrained. If, as is possible, there are mismatches between the electrical and hemodynamic signals, the solution can then be seriously misplaced (Liu et al., 1998; Liu, 2000).

Using the same principles, Babiloni et al. (2003) estimate the prior source covariance matrix using fMRI information on an individual basis.

They directly include the percentage increase of the fMRI signal in the diagonal elements of the matrix, and introduce in the non-diagonal elements the correlation of the fMRI signals between the two corresponding areas. Simulations performed with this method showed that in the case of concordant activations, results are superior to those of a standard inverse problem with no constraints—and, crucially, solutions are equivalent when active sources *do not* correspond to fMRI spots.

Recently, Ahlfors et al. (2004) formulated the problem as a geometrical problem. This is a classic interpretation of the linear model, as the least-square estimate can be viewed as the orthogonal projection of the data onto a space spanned by the columns of the model. With this view, the bias introduced by fMRI data can be seen as a non-orthogonal projection, defined by fMRI activity.

To conclude the discussion of methods with hard or soft constraints: the work of Im et al. (2005) again suggests a word of caution. They report, both in a simulation and in a lexical judgment experiment, cases where modifying the variance of the source in order to bias results towards fMRI data, may also weaken or eliminate actual MEG sources. They also suggest a technique to use in checking whether those sources are likely artifacts, or true sources. The difficulty still lies in the lack of solid ground information on the actual local coupling between MEG sources and fMRI/BOLD activity.

Finally, Daunizeau et al. (2006) have recently presented an interesting framework to test the relevance of fMRI priors in the inverse problem, using a Bayesian formalism. They constructed different priors under two different hypotheses. Under the first one, H0, there is no correspondence between fMRI and MEG/EEG sources (the priors are simply defined as a independent zero-mean Gaussian with constant variance). Under the second hypothesis, H1, a link is assumed between the fMRI activation map and the source intensities, and the corresponding prior is modified by weighting the source variance by a factor that is proportional to a function of the fMRI activation. These two hypotheses are then compared, by computing the ratio between the posterior probability of the model H0 and H1, given the MEG/EEG data M: $\log(P(H1/M)/P(H0/M))$. If this ratio is positive, then the fMRI-constrained inverse problem solution should be favored.

Fusion Model with Non-Simultaneous Acquisitions?

This line of research consists of defining large-scale neural models, generated with computer techniques, and simulating data at the neuronal level and at the system level. The neuronal-level parameters associated to the model can be estimated using single-unit electrophysiology recordings, and the system level parameters can be estimated using neuroimaging data (PET, fMRI, MEG/EEG). These models may help in understanding how interacting neural populations implement higher-level cognitive or sensorimotor activity. The ultimate goal of these models is to generate data and predict the results of both electrophysiology and multimodal imaging experiments. It is still unclear if this can be achieved in the foreseeable future. It should be noted that more and more researchers are attempting to, at least partially, address the problem. Horwitz and colleagues in particular (Horwitz & Tagamets 1999; Husain et al., 2004; Riera et al., 2005; see Horwitz & Glabus, 2005, for a review) have pursued these ideas in the context of cognitive systems interactions. Recently, Friston and colleagues (Friston et al., 2003) described a model to study effective connectivity that expresses activity at the neuronal level, but estimates the parameters using fMRI data and the Balloon model (Buxton et al., 1998).

In Babajani et al. (2005), an integrated model for MEG and fMRI is described in which the neural activity is related to the postsynaptic potentials (PSPs). In each voxel, the neural activity is modeled by a MEG ECD, and as input of extended balloon model in fMRI. The model shows that it is possible to detect fMRI activity but no MEG activity, and vice versa. The model could be used in the future to evaluate and compare different conjoint analysis methods of MEG and fMRI.

The major advantage of this approach is that one could work with a model able to reproduce the mechanism at the origin of signals—therefore, predictions, validation or refutations should be much easier to perform. In a sense, this is the grail that any neuroscientist is looking for. Unfortunately— and this constitutes a major issue in this research—there is simply no such model available at the level where it would be needed. While the balloon model sounds like a good approximation of the mechanistic aspects of the vascular properties of brain tissue, a full model that would truly permit the reproduction of even simple tasks are few, and are hardly convincing. In other words, while this direction of research seems to be the most appealing, it might not be fruitful until much more is known about how a simulated neural network can mimic brain processes and performances. At the moment, it is only too likely that those models are too restrictive, incomplete, or even wrong, and therefore will not help the fusion of data from several modalities. Nevertheless, it is worth noting the works that propose dynamic recurrent network models relating neuronal electrophysiological data to fMRI or PET (Corchs & Deco, 2002; Tagamets and Horwitz, 1998), as well as models that relate neuronal data to MEG/EEG signals (Arezzo & Vaughan, 1988, David et al., 2006).

Pros and Cons of Simultaneous EEG-fMRI versus MEG/EEG and fMRI

Simultaneous Acquisition: What Can We Gain?

First, for individual subject or group analyses, simultaneous EEG and fMRI acquisition does not have to rely on the assumption of reproducible physiological or cognitive state between two scanning sessions. Since it is not possible in general to verify this assumption, the advantage is fundamental. At the level of a group study, the additional assumptions are those necessary for fMRI alone, i.e., that there exists a common spatial and functional space in which the different subjects can be averaged.

Second, there are a number of research questions that can only be addressed by simultaneous acquisitions. For example, in the study of the vigilance state, to which alpha waves are associated (Goldman et al., 2002), simultaneous recordings are mandatory. Another clear example of this is shown in the sleep studies (Portas et al., 2000; Czisch et al., 2002; Maquet et al., 2003 & 2005) and the epileptic activation (Lemieux et al., 2001; Salek-Haddadi, 2002) for which the studied phenomenon is better defined through external measurements. In general, it is possible that simultaneous recordings are necessary for a correct interpretation of the fMRI data.

Third, joint recordings also allow one to investigate the link between the two kinds of measures, and may therefore set the basis and the limit for their combination in nonsimultaneous experiments. Here we describe further how the EEG-fMRI data covariation can be investigated locally.

Simultaneous Acquisition: What are the Drawbacks?

There are a number of difficulties inherent to EEG/fMRI measurements. They can be summarized as follows: loss of signals in EEG, loss of signals in fMRI, and experimental constraints. The high-static magnetic field of the MRI scanner necessitates special equipment such as nonmagnetic electrodes and amplifiers that may not be as sensitive as the usual MEG/EEG equipment. Second, magnetic gradients and radio-frequency pulses induce currents and generate large artifacts that have to be corrected (Allen et al., 2000; Niazy et al., 2005; Wan et al., 2006). The cardiac signal also requires special treatment. Third, because the experimental paradigm has to comply with both EEG and fMRI constraints, it cannot be fully optimized for both modalities and a trade-off has to be reached, depending on which is the most needed data for the question at stake.

In practice, a crucially important factor for the success of the combined information lies in the subject positioning, because the subject's comfort will dictate his or her movements during the acquisition (Lemieux et al., 1997). The discomfort can be such that subjects may not want to remain in the scanner for the duration of the acquisition session. Clearly, the quality of the data—EEG data mostly, but also BOLD—is highly dependent on the subject's movements. Standard cushions are usually not sufficient, and the head will eventually put too much weight on the electrodes at the back of the head (O1, O2). Many have found that vacuum cushions are necessary because they allow the pressure to be more equally shared on a greater scalp surface; they also minimize subjects' movements. Another important limiting factor is the experimental set-up time for each acquisition. This is a problem shared by conjoint EEG-MEG acquisitions.

In summary, conjoint recording can be extremely harmful to the data, can impose important constraints to the experimental protocol and limit the number of subjects scanned, and therefore should not be used unless the question under investigation cannot be answered without such data (Garreffa et al., 2004).

Acquisition Schemes

First, we define three acquisition schemes for simultaneous EEG–fMRI. We distinguish the spike-triggered acquisition—historically, the first to be developed for epilepsy, which entails waiting for an interictal spike, detecting it with a filter, and triggering the fMRI acquisition (Lemieux et al., 2001). The second kind of acquisition entails continuously recording the EEG and fMRI signals, and hoping that the artifacts generated by the fMRI can be appropriately corrected (Allen et al., 2000; Lemieux et al., 2001). The third principle is very much like a continuous acquisition, but with gaps of 1–2 seconds between BOLD volume acquisitions (Foucher et al., 2003). This leaves some time to place interesting stimulations while the gradients are not operating.

We review here the paradigm constraints that are common to all simultaneous EEG–fMRI acquisitions, and those that depend upon whether the acquisition is spike-triggered, alternate, or continuous.

- **Spike-triggered.** This requires having a good system to detect interictal spikes with sufficient sensitivity and specificity.
- **Continuous acquisition.** There are no specific constraints in addition to the usual constraints.
- **Alternate acquisitions.** This technique relies on the slow dynamic of the hemodynamic response. An example of such a paradigm is shown in Figure 11–1. In this example, the BOLD response is sampled regularly every 3 seconds, with 1.5 seconds of gradient (actual BOLD recording) and 1.5 seconds of silence (no gradient, therefore no noise and no gradient artifacts). This requires that the stimulation giving rise to the evoked potential is short enough, so that its EEG response can be captured within the time window, taking into account that 100–200 ms should elapse before stimulus triggering, to facilitate recording the baseline. It also means that the scanner electronics and acquisition sequence will be able to sample the brain in a shorter time. Soon, "SENSE" imaging should enable much quicker acquisition and/or better resolution, but multiple-canal head coils are, as yet, too small to place the EEG cap inside those coils. Specific head coils need to be developed.

Note that the same idea is used in fMRI for auditory or language paradigms, for which the gradients-generated noise is a problem, but with a much longer delay between EPI acquisitions. For instance, the scanner is triggered for a couple of seconds, 4 to 5 seconds after the auditory stimulation, at the

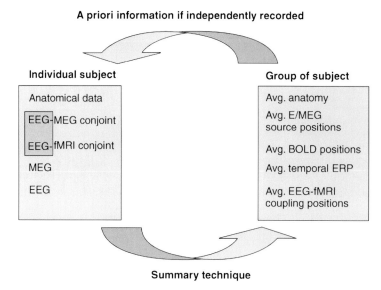

A priori information if independently recorded

Individual subject

Anatomical data
EEG-MEG conjoint
EEG-fMRI conjoint
MEG
EEG

Group of subject

Avg. anatomy
Avg. E/MEG source positions
Avg. BOLD positions
Avg. temporal ERP
Avg. EEG-fMRI coupling positions

Summary technique

Figure 11–1. Group versus individual data analysis interplay: constructing summary measures across subjects should help to provide a priori information on independently acquired data.

peak of the hemodynamic response. This is also known as "sparse event acquisition." The difficulty is that there are very few scans to be analyzed, and therefore the sensitivity is low and signals are difficult to detect (see, e.g., Belin et al., 2000 regarding fMRI, and Brunetti et al., 2005, for a design in a joint MEG-fMRI study).

Methods of Analysis (Simultaneous)

Regression Analysis

This method is the most commonly applied technique, and its principles are very simple. Since the EEG data is thought to be linked to the BOLD signal through a linear convolution with a specified hemodynamic function, in a first approximation it is customary to look for correlations between BOLD and EEG "transformed" data. The steps of the method are: (1) choose the type of EEG signal to be related to BOLD, (2) convolve with a chosen hemodynamic response, (3) subsample this signal at the resolution of the BOLD data, and (4) regress the results of step (3) onto BOLD data. In other words, a linear model such as those used in SPM, FSL, or other packages, is constructed with the explanatory variables originating from the EEG signal. The procedure is summarized in Figure 11–2.

The method has the following strengths and limitations. First, its main strength is its simplicity and applicability. Standard fMRI analysis methods

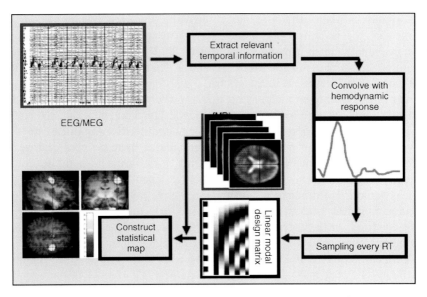

Figure 11–2. Principle of the construction of a BOLD brain volume activity from simultaneous EEG acquisitions.

can then be used for detecting regions. It is also simple to interpret, as the maps produced can be easily thought of as correlation maps. The method is flexible and has successfully been used in a number of previous works. The works of Laufs et al. (2003), Goldman et al. (2002), and others who have found regions where hemodynamic functions correlate most with increased alpha- or beta-frequency power, are based on this method. More recently, Foucher et al. (2003) show that the gamma-band power is related to BOLD activity in an oddball detection task. In Debener et al. (2005), EEG single-trial electric activity is computed as the minimum value in a temporal window, defined using the grand average of independent component analysis results. These amplitudes are convolved with the canonical hemodynamic response, and used as regressors for the fMRI analysis. This trial-by-trial EEG measure predicted the fMRI activity in the rostral cingulate zone, a brain region thought to play a key role in processing of response errors. Using the same principle, Parkes et al. (2006) investigate the post-movement beta rebound (an increased in beta-frequency power following movement) and use a time-frequency analysis of the EEG signal to construct regressors for the fMRI analysis—and, with the EEG, detect an additional region in the post-central sulcus for this task. Interestingly, signals of no interest can be treated similarly, to remove fMRI artifacts such as the cardiac beat (Liston et al., 2005). These are but very few of the examples that can be found in the literature, and it is expected that many more studies will use this method to relate the two types of information.

However, there are limitations to the technique. First, it is important to note that the hemodynamic model is not constant across the brain— for example, with epileptic patients (Kang et al., 2003; Gotman et al., 2004), and with normal subjects (Neumann et al., 2003). Therefore, the models relating the local BOLD response to the electric signals have to be estimated locally, and the relationship on a larger scale in space is yet to be investigated. Second, in optical imaging studies (near-infra red optical imaging, or NIOI) that have high spatial precision and can reveal the oxy and deoxy components of the BOLD signal, Devor et al. (2003) demonstrated that there is a nonlinear relationship between neural activity and the local evoked hemodynamic. Tuunanen et al. (2003) also observed differing dependency of the BOLD and MEG responses on interstimulus intervals. While this can be seen as invalidating the linear models that are widely used for describing the link between the two kinds of measures, it is still possible that a linear approximation is a good description for a given range of neural signal timing and magnitude. Third, the so-called silent BOLD phenomenon during registration of the MEG/EEG signals may produce poor correlations.

Coupling Detection: Local Versus Nonlocal

With the regression technique, a map is constructed. This permits the description of local phenomena and, to some extent, their interpretation. However, the actual *local* correlation of the electrical signal with the BOLD signal is never computed, and cannot be until a local estimation of the EEG signal is estimated through an inverse solution. In Lahaye et al. (2004), this local correlation is computed and the locations of high correlations are compared to the position of the highest BOLD signal and EEG signals. This is a challenging task, since the number of electrodes used for simultaneous acquisitions, and the associated signal-to-noise ratio issues, make the source reconstruction particularly difficult. In this work, a parcellation of the surface of the brain was computed to reduce the number of possible sources to 1000 per hemisphere, and the local hemodynamic responses were computed on those parcels (Ciuciu et al., 2003). The correlation could then be computed using a local regression analysis technique, by convolving the EEG source-reconstructed signal of interest by the local hemodynamic function. Because the experimental paradigm was designed as event-related, it was also possible to correlate each event BOLD-magnitude to the event EEG-summary measure. Preliminary results show that the location of the highest correlation does not coincide closely either with the location of the reconstructed sources with the strongest energy, nor to the mean maximum BOLD value across events. This confirms other findings that indirectly compared the positions of the MEG/EEG reconstructed sources and the BOLD activity.

This local coupling can then be used to constrain the inverse problem in an iterative scheme. Lahaye et al. (2004) have proposed to weight differently the source covariance matrix, using the coupling coefficient derived locally on a trial by trial basis. This allows a new estimate of an optimized spatial filter in a beamformer formalism. fMRI priors on localization are introduced only where a significant coupling is demonstrated.

Conjoint Linear Multivariate Analysis a la Martinez-Montes (2005)

One difficulty with the standard regression analysis described above is that the EEG data to be convolved and regressed must be specified, and may not be clearly known from the literature. To solve for this, Martinez-Montes (2004) proposes a multivariate linear analysis using a technique originally developed in the domain of chemometrics. Its basic idea is to extend the Partial Least Square technique for data with higher dimensions than are possible with PLS. fMRI data has dimension time and voxels, while the EEG data has dimension time (shared dimension), frequency, and electrodes. The method proposed will find the weights of a BOLD image and the weights of electrodes and frequencies, such that the correlation of the two time dimensions is maximized. In other words, the technique will find a BOLD image on the one hand, a frequency spectrum, and the topographic map on the other hand. In this way, the linear combination of the BOLD time series weighted by the found BOLD image will maximally correlate with the linear combination of the EEG time series weighted by the topographic map and frequency spectrum. The method is interesting as a means to quickly summarize the important features of the covariation of such large data. It does require that a constant model of the hemodynamic response is chosen *a priori*, and that the EEG data are preprocessed to remove muscle and motion artifacts. When applied to the data used by Goldman et al. (2002), the results show that the time dimensions are well correlated in the alpha band, less in the theta, and not in the gamma. Spatially, the alpha and gamma spatial representation is found to be in the occipital, while the theta has a pattern less clearly interpretable.

Conclusion

The combination of neuroimaging techniques is an intense research domain, which will grow in the future due to the increasing number of noninvasive imaging techniques and their technological advances. If this chapter is mainly concerned with the fusion between electromagnetic and hemodynamic signals for brain mapping, other imaging modalities or information can be considered (diffusion MRI, optical imaging, etc.) but the corresponding literature is still meager on the use of those with MEG/EEG data.

Could a MEG with good spatial localization power replace conjoint EEG-fMRI recording?

With the progress of inverse resolution techniques in MEG, one can ask the question whether sufficient spatial and temporal resolution can be reached with this technique alone, and whether performing cumbersome simultaneous or non-simultaneous recordings is helpful. The answer at the time of the writing of this text is yes. The first argument is that the MEG/EEG inverse problem has, fundamentally, not a unique solution, and fMRI provides additional means to assess the localization of active regions. However, as seen before, for a number of physiological reasons the networks seen in MEG/EEG may not be identical to those seen in fMRI, in which case fMRI is not an appropriate response to the problem of the nondetermination of MEG/EEG inverse solutions (see Babiloni [2004] for an example of study with fMRI, EEG, and MEG and the localization problem).

Nevertheless, this very observation may turn out to be the strongest argument in favor of the fusion: data recorded in both modalities do not reflect the exact same neuronal and physiological processes. The conjoint use of those modalities should reveal brain processes invisible to any single modality alone. In the course of time, when more knowledge is available on the physiological coupling, the combined recordings may allow a more complete description of the neural and metabolic brain processes. In this sense, *combination of MEG/EEG and fMRI is more informative than fusion between MEG and EEG* issued from the same neuronal signals, even if the sensitivities of these two techniques are different according to position and source orientations.

EEG can also be seen as a key measure, since it is one that can be made during both MEG and fMRI experiments. In this sense, EEG signals could define a common temporal reference linked to the experimental paradigm (for instance, using evoked potential), relating MEG and fMRI nonsimultaneous acquisitions. More specifically, the early or late components of evoked potential can be localized with both EEG/MEG and EEG/fMRI signals, establishing a precise relationship for the localization obtained with these two modalities. In this domain, the ongoing development of new acquisition systems such as simultaneous EEG/MEG recordings may provide more comfortable simultaneous recordings, yielding better spatial and time resolution than those currently available with EEG/fMRI.

The most interesting future research may come from diffusion imaging. As brain imaging moves from purely localization issues to the understanding of brain interactions and their dynamics (e.g., Babiloni et al., 2005), diffusion MRI imaging is likely to play a crucial role in determining anatomical connectivity. In conjunction with the localization power of MEG and fMRI, and the studies of functional signals interactions with MEG/EEG and fMRI via coherence or correlation analysis, one may hope that a model of function will emerge at the level of neuroimaging information. So far, little has been published on the subject (Kamada et al., 2003). Concerning MEG/EEG, DTI imaging has only been used to infer models of anisotropic conductivity from DTI diffusion tension, for the computation of forward models, but this data is shown to correlate with behavior (Tuch et al., 2005). To our knowledge, no research has been done to relate information about MEG/EEG synchronies or coherences to anatomical knowledge of the main connectivity paths in the brain.

In this domain, linking an increase or decrease of synchronization patterns in a population with an abnormal diffusion MRI pattern or fMRI activity (Mizuhara et al., 2005) will certainly be of particular interest in understanding the dysfunctions associated with some pathologies. But this requires better knowledge of the diffusion MRI pattern in the normal population.

References

Ahlfors, S. P., Simpson, G. V., Dale, A. M., Belliveau, J. W., Liu, A. K., Korvenoja, A., et al. (1999). Spatiotemporal activity of a cortical network for processing visual motion revealed by MEG and fMRI. *J Neurophysiol, 82*(5), 2545–2555.

Ahlfors, S. P., & Simpson, G. V. (2004). Geometrical interpretation of fMRI-guided MEG/EEG inverse estimates. *Neuroimage, 22*(1), 323–332.

Allen, P. J., Josephs, O., & Turner, R. (2002). A method for removing imaging artifact from continuous EEG recorded during functional MRI. *Neuroimage, 12*(2), 230–239.

Arezzo, J. C., & Vaughan, H. G. Jr. (1982). The contribution of afferent fiber tracts to the somatosensory evoked potential. *Ann N Y Acad Sci, 388*, 679–682.

Arthurs, O. J., Williams, E. J., Carpenter, T. A., Pickard, J. D., & Boniface, S. J. (2000). Linear coupling between functional magnetic resonance imaging and evoked potential amplitude in human somatosensory cortex. *Neuroscience, 101*, 803–806.

Babajani A, Nekooei MH, Soltanian-Zadeh H. Integrated MEG and fMRI model: synthesis and analysis. *Brain Topogr.* 2005 Winter;*18*(2):101–13. Epub 2005 Dec 5. PubMed PMID: 16341578.

Babiloni, F., Babiloni, C., Carducci, F., Romani, G. L., Rossini, P. M., Angelone, L. M., et al. (2003). Multimodal integration of high-resolution EEG and functional magnetic resonance imaging data: a simulation study. *Neuroimage, 19*(1), 1–15.

Babiloni, F., Cincotti, F., Babiloni, C., Carducci, F., Mattia, D., Astolfi, L., et al. (2005). Estimation of the cortical functional connectivity with the multimodal integration of high-resolution EEG and fMRI data by directed transfer function. *Neuroimage, 1*, 24(1), 118–131.

Babiloni, F., Mattia, D., Babiloni, C., Astolfi, L., Salinari, S., Basilisco, A., et al. (2004). Multimodal integration of EEG, MEG and fMRI data for the solution of the neuroimage puzzle. *Magn Reson Imaging, 22*(10), 1471–1476.

Bagshaw, A. P., Hawco, C., Benar, C. G., Kobayashi, E., Aghakhani, Y., Dubeau, F., et al. (2005). Analysis of the EEG-fMRI response to prolonged bursts of interictal epileptiform activity. *Neuroimage, 24*(4), 1099–1112.

Bagshaw, A. P., Kobayashi, E., Dubeau, F., Pike, G. B., & Gotman, J. (2006). Correspondence between EEG-fMRI and EEG dipole localisation of interictal discharges in focal epilepsy. *Neuroimage, 30*, 417–425.

Ball, T., Schreiber, A., Feige, B., Wagner, M., Lucking, C. H., & Kristeva-Feige, R. (1999). The role of higher-order motor areas in voluntary movement as revealed by high-resolution EEG and fMRI. *Neuroimage, 10*(6), 682–694.

Belin, P., Zatorre, R. J., Lafaille, P., Ahad, P., & Pike, B. (2000). Voice-selective areas in human auditory cortex. *Nature, 403*(6767), 309–312.

Benar, C., Aghakhani, Y., Wang, Y., Izenberg, A., Al-Asmi, A., Dubeau, F., et al. (2003). Quality of EEG in simultaneous EEG-fMRI for epilepsy. *Clin Neurophysiol, 114*(3), 569–580.

Benar, C. G., Grova, C., Kobayashi, E., Bagshaw, A. P., Aghakhani, Y., Dubeau, F., et al. (2006). EEG fMRI of epileptic spikes: Concordance with EEG source localization and intracranial EEG. *Neuroimage, 30,* 1161–1170

Bonmassar, G., Schwartz, D. P., Liu, A. K., Kwong, K. K., Dale, A. M., & Belliveau, J. W. (2001). Spatiotemporal brain imaging of visual-evoked activity using interleaved EEG and fMRI recordings. *Neuroimage, 13*(6–1),1035–1043.

Brunetti, M., Belardinelli, P., Caulo, M., Del Gratta, C., Della Penna, S., Ferretti, A., et al. (2005). Human brain activation during passive listening to sounds from different locations: an fMRI and MEG study. *Hum Brain Mapp, 26*(4), 251–261.

Buxton, R. B., Wong, E. C., & Frank, L. R. (1998). Dynamics of blood flow and oxygenation changes during brain activation: the balloon model. *Magn Reson Med, 39*(6), 855–864.

Ciuciu, P., Poline, J.-B., Marrelec, G., Idier, J., Pallier, Ch., & Benali, H. (2003). Unsupervised robust non-parametric estimation of the hemodynamic response function for any fMRI experiment. *IEEE Trans Med Imag, 22*(10), 1235–1251.

Corchs, S., & Deco, G. (2002). Large-scale neural model for visual attention: integration of experimental single-cell and fMRI data. *Cereb Cortex, 12*(4), 339–48.

Czisch, M., Wetter, T. C., Kaufmann, C., Pollmacher, T., Holsboer, F., & Auer, D. P. (2002). Altered processing of acoustic stimuli during sleep: reduced auditory activation and visual deactivation detected by a combined fMRI/EEG study. *Neuroimage, 16*(1), 251–258.

Dale, A. M., Liu, A. K., Fischl, B. R., Buckner, R. L., Belliveau, J. W., Lewine, J. D., et al. (2000) Dynamic statistical parametric mapping: combining fMRI and MEG for high-resolution imaging of cortical activity. *Neuron, 26*(1), 55–67.

Daunizeau, J., Mattout, J., Clonda, D., Goulard, B., Benali, H., & Lina, J. M. (2006) Bayesian spatio-temporal approach for EEG source reconstruction: conciliating ECD and distributed models. *IEEE transactions on bio-medical engineering* 53, 503–516.

David, O., Kiebel, S. J., Harrison, L. M., Mattout, J., Kilner, J. M., & Friston, K. J. (2006). Dynamic causal modeling of evoked responses in EEG and MEG. *Neuroimage, 30,* 1255–1272.

Debener, S., Ullsperger, M., Siegel, M., Fiehler, K., von Cramon, D. Y., Engel, A. K. (2005) Trial-by-trial coupling of concurrent electroencephalogram and functional magnetic resonance imaging identifies the dynamics of performance monitoring. *J Neurosci, 25,* 11730–11737.

Dehaene, S., Naccache, L., Le Clec, H. G., Koechlin, E., Mueller, M., Dehaene-Lambertz, G., et al. (1998). Imaging unconscious semantic priming. *Nature, 395,* 597–600.

Del Gratta, C., Della Penna, S., Ferretti, A., Franciotti, R., Pizzella, V., Tartaro, A., et al. (2002). Topographic organization of the human primary and secondary somatosensory cortices. comparison of fMRI and MEG findings. *Neuroimage, 17*(3), 1373–1383.

Devor, A., Dunn, A. K., Andermann, M. L., Ulbert, I., Boas, D. A., & Dale, A. M. (2003). Coupling of total hemoglobin concentration, oxygenation, and neural activity in rat somatosensory cortex. *Neuron, 39*(2), 353–359.

Downing, P., Liu, J., & Kanwisher, N. (2001). Testing cognitive models of visual attention with fMRI and MEG. *Neuropsychologia, 39*(12), 1329–1342.

Duong, T, Q., Kim, D. S., Ugurbil, K., & Kim S. G.(2000). Spatiotemporal dynamics of the BOLD fMRI signals: toward mapping submillimeter cortical columns using the early negative response. *Magn Reson Med*, *44*(2), 231–242.

Foucher, J. R., Otzenberger, H., & Gounot, D. (2003). The BOLD response and the gamma oscillations respond differently than evoked potentials: an interleaved EEG-fMRI study. *BMC Neurosci*, *4*, 22.

Foucher, J. R., Otzenberger, H., & Gounot, D. Where arousal meets attention: a simultaneous fMRI and EEG recording study. *Neuroimage*, *22*(2), 688–697.

Friston, K. J., Harrison, L., & Penny, W. (2003). Dynamic causal modelling. *Neuroimage*, *19*(4), 1273–1302.

Fujimaki, N., Hayakawa, T., Nielsen, M., Knosche, T. R., & Miyauchi, S. (2002). An fMRI-constrained MEG source analysis with procedures for dividing and grouping activation. *Neuroimage*, *17*(1), 324–343.

Garreffa, G., Bianciardi, M., Hagberg, G. E., Macaluso, E., Marciani, M. G., Maraviglia, B., et al. (2004). Simultaneous EEG-fMRI acquisition: how far is it from being a standardized technique? *Magn Reson Imaging*, *22*(10), 1445–1455.

Goldman, R. I., Stern, J. M., Engel, J. Jr., & Cohen, M. S. (2002). Simultaneous EEG and fMRI of the alpha rhythm. *Neuroreport*, *13*(18), 2487–2492.

Goncalves, S. I., de Munck, J. C., Pouwels, P. J., Schoonhoven, R., Kuijer, J. P., Maurits, N. M., et al. (2005). Correlating the alpha rhythm to BOLD using simultaneous EEG/fMRI: Inter-subject variability. *Neuroimage*, *30*, 203–213.

Gotman, J., Benar, C. G., & Dubeau, F. (2004). Combining EEG and FMRI in epilepsy: methodological challenges and clinical results. *J Clin Neurophysiol*, *21*(4), 229–240.

Guy, C. N., ffytche, D. H., Brovelli, A., & Chumillas, J. fMRI and EEG responses to periodic visual stimulation. *Neuroimage*, *10*(2), 125–148.

Halchenko, Y.O., Hanson, S.J. & Pearlmutter, B. A. (2005). MultimodalIntegration: fMRI MRI, EEG, MEG, in Advanced Image Processing. In: Dekker (Ed.), *Magnetic Resonance Imaging*. Boston, MA:MIT Press. (pp. 223–266).

Horwitz, B., & Glabus, M. F. (2005). Neural modeling and functional brain imaging: the interplay between the data-fitting and simulation approaches. *Int Rev Neurobiol*, *66*, 267–290.

Horwitz, B., & Poeppel, D.(2002). How can EEG/MEG and fMRI/PET data be combined? *Hum Brain Mapp*, *17*(1), 1–3.

Horwitz, B., Tagamets, M. A., & McIntosh, A. R. (1999). Neural modeling, functional brain imaging, and cognition. *Trends Cogn Sci*, *3*(3), 91–98.

Horwitz, B., & Tagamets, M. A. (1999). Predicting human functional maps with neural net modeling. *Hum Brain Mapp*, *8*(2–3), 137–142.

Horwitz, B., Warner, B., Fitzer, J., Tagamets., M. A., Husain, F.T., & Long, T. W. (2005). Investigating the neural basis for functional and effective connectivity. Application to fMRI. *Philos Trans R Soc Lond B Biol Sci*, *360*(1457), 1093–1108.

Husain, F. T., Tagamets, M. A., Fromm, S. J., Braun, A. R., & Horwitz, B. (2004). Relating neuronal dynamics for auditory object processing to neuroimaging activity: a computational modeling and an fMRI study. *Neuroimage*, *21*(4), 1701–1720.

Im, C. H., Jung, H. K., & Fujimaki, N. (2005). fMRI-constrained MEG source imaging and consideration of fMRI invisible sources. *Hum Brain Mapp*, *26*(2), 110–118.

Ioannides, A. A. (1999). Problems associated with the combination of MEG and fMRI data: theoretical basis and results in practice. In: Yoshimoto, T., Kotani, M., Kuriki, S.,

Karibe, H., Nakasato, N. (eds.). *Recent Advances in Biomagnetism*. Sendai: Tohoku University Press, pp. 133–136.

Joliot, M., Crivello, F., Badier, J. M., Diallo, B., Tzourio, N., & Mazoyer, B. (1998). Anatomical congruence of metabolic and electromagnetic activation signals during a self-paced motor task: a combined PET-MEG study. *Neuroimage, 7*(4–1), 337–351.

Kamada, K., Houkin, K., Takeuchi, F., Ishii, N., Ikeda, J., Sawamura, Y., et al. (2003). Visualization of the eloquent motor system by integration of MEG, functional, and anisotropic diffusion-weighted MRI in functional neuronavigation. *Surg Neurol, 59*(5), 352–361; discussion 361–362.

Kang, J. K., Benar, C., Al-Asmi, A., Khani, Y. A., Pike, G. B., Dubeau, F., et al. (2003). Using patient-specific hemodynamic response functions in combined EEG-fMRI studies in epilepsy. *Neuroimage, 20*(2), 1162–1170.

Kim, D. S., Duong, T. Q., & Kim, S. G. (2000). High-resolution mapping of iso-orientation columns by fMRI. *Nat Neurosci, 3*, 164–169.

Kircher, T. T., Rapp, A., Grodd, W., Buchkremer, G., Weiskopf, N., Lutzenberger, W., et al. (2004). Mismatch negativity responses in schizophrenia: a combined fMRI and whole head MEG study. *Am J Psychiatry, 161*(2), 294–304.

Kober, H., Nimsky, C., Moller, M., Hastreiter, P., Fahlbusch, R., & Ganslandt, O. Correlation of sensorimotor activation with functional magnetic resonance imaging and magnetoencephalography in presurgical functional imaging: a spatial analysis. *Neuroimage, 14*(5), 1214–1228.

Krakow, K., Allen, P. J., Lemieux, L., Symms, M. R., & Fish, D. R. (2000b). Methodology: EEG-correlated fMRI. *Adv Neurol, 83*, 187–201.

Krakow, K., Allen, P. J., Symms, M. R., Lemieux, L., Josephs, O., & Fish, D. R. (2000a). EEG recording during fMRI experiments: image quality. *Hum Brain Mapp, 10*(1), 10–15.

Lahaye, P.-J., S. Baillet, J.-B. Poline, & Garnero, L. (2004). Fusion of simultaneous fMRI/EEG data based on the electro-metabolic coupling. In: *Proc. 2th Proc. IEEE ISBI*, Arlington, VA. pp. 864–867.

Laufs, H., Kleinschmidt A., Beyerle, A., Eger, E., Salek-Haddadi, A., Preibisch, C., & Krakow, K. (2003). EEG-correlated fMRI of human alpha activity. *Neuroimage, 19*(4), 1463–1476.

Leahy, R. M., Mosher, J. C., Spencer, M. E., Huang, M. X., & Lewine, J. D. (1998). A study of dipole localization accuracy for MEG and EEG using a human skull phantom. *Electroencephalogr Clin Neurophysiol, 107*(2), 159–173.

Lemieux, L., Allen, P. J., Franconi, F., Symms, M. R., & Fish, D. R. (1997). Recording of EEG during fMRI experiments: patient safety. *Magn Reson Med, 38*(6), 943–952.

Lemieux, L., Krakow, K., & Fish, D. R. (2001). Comparison of spike-triggered functional MRI BOLD activation and EEG dipole model localization. *Neuroimage, 14*(5), 1097–1104.

Lemieux, L., Salek-Haddadi, A., Josephs, O., Allen, P., Toms, N., Scott, C., et al. (2001). Event-related fMRI with simultaneous and continuous EEG: description of the method and initial case report. *Neuroimage, 14*(3), 780–787.

Liston, A. D, Lund, T. E., Salek-Haddadi, A., Hamandi, K., Friston, K. J., & Lemieux, L. (2005). Modelling cardiac signal as a confound in EEG-fMRI and its application in focal epilepsy studies. *Neuroimage, 30*, 827–834.

Logothetis, N. K., Pauls, J., Augath, M., Trinath, T., & Oeltermann, A. (2001). Neurophysiological investigation of the basis of the fMRI signal. *Nature, 412*(6843), 150–157.

Logothetis, N. K., & Pfeuffer, J. (2004). On the nature of the BOLD fMRI contrast mechanism. *Magn Reson Imaging, 22*(10), 1517–1531.

Logothetis, N. K. (2003). The underpinnings of the BOLD functional magnetic resonance imaging signal. *J Neurosci, 23*(10), 3963–3971.

Maquet, P., Peigneux, P., Laureys, S., Boly, M., Dang-Vu, T., Desseilles, M., et al. (2003). Memory processing during human sleep as assessed by functional neuroimaging. *Rev Neurol (Paris), 159*(11 Suppl), 6S27–6S29.

Maquet, P., Ruby, P., Maudoux, A., Albouy, G., Sterpenich, V., Dang-Vu, T., et al. (2005). Human cognition during REM sleep and the activity profile within frontal and parietal cortices: a reappraisal of functional neuroimaging data. *Prog Brain Res, 150*, 219–227.

Martinez-Montes, E., Valdes-Sosa, P. A., Miwakeichi, F., Goldman, R. I., & Cohen, M. S. (2004). Concurrent EEG/fMRI analysis by multiway Partial Least Squares. *Neuroimage, 22*(3), 1023–34. Erratum in: (2005) *Neuroimage, 26*(3), 973.

Mizuhara, H., Wang, L. Q., Kobayashi, K., & Yamaguchi, Y. (2005). Long-range EEG phase synchronization during an arithmetic task indexes a coherent cortical network simultaneously measured by fMRI. *Neuroimage, 27*(3), 553–563.

Moradi, F., Liu, L. C., Cheng, K., Waggoner, R. A., Tanaka, K., Ioannides, A. A. (2003) Consistent and precise localization of brain activity in human primary visual cortex by MEG and fMRI. *Neuroimage, 18*(3), 595–609.

Neumann, J., Lohmann, G., Zysset, S., & von Cramon, D. Y. (2003). Within-subject variability of BOLD response dynamics. *Neuroimage, 19*(3), 784–796.

Niazy, R. K., Beckmann, C. F., Iannetti, G. D., Brady, J. M., & Smith, S. M. (2005). Removal of FMRI environment artifacts from EEG data using optimal basis sets. *Neuroimage, 28*(3), 720–737.

Northoff, G., Witzel, T., Richter, A., Gessner, M., Schlagenhauf, F., Fell, J., et al. (2002). GABA-ergic modulation of prefrontal spatio-temporal activation pattern during emotional processing: a combined fMRI/MEG study with placebo and lorazepam. *J Cogn Neurosci, 14*(3), 348–370.

Nunez, P. L., & Silberstein, R. B. (2000). On the relationship of synaptic activity to macroscopic measurements: does co-registration of EEG with fMRI make sense? *Brain Topogr, 13*(2), 79–96.

Parkes, L. M., Bastiaansen, M. C., & Norris, D. G. (2006). Combining EEG and fMRI to investigate the post-movement beta rebound. *Neuroimage, 29*(3), 685–696.

Portas, C. M., Krakow, K., Allen, P., Josephs, O., Armony, J. L., & Frith, C. D. (2000). Auditory processing across the sleep-wake cycle: simultaneous EEG and fMRI monitoring in humans. *Neuron, 28*(3), 991–999.

Pouthas, V., Garnero, L., Ferrandez, A. M., & Renault, B. (2000). ERPs and PET analysis of time perception: spatial and temporal brain mapping during visual discrimination tasks. *Hum Brain Mapp, 10*(2), 49–60.

Riera, J., Aubert, E., Iwata, K., Kawashima, R., Wan, X., & Ozaki, T. (2005). Fusing EEG and fMRI based on a bottom-up model: inferring activation and effective connectivity in neural masses. *Philos Trans R Soc Lond B Biol Sci, 360*(1457), 1025–1041.

Rossini, P. M., Caltagirone, C., & Castriota-Scande, O. K. (1998). Hand motor cortical area reorganization in stroke: a study with fMRI, MEG and TCS maps. *Neuroreport, 9*(9), 2141–2146.

Salek-Haddadi, A., Merschhemke, M., Lemieux, L., & Fish, D. R. (2002). Simultaneous EEG-Correlated Ictal fMRI. *Neuroimage, 16*(1), 32–40.

Sammer, G., Blecker, C., Gebhardt, H., Kirsch, P., Stark, R., & Vaitl, D. (2005). Acquisition of typical EEG waveforms during fMRI: SSVEP, LRP, and frontal theta. *Neuroimage, 24*(4), 1012–1024.

Sanders, J. A., Lewine, J. D., & Orrison, W. W. (1996). Comparison of primary motor cortex localization using functional magnetic resonance and magnetoencephalography, *Human Brain Mapping, 4*, 47–57

Schulz, M., Chau, W., Graham, S. J., McIntosh, A. R., Ross, B., Ishii, R., et al. (2004). An integrative MEG-fMRI study of the primary somatosensory cortex using cross-modal correspondence analysis. *Neuroimage, 22*(1), 120–133.

Shmuel, A., Yacoub, E., Pfeuffer, J,. Van de Moortele. P. F., Adriany, G., Hu, X., et al. (2002). Sustained negative BOLD, blood flow and oxygen consumption response and its coupling to the positive response in the human brain. *Neuron, 36*(6), 1195–1210.

Singh, K. D., Barnes, G. R., Hillebrand, A., Forde, E. M., & Williams, A. L. (2002). Task-related changes in cortical synchronization are spatially coincident with the hemodynamic response. *Neuroimage, 16*(1), 103–114.

Singh, M., Kim, S., & Kim, T. S. (2003). Correlation between BOLD-fMRI and EEG signal changes in response to visual stimulus frequency in humans. *Magn Reson Med, 49*(1), 108–114.

Stippich, C., Freitag, P., Kassubek, J., Soros, P., Kamada, K., Kober, H., et al. (1998). Motor, somatosensory and auditory cortex localization by fMRI and MEG. *Neuroreport, 9*(9), 1953–1957.

Symms, M. R., Allen, P. J., Woermann, F. G., Polizzi, G., Krakow, K., Barker, G. J., et al. (1999). Reproducible localization of interictal epileptiform discharges using EEG-triggered fMRI. *Phys Med Biol, 44*(7), N161–N168.

Tagamets, M. A., & Horwitz, B. (1998). Integrating electrophysiological and anatomical experimental data to create a large-scale model that simulates a delayed match-to-sample human brain imaging study. *Cereb Cortex, 8*(4), 310–320.

Takanashi, Y., Yoshikawa, K., Iwamoto, K., Yoshida, Y., Ueda, M., Tanaka, C., et al. (1996). Comparison of functional localization in human visual cortices using MEG and fMRI: a preliminary report. Electroencephalogr *Clin Neurophysiol Suppl. 4*, 59–63.

Toma, K., Matsuoka, T., Immisch, I., Mima, T., Waldvogel, D., Koshy, B., et al. (2002) Generators of movement-related cortical potentials: fMRI-constrained EEG dipole source analysis. *Neuroimage, 17*(1), 161–173.

Torquati, K., Pizzella, V., Babiloni, C., Del Gratta, C., Della Penna, S., Ferretti, A., et al. (2005). Nociceptive and non-nociceptive sub-regions in the human secondary somatosensory cortex: an MEG study using fMRI constraints. *Neuroimage, 26*(1), 48–56.

Tuch, D. S., Salat, D. H., Wisco, J. J., Zaleta, A. K., Hevelone, N. D., & Rosas, H. D. (2005). Choice reaction time performance correlates with diffusion anisotropy in white matter pathways supporting visuospatial attention. *Proc Natl Acad Sci U S A, 102*(34), 12212–12217.

Tuunanen, P. I., Kavec, M., Jousmaki, V., Usenius, J. P., Hari, R., Salmelin, R., et al. (2003). Comparison of BOLD fMRI and MEG characteristics to vibrotactile stimulation. *Neuroimage, 19*(4), 1778–1786.

Waites, A. B., Shaw, M. E., Briellmann, R. S., Labate, A., Abbott, D. F., & Jackson, G. D. (2005). How reliable are fMRI-EEG studies of epilepsy? A nonparametric approach to analysis validation and optimization. *Neuroimage, 24*(1), 192–199.

Wan, X., Iwata, K., Riera, J., Ozaki, T., Kitamura, M., & Kawashima, R. (2006). Artifact reduction for EEG/fMRI recording: Nonlinear reduction of ballistocardiogram artifacts. *Clin Neurophysiol, 117*, 668–680.

12

Somatosensory and Motor Function

Ryusuke Kakigi and Nina Forss

- MEG is well-suited for studies of pain-related cortical areas
- Various stimulation methods can be used to record pain-related activity with MEG, but painful laser stimulation and intracutaneous epidermal electrical stimulation are recommended
- With MEG's excellent temporal resolution, it is possible to separate nociceptive activation mediated by the two fiber systems, Aδ- and C-fibers

Somatosensory Function

Introduction

In the twenty years since the averaged MEG values following somatosensory stimulation, i.e., the somatosensory evoked magnetic field (SEF), were first reported (Brenner et al., 1978; Kaufman et al., 1981; Hari et al., 1983, 1985; Wood et al., 1985; Sutherling et al., 1988), many studies have been conducted, and their number continues to increase. In this chapter, therefore, we will introduce basic methods for the beginner; that is, how to record a clear SEF. In addition, we will introduce basic information and findings related to SEF, particularly unique and interesting aspects.

Since the landmark studies of Foerster (1936) and Penfield and Boldrey (1937) on the motor and sensory representations in the human cerebral cortex based on direct electrical stimulation of the cortical surface, it has been established that the primary sensorimotor cortex is organized in an orderly somatotopic way, which has been termed the 'homunculus' representation of the cutaneous body surface. SEFs following stimulation applied to various parts of the body in normal subjects have been reported to examine the homunculus noninvasively.

MEG detects only a specific orientation of brain current tangential to the skull. Therefore, dipoles generated in area 3b of the primary somatosensory cortex (SI) and/or 4 of the primary motor cortex (MI), each of which is located on the posterior and anterior bank of the central sulcus, respectively, are easily detected—but dipoles in area 1 or 3a in SI, which is located on the crown and the bottom of the central sulcus, respectively, are not (Figure 12–1).

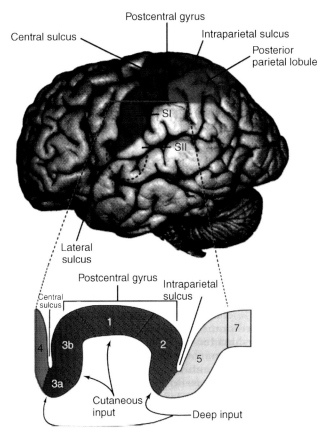

Figure 12–1. Anatomy of the primary somatosensory and motor cortex. Signals following electrical and mechanical stimulation (cutaneous input) reach mainly area 3b, and signals following passive movement (deep input) reach mainly area 3a.
From Kandel, & Jessel (1991).

Methods (Key Points for Recording a Clear SEF)

SEFs are usually recorded following electrical or mechanical stimulation. Since the signal-to-noise (S/N) ratio is much larger following electrical stimulation than mechanical stimulation, most SEF studies have been performed using electrical stimulation. However, the first major problem which researchers face when recording SEFs is the presence of stimulus artifacts caused by the stimulator. In our experience, the stimulus artifacts from an electric stimulator used for animal studies were too large to record clear SEF. We eventually selected a stimulator in a commercially available machine used for recording evoked potentials (EPs), which was designed for recording clear EPs in surgical theaters—that is, monitoring during surgery (intraoperative recording)—i.e., Nihon-Kohden MEB series. However, even using such a good stimulator, one has to be careful of various factors. When a high-intensity electrical stimulation is applied from the beginning of recording SEFs, many coils may be greatly affected, and their baseline not stable for some period. Therefore, we slowly and gradually increase the intensity until the necessary strength, which is slightly over the motor threshold of the corresponding muscles. When we cannot avoid stimulus artifacts despite being very careful of the stimulus described above, we have to reduce the intensity. In such a case, we try to prolong the stimulus duration to some degree; for example, 1 or 2 ms (usually 0.1 or 0.2 ms), to get enough strength for producing muscle contraction. However, the SEF has a great advantage with regard to stimulus artifacts compared to the averaged electroencephalogram (EEG) somatosensory evoked potentials (SEPs). That is, a very short duration (period) of stimulus artifacts, usually less than 5 ms following stimulation, to return to the baseline of the waveform. For example, when we try to record SEPs following stimulation of the face (lip, tongue, ear or facial skin), we cannot identify the short-latency subcortical and cortical components within 20 ms following the stimulation, due to long-lasting large stimulus artifacts. However, we can record clear short-latency SEFs following stimulation of those parts, due to short-lasting stimulus artifacts (see below on SEF following stimulation of various parts of the body).

Even if the duration of stimulus artifacts of SEF is shorter than that of SEP, however, when we stimulate sites very close to the magnetic coils, for example, facial skin (Nguyen et al., 2004; 2005) and tongue (Sakamoto et al., 2008a,b), it is frequently impossible to record clear SEFs due to large stimulus artifacts. In such a case, mechanical stimulation is frequently used. The most popular method of mechanical stimulation is the use of a pressure-induced device, which consists of a small balloon attached to the site to be stimulated (Figure 12–2). Air pressure is needed to inflate the small balloon. This device elicits a clear tactile sensation (Hoshiyama et al., 1995; Nguyen et al., 2004; 2005). When using mechanical stimulation, one has to note the following two points:

(1) Since the S/N ratio following mechanical stimulation is smaller than that for electrical stimulation, the recorded waveforms are noisy and not very sharp.

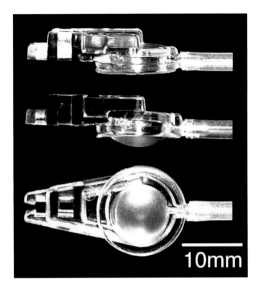

10mm

Figure 12–2. A sensory output device (mechanical stimulator) consisting of a small balloon (1 cm in diameter) attached to the stimulation site. The air pressure inflates the small balloon.

(2) It is difficult to record short-latency components such as N20m and P30m following electrical stimulation. The peak latency of the first recognizable component is 20 – 40 ms longer following mechanical stimulation than electrical stimulation (Nakamura et al., 1998).

SEFs Following Stimulation of Various Parts of the Body

There are many important reports on the receptive sites following stimulation of the lower limb (Hari et al., 1984; Kaukoranta et al., 1986; Huttunen et al., 1987; Rogers et al., 1994; Kakigi et al., 1995a; Hari et al., 1996; Shimojo et al., 1996a), the urogenital organs (Nakagawa et al. 1998), the truncus (Itomi et al., 2000a), the neck and shoulder (Itomi et al., 2000b), the upper limb (Huttunen et al., 1987; Tiihonen et al., 1989; Rossini et al., 1989, 1994; Baumgartner et al., 1991; Suk et al., 1991; Gallen et al., 1994; Buchner et al., 1994; Akhtari et al., 1994; Schnitzler et al., 1995a,b; Kawamura et al., 1996; Mauguiere et al., 1997a,b; Xiang et al., 1997a; Shimizu et al., 1997; Tecchio et al., 1998; Jousmaki and Hari, 1999; Wasaka et al., 2003, 2005; Inui et al., 2004), face (Karhu et al., 1991; Mogilner et al., 1994; Hoshiyama et al., 1995, 1996; Nihashi et al., 2001, 2003; Nguyen et al., 2004, 2005; Sakamoto et al., 2008a,b) and multiple sites (Narich et al., 1991; Yang et al., 1993; Gallen et al., 1994; Nakamura et al., 1998; Inoue et al., 2005).

For example, we made a complete homunculus in 5 normal subjects (Nakamura et al., 1998). We recorded SEF following stimulation of 19 sites—tongue, lower lip, upper lip, thumb, index finger, middle finger, ring finger,

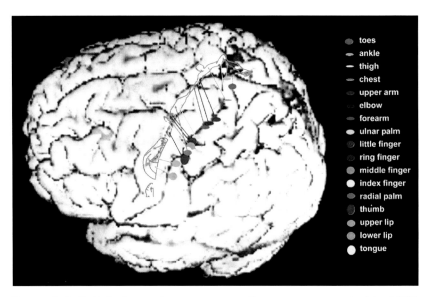

Figure 12–3. Detailed somatosensory receptive map represented by MEG. The 3D brain image was reconstructed using MRI of this subject. Each receptive area, which was estimated to be located in the posterior bank of the central sulcus, was projected onto the cortical surface. The size of each ellipse reflects the presumed size of the activated cortical area. Note that the receptive area for the toes is on the medial side of the left hemisphere.
Adapted from Nakamura et al. (1998).

little finger, radial palm, ulnar palm, forearm, elbow, upper arm, chest, thigh, ankle, big toe, second toe and fifth toe—and put their ECD on the MRI of each subject (Figure 12–3). These representative areas were generally arranged in the above order from inferior to superior, lateral to medial, and anterior to posterior. The changes in the coordinates were compatible with the anatomy of the central sulcus and the homunculus. The location of the ECD for the upper lip could be distinguished from that on the lower lip, with the former positioned more superior than the latter in all subjects. Each representation of the thumb, index finger, middle finger, ring finger and little finger was distinguishable. They were represented sequentially from thumb to little finger, ascending the postcentral sulcus. Next, we introduce some interesting findings.

The Lower Limb Stimulation

We recorded SEFs following the stimulation of various nerves of the lower limb—the posterior tibial (PT), and sural (SU) nerves at the ankle, the peroneal nerve (PE) at the knee, and the femoral nerve (FE) overlying the inguinal ligament—in 7 normal subjects (14 limbs; see Figure 12–4 and Shimojo et al., 1996b). The ECDs of the 14 limbs were classified into two types according to the distance of ECD between PT and FE; Type 1 (>1 cm, nine limbs) and Type 2 (<1 cm, five limbs) (Figure 12–5). The ECD following FE stimulation was located on the crown of the postcentral gyrus or at the edge of the interhemispheric fissure in Type 1, and was close to the ECDs following PT and SU stimulation along the interhemispheric fissure in Type 2. The ECD following PE stimulation was located along the interhemispheric fissure in all 14 limbs, as for PT and SU. Its location was slightly but significantly higher than that of PT and SU stimulation in Type 1, and was close to the ECDs following PT and SU stimulation in Type 2. The present findings indicated that approximately 65 % (9 of 14) of the limbs showed particular receptive fields compatible with the homunculus. The large inter- and intraindividual (left-right) differences found in this study indicated significant anatomical variations in the area of the lower limb in the sensory cortex in humans.

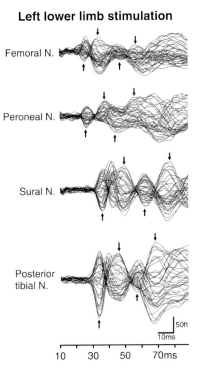

Left lower limb stimulation

Figure 12–4. Chart showing SEFs following stimulation of the posterior tibial and sural nerve at the ankle, the peroneal nerve at the knee, and the femoral nerve overlying the inguinal ligamentum of the right lower limb in one subject. Waveforms recorded at 37 channels are superimposed. Four components indicated by arrows are identified in each waveform. Adapted from Shimojo et al. (1996a).

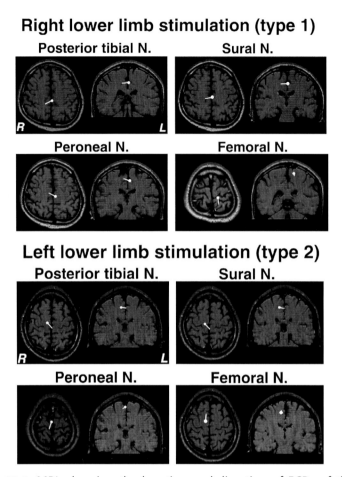

Figure 12–5. MRIs showing the location and direction of ECDs of the 1M following stimulation of 4 nerves of the right lower limb in 2 subjects. In Subject 1, the ECD following the femoral nerve stimulation is located on the crown of the postcentral gyrus, directed to the inferior and posterior sides. In contrast, the ECDs following stimulation of the other nerves are located along the interhemispheric fissure directed to the right hemisphere. The ECDs of the other nerves are located very close together, but that following peroneal nerve stimulation is slightly higher than that following the stimulation of the other two nerves. This type of receptive field is classified as Type 1. In Subject 2, the ECDs following the stimulation of each nerve are located close together, along the interhemispheric fissure. Those following stimulation of the posterior tibial and sural nerve were directed to the right hemisphere horizontally, but those following stimulation of the peroneal and femoral nerves were directed anteriorly and posteriorly, respectively. This type of receptive field is classified as Type 2. L = left, R = right.
Adapted from Shimojo et al. (1996a).

Upper Limb Stimulation

There have been a great number of reports on SEFs following stimulation of the upper limb. Although numerous anatomical and electrophysiological findings in animal studies have supported a hierarchical scheme of somatosensory processing, the precise activation timing of each cortical area in humans is not known. Therefore, we examined the temporal relationship of activities among multiple cortical areas in detail using a multidipole model, brain electric source analysis (BESA) established by Scherg et al. (1995, MEGIS Software GmbH, Munich, Germany). We found activations in Brodmann's areas 3b, 4, 1, and 5, and in the secondary somatosensory cortex (SII) region in the right hemisphere following transcutaneous electrical stimulation of the dorsum of the left hand (Figure 12–6). The mean onset latencies of each cortical activity were 14.4, 14.5, 18.0, 22.4 and 21.7 ms, respectively. The differences of onset latencies among these activations indicated the serial mode of processing both through the postcentral gyrus and through the SI and SII.

Kanno et al. (2003) reported that SEFs following stimulation of the median nerve detected responses in ipsilateral area 3b in 18 hemispheres of 14 individuals (1 normal subject and 13 patients with brain diseases) among 482 consecutive subjects. The three major peaks in the ipsilateral response were named iP50m, iN75m, and iP100m, based on the current orientation in the posterior, anterior, and posterior directions and a latency of 52.7 +/− 6.2, 74.1 +/− 9.4, and 100.2 +/− 15.8 ms (mean +/− standard deviation), respectively. Dipoles of iP50m and cN20m were similarly located on the posterior bank of the central sulcus. Therefore, the somatosensory afferent pathway from the hand may directly reach ipsilateral area 3b, at least in part of the human population. These ipsilateral responses were also reported using fMRI (Nihashi et al., 2005).

Ear Stimulation

The somatotopic representation of the ear in the SI is not clarified in the homunculus, though it may be located near the representation of the face or neck. We stimulated three parts of the left ear: the helix, lobulus, and tragus (Nihashi et al., 2001; 2003). SEFs were successfully measured in 7 of 13 subjects, since the regions stimulated are very close to the magnetic coils. Short-latency responses were analyzed using both single dipole and multidipole models (BESA). From the single dipole model, the ECD following the helix's stimulation was estimated to be near the neck area of SI in all the subjects. On stimulation of the lobulus, the ECDs were estimated to lie around the neck area of SI in four subjects, in the face area in one subject, and in the deep white matter in two subjects. On stimulation of the tragus, the ECDs were estimated to lie around the neck area of SI in three subjects, in the hand area of SI in two subjects, and in the deep white matter in two subjects. When the ECDs were estimated to be located in unlikely sites (hand area and deep white

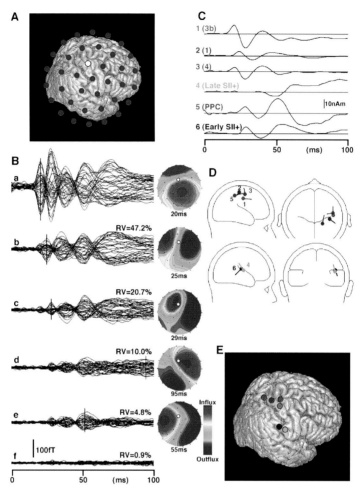

Figure 12-6. Procedures and results of the data analysis. (A) Sensor layout. (B) Superimposed waveforms recorded from 37 channels (a), residual magnetic fields obtained by a subtraction of those due to one (b), two (c), three (d), four (e) and six (f) sources determined from the recorded data. Isocontour maps at the peak latency of a selected deflection (vertical bars) are shown on the right side of each trace. (C) Time course of each strength. (D) Schematic drawings of the location and orientation of each source. Bars indicate the direction of upward deflections of the corresponding waveforms in (C). (E) Superimposition of sources on a subject's brain surface image. White circles in (A) and isocontour maps indicate the position of the sensor (channel 3) that is just on the central sulcus. SII+, secondary somatosensory cortex plus adjoining areas; PPC, posterior parietal cortex; RV, residual variance.

Adapted from Inui et al. (2004).

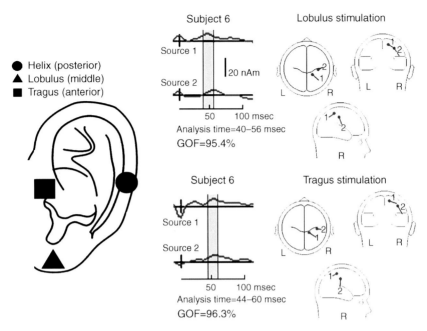

Figure 12–7. Two-dipole model calculated by BESA for the responses to the electrical stimulation of the lobulus and tragus in Subject 6. Source 1 and 2 were located near the neck and facial areas of the SI, respectively. Sources 1 and 2 corresponded to the M40 component and the gray area shows the window for BESA.
Adapted from Nihashi et al. (2001).

matter), a two-dipole model—(1) the neck area of SI and (2) face area of SI—was found to be the most appropriate (Figures 12–7, 12–8, 12–9). These results indicated that receptive fields of some parts of the ear, such as the lobulus and tragus, might be present in both the neck and face areas of SI. These findings suggested that the "ear area" of SI has variability between subjects, unlike the other areas of SI, possibly because the ear is located on the border between the neck and face. We confirmed this finding by fMRI (Nihashi et al., 2002)

Shoulder, Posterior Neck and Lower Part of Head Stimulation

The shoulder, posterior neck and lower part of the head occupied a strange area of the homunclus between the trunk and arm, separate from the face area of the homunclus. We recorded SEF following stimulation of the lower part of the posterior head around the mastoid and shoulder (Itomi et al., 2000b). In most subjects, the ECDs on stimulation of the mastoid and shoulder were located in an area slightly lateral and inferior to the ECD for the trunk's stimulation. However, in a small number of subjects, the ECD for the mastoid

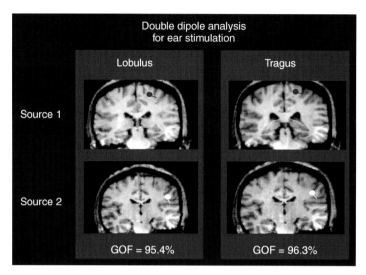

Figure 12–8. Two sources of M40 in a representative subject overlapping on MRI.
Adapted from Nihashi et al. (2001).

stimulation was located near that of the face stimulation (Figure 12–9). This may be due to anatomical variations in the subjects.

Face Stimulation

Since Penfield and Boldrey (1937) revealed the somatotopic body surface representation in the primary somatosensory cortex (SI), many studies using various methods have confirmed this somatosensory homunculus. Regarding the representation of the face in the SI, the face area drawn by Penfield and Boldrey (1937) is organized along the central sulcus with the forehead in the superiomedial region adjacent to the hand area, and the chin in the inferiolateral region. Many authors have reported the locations in the SI of the lip (Nakamura et al., 1998, Hoshiyama et al., 1995; Mogilner et al., 1994), tongue (Karhu et al., 1991; Sakamoto et al., 2008a,b), oral cavity (Hari et al., 1993), and ear (Nihashi et al., 2003, Nihashi et al., 2002, Nihashi et al., 2001). However, there are only a few reports (Servos et al., 1999 and Yang et al., 1994) on skin-covered areas of the face such as the forehead, cheek and chin in humans. Interestingly, some results showed the representation of an inverted face along the central sulcus of the human brain (Servos et al., 1999, Yang et al., 1994, Pons et al., 1991), which is not consistent with the homunculus map drawn by Penfield and Boldrey (1937). Therefore, to investigate the representation of facial skin areas in SI, we recorded magnetic fields evoked by air-pressure-induced tactile stimulation applied to six points on the face, lower lip and thumb (Figure 12–10). The thumb area in the SI was located more medial and superior to the lip area, which was consistent with

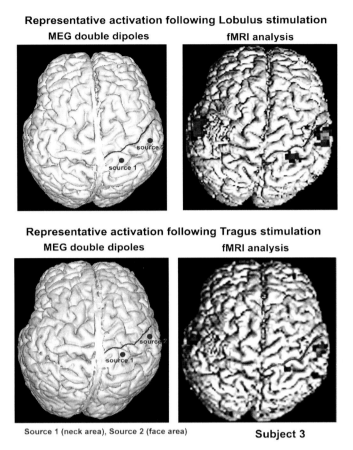

Figure 12–9. ECD location following stimulation of various sites in a representative subject, using results of the present study as well as our previous reports.
Adapted from Nihashi et al. (2001).

Penfield's homunculus. However, the representations of all skin-covered areas including forehead, cheek, nose and chin in the SI were located between the thumb and lower lip area (Figure 12–11). There was no significant difference in location among the six facial points. Our results imply that lips occupy a large area of the face representation in the SI, whereas only a small area located between the thumb and lip areas is devoted to skin-covered surfaces. This is the first study showing that the facial skin areas in the human SI are located between the thumb and lower lip areas and close together.

Topography of SII

One of the major advantages of SEF is that it easily records activities in the SII, where it is difficult for SEP to detect activities due to the location and direction

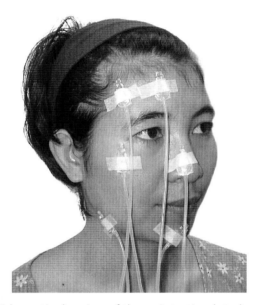

Figure 12–10. Schematic drawing of the points stimulated on the face – six sites were stimulated as shown in the figure.
Adapted from Nguyen et al. (2004).

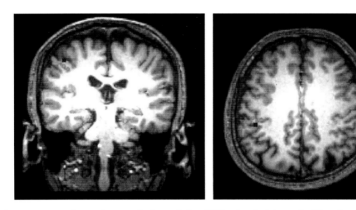

Figure 12–11. Locations of the eight ECDs in Subject 1. The locations of all sources are superimposed on a single axial and coronal MRI slice, with which the ECD for stimulation of the lip was estimated, to show their relative relationships. The ECD location for the thumb is illustrated by a square, that for the lip by a triangle, and that for the six points of facial skin by dots.
Adapted from Nguyen et al. (2004).

of dipole sources (Hari et al., 1983, 1990, 1993; Elbert et al., 1995a; Forss et al., 1995, 1998; Mima et al., 1997, 1998a). A random or long interstimulus interval stimulation rate (Wikstrom et al., 1996; Nagamine et al., 1998), and the oddball paradigm, using rare and frequent, or target and non-target stimuli, (Hari et al., 1990, 1993; Forss et al., 1995; Mima et al., 1998a) cause the SII components to increase in amplitude. This finding suggested that SII activities are more affected by volitional or attention effects than SI activities.

We analyzed the topography of SII on somatosensory stimulation applied to various parts of the body of normal subjects using SEF (Maeda et al., 1999; Nguyen et al., 2005; Sakamoto et al., 2008a,b). SII components were found about 80-100 ms after the stimulation as middle-latency components. SII in the bilateral hemisphere was activated on stimulation of the unilateral side of the body; that is, SII in humans has a "bilateral function." Although there were large interindividual differences, the receptive fields ranked (Figure 12–12) as follows: (1) Anterior–posterior direction; lower lip – upper lip – thumb – middle finger – foot; (2) Medial–lateral direction; foot – middle finger – thumb – upper lip – lower lip; and (3) Lower–upper direction; lower lip – upper lip – thumb – middle finger – foot. In general, these findings are similar to those obtained in studies of animals (Whitzel et al., 1969) and humans (Hari et al., 1993). However, the differentiation was not as clear as that seen in the homunculus in the SI. The SII is located anterior to, medial to, and above the auditory cortex.

SEF Studies on Plasticity in SI

Plasticity of the SI is one of the most interesting topics in the study of SEF. A change of homunculus is reported to be due to limb deafferentation after amputation (Yang et al., 1994; Elbert et al., 1994, 1997; Flor et al., 1995; Knecht et al., 1995, 1996, 1998; Weiss et al., 1998). Yang et al. (1994) and Elbert et al. (1994) first reported the marked intrusion of facial representations into the digit and hand area after upper limb amputation. Further, Knecht et al. (1996) reported that phantom sensations could be evoked from sites on the face and the trunk ipsilateral, but also contralateral to the amputation, and that the amount of reorganization strongly correlates with the number of sites, be it ipsi- or contralateral, from where painful stimuli evoked the referred sensation. These findings suggested the involvement of bilateral pathways, and demonstrated that the perceptual changes go beyond what can be explained by shifts in neighboring cortical representational zones.

Mogilner et al. (1993) reported somatosensory cortical plasticity in patients who were studied before and after surgery for webbed fingers (syndactyly). The presurgical maps displayed shrunken and nonsomatotopic representations of the hand. Within weeks of the surgery, cortical reorganization occurring over distances of 3–9 mm was evident, correlating with the new functional status of the separated digits. Such a reorganization of the SI was also reported in patients with stroke and neoplasm (Rossini et al., 1998a,b).

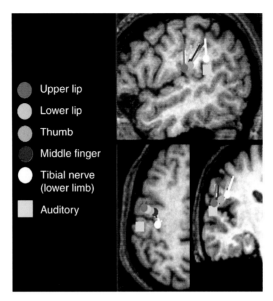

- Upper lip
- Lower lip
- Thumb
- Middle finger
- Tibial nerve (lower limb)
- Auditory

Figure 12–12. ECD location in SII following somatosensory stimulation applied to various parts of the body and auditory stimulation overlapped on MRI in a representative subject. All ECD are projected to a slice in which the ECD for the thumb stimulation was found, since it is easily understood by this procedure, and since it is impossible to show all slices in which each ECD is located. The relationship of each ECD was easily found with these figures. There was a large interindividual topographic difference in the SII, but no clear topographic order in the SII, unlike the homunculus in the SI. However, there was a tendency for a topographic order as follows: *Anterior-posterior direction:* Lower lip–upper lip–thumb–middle finger–tibial nerve (lower limb). *Medial–lateral direction:* Tibial nerve (lower limb)–middle finger–thumb–upper lip–lower lip, *Lower–upper direction:* Lower lip–upper lip–thumb–middle finger–tibial nerve (lower limb). The auditory cortex is located at a site more posterior, lateral and lower than the SII. Adapted from Maeda et al. (1999).

Elbert et al. (1995b) reported an interesting study. They examined SEFs following stimulation of the thumb and little finger of the left hand in string players, and compared their results with controls. They found that the cortical representation of the digits of the left hand of string players was larger than that in controls, and that the amount of cortical reorganization in the representation of the digits correlated with the age at which the person had begun to play. These results suggest that the representation of different parts of the body in the SI of humans depends on use, and changes to conform to the current needs and experiences of the individual. Sterr et al. (1998a,b) studied SEFs in blind multifinger Braille readers. They found that the cortical somatosensory representation of the fingers was frequently topographically disordered in these subjects; in addition, the subjects frequently misperceived which of their fingers was being touched by a light tactile stimulus. Therefore, use-dependent cortical reorganization can be associated with functionally relevant changes in the perceptual and behavioral capacities of the individual.

Plasticity and Pain

Flor and her coauthors showed that the extent of the reorganization after limb amputation was positively correlated with the perceived strength of phantom limb pain; i.e., the stronger the pain, the larger plastic changes are observed at the cortex (Flor et al., 1995). Reorganization of the somatosensory cortex has also been observed in chronic pain syndromes without any evidence of peripheral nerve lesions. For example, in CRPS (Complex Regional Pain Syndrome) Type 1 patients with unilateral persistent upper limb pain, the distance between the thumb and the little finger representations was significantly shorter in the affected hemisphere (contralateral to the painful upper extremity) compared with the healthy side (Juottonen et al., 2002). These results indicated, for the first time, that plastic changes occur in the somatosensory cortex in association with chronic pain without nerve deafferentation. These findings have been later on confirmed and extended by several other groups (Maihofner et al., 2003; Pleger et al., 2004) and they have clinically important implications. Objectively measurable changes of the representation areas underlines the role of the central nervous system in chronic pain disorders. The above-mentioned studies have also indicated that the observed plastic changes are at least to some extent reversible, suggesting that rehabilitation should be targeted to "turn back the clock" for regaining the orderly somatotopic arrangement at the SI cortex (Maihofner et al., 2004).

Clinical Application of SEF

The clinical application of MEG including SEFs is an important subject. However, the number of papers on it is still small. SEF is used for neurosurgery (Kamada et al., 1993; Gallen et al., 1993; Sobel et al., 1993; Nakasato et al., 1996, 1999). SEF before surgery is used to localize the central sulcus, since space occupying lesions such as tumors frequently shift the central sulcus. As compared with a direct recording of SEP from the cortex using subdural electrodes, a noninvasive SEF recording is much safer.

In the field of neurology, SEF is useful to detect functional abnormalities in patients with cerebrovascular diseases (Makela et al., 1992; Maclin et al., 1994; Wikstrom et al., 1996; Rossini et al., 1998a, 2001; Gallien P et al., 2003, Huang et al., 2004). Wikstrom et al. (1996) reported SEF findings in 15 patients in the acute stage of stroke involving sensorimotor cortical and/or subcortical structures in the area of the middle cerebral artery. Patients with pure motor stroke showed no alterations in SEFs, but patients with pure sensory stroke showed markedly attenuated or absent SEFs. Abnormal SEF findings were more clearly correlated with an impairment of two-point discrimination than of joint-position or vibration senses.

A SEP of large amplitude (giant SEP) is recorded in patients with cortical reflex myoclonus. We reported that giant SEPs are generated in area 3b of the SI (Kakigi et al., 1987). Recent SEF studies confirmed this hypothesis (Uesaka et al., 1993, 1996; Karhu et al., 1994; Mima et al., 1998b). In addition, Mima et al. (1998b) found other components located in the anterior bank of the central sulcus, and suggested the importance of the motor cortex for generation of the cortical reflex myoclonus.

Karhu et al. (1992) reported SEFs in 10 patients with multiple sclerosis. Seven patients showed SEFs of abnormally large amplitude at 60–80 ms; 5 of them had multiple lesions around lateral ventricles. In 2 patients with plaques at the level of the 3rd and 4th ventricles and medulla, the 30-ms responses were enlarged. The results suggest that early- and middle-latency SEF components reflect the parallel processing of somatosensory inputs. Significant changes not only in the SI but also in the SII responses has been also reported in patients with genetically verified progressive myoclonus epilepsy (Forss et al., 2001).

High-frequency Oscillations (HFOs)

One of the recent topics of SEF study is high-frequency oscillations (HFOs) (>300 Hz) whose latency was almost the same as that of the primary component of SEF (Curio et al., 1994; Hashimoto et al., 1996; Sakuma et al. 1999a,b; Tanosaki et al., 2002; Inoue et al., 2004). They were generated in the SI, and much reduced in amplitude during sleep (Hashimoto et al., 1996). Hashimoto et al. (1996) hypothesized that the somatic evoked high-frequency oscillations represent the activity of GABAergic inhibitory interneurons, controlling output pyramidal cells in the cortex.

Pain Processing

Recently a number of studies have appeared where MEG has been applied in studies of the human nociceptive system. The results have shown that MEG is very suitable to study pain-related cortical areas, especially the cortical areas processing the sensory aspects of the nociceptive signal. Prior MEG studies have observed activation of the SII, PPC and SI to painful electric or laser stimuli (Kakigi et al., 1995, 2003, 2005; Bromm 1996, Ploner et al., 1999, 2000; Forss et al., 2005). In contrast, activation of deep brain structures that are more related to emotional aspects of the pain processing (like anterior cingulated cortex, anterior insula and amygdala) may be difficult to detect in MEG measurements because of the methodological limitations. However, by applying different analysis methods, or by using grand average data instead of individual data sets, activation of some of these areas may be detected (Ploner et al., 2002).

Various stimulation methods have been used to record pain-related evoked fields such as high-intensity electrical nerve stimulation (Kitamura et al., 1995, 1996), dental pulp stimulation (Hari et al., 1983), CO_2 gas applied to the nasal mucosa (Huttunen et al., 1986; Hari et al., 1997), painful impact stimulation (Arendt-Nielsen et al., 1999) and intracutaneous epidermal electrical stimulation (Inui et al., 2002a,b; 2003a,b; Wang et al., 2004; Inui et al., 2006).

Although each stimulation method has its own advantages and disadvantages, many of the abovementioned methods are problematic in MEG measurements because of their very long rise time and/or stimulus duration, which does not allow studies of the temporal aspects of cortical pain processing. The ideal painful stimulation for MEG measurements should be pain-specific, controllable, safe and reproducible. At present, two methods seem appropriate for recording pain-related SEFs—painful laser stimulation and intracutaneous epidermal electrical stimulation.

Painful Laser Stimulation

Thulium laser stimulates selectively nociceptive fibers, and has fast rise time and short duration (typically 0.5 ms). Commercially available laser stimulation equipment is nowadays safe and easy to use. Short laser pulses to skin provide highly selective and temporally precise noxious stimuli that evoke prominent EEG and magnetoencephalographic (MEG) responses. In MEG measurements we have used laser stimuli (1 msec in duration, 2,000 nm in wavelength) that were produced by a thulium-YAG stimulator (BLM 1000 Tm:YAG; Baasel Lasertech, Starnberg, Germany), and the laser beam was conducted to the magnetically shielded room via an optic fiber. To keep the distance stable between the optic fiber and the stimulated skin area, the hand piece can be connected by a wire to the top of the neuromagnetometer.

An assistant directs the laser beam of approximately 10 mm^2 to the skin. To avoid skin burns and adaptation, the stimulus site should be moved after each pulse to a random direction in the skin area of approximately 5 cm in diameter. Stimulus intensity can be adjusted individually to equal twofold the subjective pain threshold.

Stimulation of Aδ- and C-fibers

The majority of functional brain imaging studies on pain have described cortical activation to Aδ-fiber mediated pain, or to a combination of Aδ-and C-fiber pain, because it has been difficult to selectively stimulate the C-fiber system without significant activation of the Aδ-fibers. For example, Ploner and his coworkers 1999 showed that brief painful laser stimuli evoke sustained cortical activity corresponding to sustained pain perception, comprising early first pain-related and late second pain-related components.

Cortical responses to selective C-fiber stimulation have been recorded by using conduction blockade of Aδ-fibers (Bromm & Treede, 1987) or temperature-controlled laser heat stimuli (Magerl et al. 1999). Bragard et al. (1996) directly and selectively activated C-fibers by delivering the stimuli to a tiny area (0.15 mm²) of skin. In contrast, stimulation of a larger area (15.5 mm²) with high-energy pulses elicited cortical responses related to Aδ-fiber activity. C-fiber-related responses were also obtained if large-area stimuli were given with the lower stimulus intensity. The physiological basis for this stimulus selectivity is the higher density and lower activation threshold of the C-fibers than the Aδ-fibers of the skin (Ochoa & Mair, 1969; Scmidt et al. 1994; Treede et al., 1994). Therefore, laser stimulation delivered to a tiny skin area with low total energy is likely to activate predominantly the unmyelinated C-fibers. Recently, the first reports describing cortical activation patterns to selective C-fiber stimulation have appeared (Opsommer et al., 2001; Tran et al., 2002; Kakigi et al., 2003 Tran et al., 2001, 2002a,b; Qiu et al., 2001, 2004, 2002, 2003; Forss et al., 2005).

Prior studies have introduced two different ways to reduce the size of the laser beam to activate the C-fibers. We used a thin (0.1 mm in depth) aluminum plate (40 mm in length and 60 mm in width). In a 25×25 mm square on this plate, 26 parallel lines were drawn every 1 mm, so that there were 26×26 intersections. A total of 676 (26×26) tiny holes were drilled at these intersections, each with a diameter of 0.4 mm, corresponding to an area of 0.125 mm² for each hole. This thin plate was used as a spatial filter and placed on the skin at the site of stimulation. The stimulus intensity was approximately 2–4 Watts, which was much smaller than that used for recording the late LEP relating to Aδ-fibers, approximately 6–8 Watts. Following the stimulation, some subjects felt that it was similar to so-called second or burning pain, but others only felt pressure, touch, or slight pain. Selective activation of the C-fibers was confirmed by using microneurography (Qiu et al., 2003) and EEG (Tran et al., 2001, 2002a; Qiu et al., 2001, 2002, 2003; Kakigi et al., 2003). The conduction velocity (CV) of C-fibers using this method is approximately 1 m/sec (Tran et al., 2001) and the CV ascending through the spinal cord, probably the spinothalamic tract, is 1–3 m/sec (Tran et al., 2002a, Qiu et al., 2001). The ultra-late LEFs were measured and two components—1M and 2M, whose peak latency was approximately 750 and 950 ms, respectively—were identified (Tran et al., 2002b; Qiu et al., 2004). They were clearly identified in both hemispheres ipsilateral and contralateral to the side stimulated, but the shorter-latency small component generated in the SI, which was recorded by ES (Inui et al., 2003a,b), was not consistently recorded following the stimulation of C-fibers. The generators for 1M and 2M were almost the same as those following Aδ stimulation.

Another possibility is to attach a small diaphragm to the handpiece of the laser stimulator and direct the laser beam through a tiny hole made to the diaphragm. The benefit is that this method allows flexible usage of the C-fiber stimulation to any part of the body. Using this method, the Aδ- and C-fiber responses were compared in 10 healthy subjects (Forss et al., 2005). Laser evoked fields were measured to 1-ms thulium-laser stimuli delivered to the dorsum of the subject's left hand. The earliest cortical responses peaked at 165 ± 7 ms, agreeing with the conduction velocity of Aδ-fibers. To stimulate unmyelinated C-fibers, the total energy of the laser beam was decreased and the size of the stimulated skin area was restricted to 0.2–0.3 mm^2. The earliest cortical responses to these stimuli peaked at 811 ± 14 ms. In addition to the consistent activation of the SII cortices, activation was observed in the posterior parietal cortex (PPC). Activation of PPC to painful stimuli could be related to the sensorimotor coordination that is needed to precisely define the site of the painful stimuli with respect to other parts of the body, and the outer space to reduce or prevent the pain. In contrast to some earlier studies, our data did not indicate participation of the primary somatosensory cortex (SI) in processing of the painful laser stimuli. The results imply that the nociceptive inputs mediated by the two fiber systems are processed in a common cortical network in different time windows. Characterization of cortical responses to first and second pain offers a practical tool for clinical neuroscience to study the two distinctive pain fiber systems.

ISI and Number of Averages

In order to obtain clear and replicable cortical responses to painful stimuli, it is important to remember a couple of important points. Measurement noise decreases proportional to the square root of the number of averaged responses, but the number of averages must be limited in order to shorten measurement time as much as possible; like most long-latency responses, pain responses are very vulnerable to changes in vigilance and attentional state. On the other hand, interstimulus interval (ISI) affects response amplitudes; the responses increase along with increasing ISI to a certain extent. Thus the optimal signal-to-noise ratio during a fixed measurement time is achieved by using optimal ISI. For Aδ stimuli, a recent study indicated that the SII response amplitudes increase strongly with ISIs from 0.5 s to 4s, and saturated at ISIs of 8 to 16 s (Raij et al., 2003). Typically, 40–50 averaged responses are enough for good signal-to-noise ratio. The "ultra-late" C-fiber responses habituate even faster; according to Tran et al. (2001), the optimal number of averages is 10 in one session to avoid attenuation of responses due to habituation. Sessions can then be repeated after a break that exceeds the recovery cycles of the responses. Alternatively, ISI may be increased but this, of course, results in extended measurement times. So far, exact recovery cycles for C-fiber responses have not been reported.

Not only attention and vigilance but also anticipation of pain may affect pain-evoked responses. Therefore, it may be necessary to use random ISIs (for example, between 4–6 s) to avoid time-locked anticipation effects on cortical responses.

Intracutaneous Epidermal Electrical Stimulation

The nociceptive fiber terminals are located in the epidermis and superficial layer of the dermis (Kruger et al., 1985; Novotny & Gommert-Novotny, 1988), while other fibers run more deeply in the dermis (Munger & Halata, 1983). Therefore, we have recently developed a method utilizing a pushpin-like needle electrode to stimulate the epidermal area for activating Aδ-fibers (epidermal electrical stimulation, ES) (Inui et al., 2002a b, 2003a b, 2006) (Figure 12–13). The soft stop device protrudes 1.0 mm from the plate, and the tip of the needle, in turn, protrudes 0.2 mm from the soft stop device. By pressing the electrode plate against the skin gently, the needle tip is inserted adjacent to the free nerve endings of the thin myelinated fibers in the epidermis and superficial part of the dermis. The insertion of the needle electrode causes no bleeding or visible damage to the skin. The stimulus intensity is very small, approximately 0.2–0.3 mA. Compared with other stimuli, such as laser stimulation and CO_2 gas stimulation of the nasal mucosa, time locking of the ES method is much better, since it is an electrical stimulus. Recently, we developed a system to produce this ES needle with Nihon Kohden, Inc., and can now offer the needle on request.

The early processing of pain perception can be analyzed in detail using the ES needle. We used a multidipole model, BESA (MEGIS Software GmbH, Munich, Germany, 1995). We recorded MEG in detail following not only ES stimulation (see Chapter 3) but also TS (transcutaneous electrical) stimulation to compare the results (Inui et al., 2003a,b). The TS was a conventional SEP, with signals ascending through cutaneous (Aβ) fibers. TS activated two sources sequentially within the SI, areas 3b and 1. ES (Aδ fibers) activated one source within the SI, whose location and orientation were similar to those of

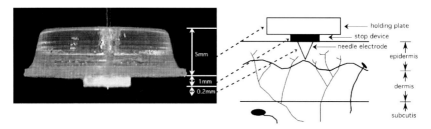

Figure. 12–13. Picture of a needle electrode (left) and a schematic drawing of its insection in the epidermis (right). In the most superficial layers, there are only free nerve endings, which emerge from the subepidermal nerve plexus of the Aδ– and C-fibers (Novotony & Gommert-Novotony, 1988). Encapsulated endings and myelinated Aβ afferents are situated in the deepest papillae of the epidermis or in the deeper structures. Note that the intracutaneous area is enlarged ten times.
Adapted from Inui et al. (2002a).

the TS-activated area-1 source (Figure 12–14). Activities from this source consisted of three components peaking at 88, 98 and 109 ms, before the SI activity reported in previous MEG studies (Ploner et al., 2000, Kanda et al., 2000). The reason these studies failed to identify the early SI components largely lies in the fact that early SI components are very weak and easily overlooked.

Then, a clear and large component, 1M, whose peak latency was approximately 160 msec, was identified in both hemispheres. The generators for 1M were the SI, SII and insula—mainly the SII and insula. The 1M recorded from the ipsilateral hemisphere was significantly longer in latency in all the subjects, and the interhemispheric difference in latency was approximately 10-20 ms. This difference probably indicates transcallosal transmission. We found that the dipole for insular activity was located more anterior following ES than TS, though SII activity showed no significant difference between the two (Figure 12–15). The results suggested that cortical processing was similar between noxious and innocuous stimulation in the SII, but different in the insular cortex. The anterior location of pain-related activation in the insula was consistent with the results of most functional imaging studies (for review, see Schnitzler & Ploner, 2000). Neuroimaging studies have reported that vibrotactile stimulations activated more posterior parts of the insula (Coghill et al., 1994; Davis et al., 1998) in human studies, supporting our results.

Following 1M, a rather complicated component, 2M, whose peak latency was approximately 250 ms, was identified. The main generators for 2M were the cingulate cortex and midtemporal region (MT) around the amygdala and/or hippocampus. Neuroimaging techniques such as positron emission tomography (PET) and functional magnetic resonance imaging (fMRI) have found extensive activity in the cingulate cortex following laser stimulation (Xu et al., 1997, Svensson et al., 1997; Sawamoto et al., 2000; Peyron et al., 2002; Qiu et al., 2006). Intracranial EEG recordings also clearly identified strong activity there (Lenz et al., 1998). However, it has been rather difficult for the MEG to detect it (Bromm et al., 1996; Watanabe et al., 1998; Yamasaki et al., 1999; Ploner et al., 1999; Kanda et al., 2000; Nakata et al., 2004; Kakigi et al., 1995b, 1996) with some exceptions (Kitamura et al., 1995, 1997, Inui et al., 2003a,b and Figure 12–16, 12–17). This is probably due to the fact that the dipoles generated in the right and left cingulate cortex cancel each other out, which is inconvenient for MEG. In addition, a dipole generated in a deep region such as the cingulate cortex is not easily detected by MEG.

The role of the MT region around the amygdala and hippocampus is still controversial. Watanabe et al. (1998) and Inui et al. (2003a & 2000b),detected it using MEG (Figure 12–16, 12–17). Garcia-Larrea et al. (2003) agreed with the possibility that this region is activated by painful stimulation, since the amygdala is thought to contribute to the emotional processing (i.e., aversive nature) of painful events, rather than the sensory-discriminative aspects of pain (Büchel et al., 1998 and Bornhövd et al., 2002), while activation of the hippocampal formation seems to be enhanced when the pain is not expected

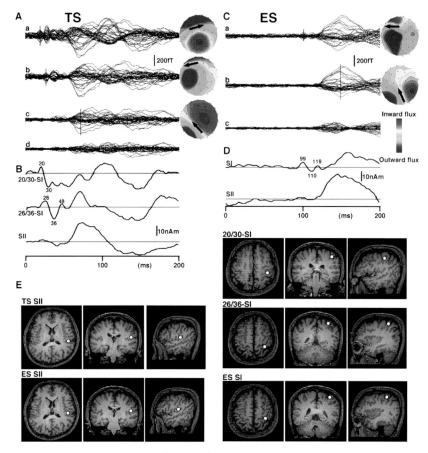

Figure 12–14. Comparison of cortical responses to noxious (ES) and innocuous (TS) stimulation in a single subject. A: magnetic fields following TS
(transcutaneous stimulation); Aa, superimposed waveform recorded
from 37 channels; Ab-d, residual magnetic fields obtained by subtraction of those due to the 20/30-SI source (b), 20/30-SI and 26/36-SI sources
(c) and all three sources (d) from the recorded data. Isocontour maps at
the peak latency of a selected deflection (vertical bars) are shown on
the right side of each trace. B: time course of the source strengths in TS.
C: magnetic fields following ES (epidermal stimulation); Ca, recorded
data; Cb, c, residual magnetic fields obtained by a subtraction of those
due to the SI source (b) and SI and SII sources from the recorded data.
D: time course of the source strengths in ES. E: source locations overlaid on
MR images. SI, primary somatosensory cortex; SII, secondary somatosensory cortex; 20/30-SI, the first SI source in TS whose activity peaked at
21 and 30 ms; 26/36-SI, the second SI source in TS whose activity peaked
at 26 and 36 ms.
Adapted from Inui et al. (2003b).

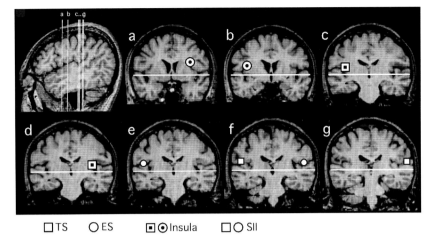

□ TS   ○ ES   ▣ ⊙ Insula   □ ○ SII

Figure 12–15. Locations of activation in the secondary somatosensory cortex (SII) and insula. A representative case for locations of cortical activations in the secondary somatosensory cortex (SII) and insula (Subject 1). Vertical lines, a–g, in a sagital image indicate positions A–P of corresponding coronal images. Horizontal lines in coronal images indicate the level 6 cm superior to the interaural line.
Adapted from Inui et al. (2003a).

(Ploghaus et al., 2000) or when the painful stimulus is associated with anxiety (Ploghaus et al., 2001).

Problems with MEG Studies on Human Pain Perception

A thorough evaluation of pain using phased painful stimuli has been performed with MEG. The biggest advantage of MEG is that one is able to clarify the temporal information on pain processing, in the order of ms. However, MEG cannot be used to evaluate continuous tonic pain such as cancer pain. Neuroimaging techniques such as PET and fMRI may be more useful in this respect, but physiological functions cannot be evaluated by neuroimaging. One promising method in electrophysiological studies for this particular problem is to analyze a change of frequency band using the fast Fourier transform (FFT) during some period, for example, the alpha wave power change in each region between a nonpainful state and painful state (Stancak et al., 2005). This method will probably be used for not only basic research but also clinical studies in the near future.

Safety Issues

Although thulium laser is probably safer than CO_2 laser as a pain stimulus, it may cause skin burns if the stimulator is too close to the skin or, alternatively,

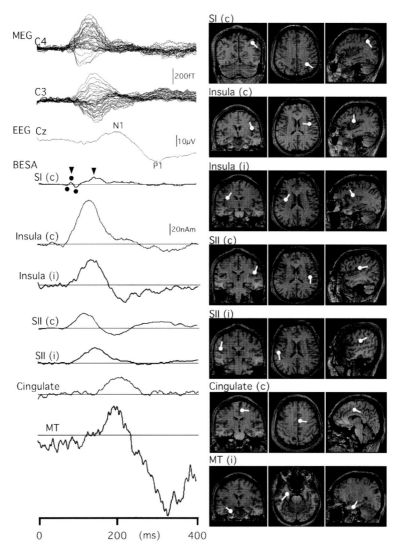

Figure 12–16. Temporal profile of cortical activities following painful epidermal stimulation (ES). Cortical responses to ES in a subject. The upper three traces are superimposed waveforms recorded from 37 channels in both hemispheres, and evoked potentials recorded at Cz. The lower seven traces are temporal profiles of each source strength. Filled circles indicate a group of early SI activities. Arrowheads indicate the peak latency of early and late SI activity. (Right) Locations of source generators overlaid on MRI scans. Magnetic fields were recorded from two probes that were centered on the C4 (hemisphere contralateral to the stimulation) and C3 (hemisphere ipsilateral to the stimulation) positions based on the International 10–20 system.
Adapted from Inui et al. (2003a).

324

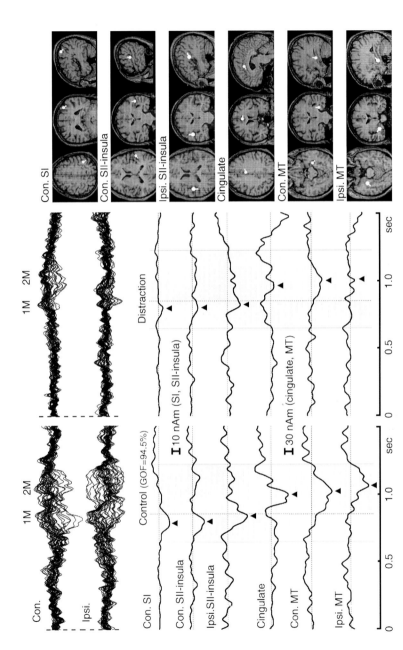

Figure 12-17. Source generators analyzed by BESA following C fiber stimulation during Control and Distraction in one subject. SI and SII-insula seem to be the main generators for 1M, while MT and cingulate cortex seem to be the main generators for 2M. During Distraction, the activities of the SI, SII-insula, MT and cingulate cortex were much reduced. Note the difference in current-strength scale—10 nA for SI and SII-insula and 30 nA for MT and Cingulate. These source locations overlapped on MRI. Adapted from Qiu et al. (2004).

stimulus intensity or frequency is too high. For example, we have noticed that it is safe to use on average 52mJ/mm^2 intensity to a skin area of 10 mm^2 for Aδ-stimulation (total energy 500 mJ), whereas for C-stimuli, in which the area is restricted to 0.2-0.3 mm^{2,} suitable energy is about 190 mJ/mm^2 (total energy 50 mJ). To avoid skin burns, the stimulus site can be slightly moved after each stimulus to a random direction within a limited area, for example 10 cm^2. In addition, the eyes of the subject and of the researcher handling the stimulator need to be protected with goggles to avoid possible damage if the laser beam is accidentally reflected toward the eye.

Motor Function

When motor function is examined by MEG, movement related cortical fields (MRCFs) or background activities (brain rhythm) related to movement are recorded.

MRCFs

MRCFs correspond to the movement-related cortical potential (MRCP) that is recorded by averaging EEG. However, since it is much more difficult to record MRCFs than MRCPs, the number of MRCF studies is relatively small (Cheyne et al., 1989; Kristeva et al.,1991; Kristeva-Feige et al., 1994; Nagamine et al., 1994; Praamstra et al., 1999; Erdler et al., 2000; Huang et al., 2004; Mayville et al., 2005).

MRCPs are recorded before and after voluntary movement, mainly finger extension or flexion (Figure 12–18). An MRCP consists of three main components (Shibasaki et al., 1980; Neshige et al., 1988; Ikeda et al., 1992): (1) *Readiness Potential* (Bereitschaftspotential). It starts approximately 2 or 3 sec before movement onset, and its amplitude gradually increases. The generator for this is mainly the supplementary motor area (SMA) in both hemispheres and M1 in the hemisphere contralateral to movement, but mainly the former. (2) *Negative Slope*. It starts approximately 0.3 sec before movement onset and its amplitude steeply increases overlapping Readiness Potential. The generators for this are mainly the bilateral SMA and M1 in the hemisphere contralateral to movement, mainly the latter. (3) *Motor Potential*. It starts just before the movement, overlapping Readiness Potential and Negative Slope. The generator for this is mainly M1 in the hemisphere contralateral to movement. Since Readiness potential is a very slow potential, a very wide high-pass filter, 0.001 sec or DC, is needed to record it clearly. However, if such a wide filter is used when recording MRCFs, the baseline will fluctuate and an accurate analysis of the results cannot be performed. Therefore, we have to use a relatively narrow bandpass filter, 0.01 or 0.1 Hz for recording MRCF, so Readiness Potential cannot be clearly recorded. In addition, the fact that ECDs generated in the right and left SMA, which is the main generator

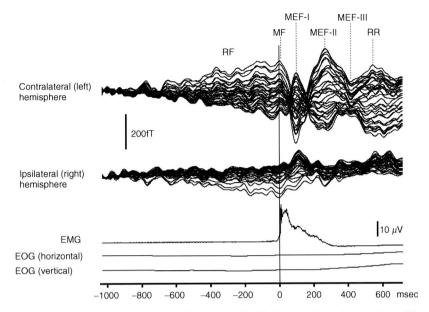

Figure 12–18. Movement-related cortical fields (MRCFs) during right middle finger movement recorded from the C3 and C4 position (hemisphere contralateral and ipsilateral to the moved side, respectively). Thirty-seven superimposed waveforms for one subject are shown to illustrate the nomenclature for each identifiable component. RF: readiness field. MF: motor field. MEF: motor evoked field. RR: reafferent response. Although the RF was recorded in each hemisphere, the subsequent responses were obtained dominantly in the hemisphere contralateral to the moved side.

for Readiness Potential cancel each other out, is inconvenient for MRCF. However, Erdler et al. (2000) succeeded in detecting activity in the SMA using an elegant analytical method.

We investigated MRCFs to identify the motor and sensory brain activities at the instant of a unilateral finger movement (Hoshiyama et al., 1997). We focused on the source of the events tightly linked to movement onset, and used BESA to model the sources generating MRCFs during the interval from 200 ms before to 150 ms after the movement onset (Figures 12–19 and 12–20). Four sources provided satisfactory solutions for MRCF activities in this interval (Figures 12–19 and 12–20). Sources 1 and 2—which were located in the pre central regions in the hemisphere contralateral and ipsilateral to the moved finger, respectively—generated readiness fields (RF), but Source 1 was predominant just before movement onset. The motor field (MF), the peak of which was just after movement onset, was mainly generated by Source 1. Sources 3 and 4 were located in the post-central regions in the hemisphere contralateral and ipsilateral to the moved finger, respectively. The first motor evoked field (MEF-I), the peak of which was about 80 ms after the movement, was mainly generated by Source 3, but with the participation of Sources 1, 2 and 4. The results indicated that the activities of both pre- and post-central regions in both hemispheres were related to voluntary movements, although the predominant areas varied over time.

We also investigated the vocalization-related cortical fields (VRCFs) following the vocalization of vowels (Gunji et al., 2000, 2001). A multiple-source model, BESA, was used to elucidate the mechanism generating VRCF in the period from 150 ms before to 150 ms after the onset of vocalization (Figure 12–21). Six sources provided satisfactory solutions for VRCF activities during that period (Figure 12–21). Sources 1 and 2, which were activated

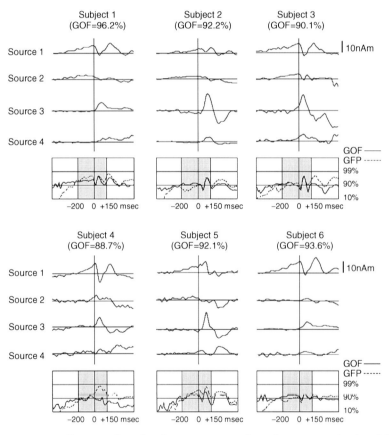

Figure 12–19. Temporal activation patterns of each source obtained by spatiotemporal source analysis in six subjects. The horizontal bar indicates the time axis (extending from –1000 to +700 ms). Dashed and continuous lines in the lower part of each column show the average global field power (GFP) and goodness-of-fit (GOF), respectively, on a logarithmic scale over the fitted interval (-200 to + 150 ms, gray area).
Adapted from Hoshiyama et al. (1997).

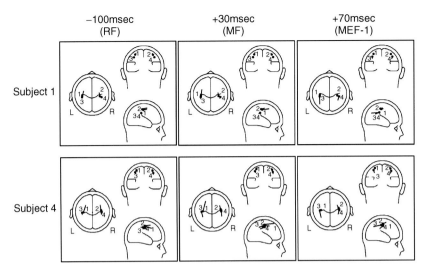

Figure 12–20. Head diagram indicating the locations of the dipole sources of two subjects. The line and its length from each point indicate the direction and magnitude of the dipole current, respectively.
Adapted from Hoshiyama et al. (1997).

from approximately 150 ms before the vocalization onset, were located in laryngeal motor areas of the left and right hemispheres, respectively. Sources 5 and 6 were located in the truncal motor area in each hemisphere, and were very similar to Sources 1 and 2 in terms of temporal change of activities. Sources 3 and 4 were located in the auditory cortices of the left and right hemispheres, respectively, and appeared to be activated just after the vocalization onset. However, all six sources temporally overlapped in the period approximately 0-100 ms after the vocalization onset. The present results suggested that the bilateral motor cortices, probably laryngeal and truncal areas, were activated just before the vocalization. We considered that the activities of the bilateral auditory areas after the vocalization were the response of the subject's central auditory system to his/her own voice. The motor and auditory activities temporally overlapped, and BESA was very useful for separating the activities of each source.

MRCFs relating to movement of the foot (Endo et al., 2004) and tongue (Nakasato et al., 2001; Loose et al., 2001) were also reported, and the results were almost the same as for the MRCF related to finger movement.

Background Activity Related to Motor Function

Mu Rhythm

The human cortical mu rhythm, prominent in the rolandic areas both in electoencephalographic (EEG) and magnetoencephalographic (MEG) recordings, consists of dominant ~10 and ~20 Hz frequency bands (for a review

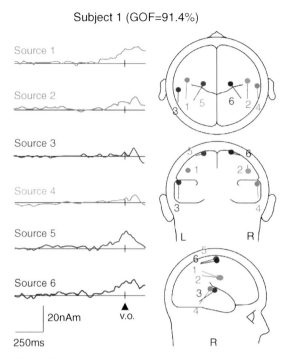

Subject 1 (GOF=91.4%)

Figure 12–21. The MEG waveforms and the results of the source analysis of Subject 1. *Upper right*: the VRCF following the vocalization at the left and right hemispheres (around C3 and C4) in Subject 1. The waveforms recorded from 37 channels were superimposed. *Left*: temporal activity of each source obtained by spatiotemporal source analysis (BESA). *Lower right:* the localization and orientation of the dipole on the spherical head model. The line from each point indicates the direction of the dipole current. Sources 1 and 2 were located in the laryngeal motor areas. Sources 3 and 4 were located in the auditory areas, and sources 5 and 6 were in the truncal motor areas. The sources in the motor areas (sources 1, 2, 5, 6) were activated approximately 100 ms prior to the vocalization onset, while the activity of the auditory sources (sources 3 and 4) appeared after the vocalization onset. All six sources temporally overlapped after the onset of vocalization.
Adapted from Gunji et al. (2000).

see Hari & Salmelin, 1997). Reactivity of the cortical mu rhythm to external stimuli can be studied with TSE-method (Temporal Spectral Evolution, see page.x). For example, electric median nerve stimuli result in an initial decrease of the mu rhythm level, followed by strong rebound within 1000 ms after stimuli. The rebound is suppressed during finger movements (Salenius et al. 1997), motor imagery (Schnitzler *et al.* 1997), and even by viewing another person making movements (Hari et al. 1998). Previous MEG and TMS studies have suggested that increase of the 20-Hz rhythm after stimuli ("rebound") may reflect decreased excitability of the motor cortex (Salmelin and Hari, 1994; Chen et al. 1999). Therefore, reactivity of the 20 Hz rhythm has been used as a tool to study the functional state of the motor cortex. For example, analysis of the reactivity of the 20-Hz rhythm in patients with progressive myoclonus epilepsy revealed abnormal excitation of the motor cortex (Silen et al., 2000).

Pain and Motor Cortex

Many chronic pain patients show signs of motor dysfunction, such as decreased muscle strength and restriction of the active range of movement. Further, a motor cortex stimulator has been used to alleviate chronic pain, suggesting that the pain and the motor systems are functionally coupled.

A recent study showed with 10 healthy subjects that acute pain modulates the functions of the motor cortex (Raij *et al.* 2004); laser stimuli delivered to the dorsum of the hand elicited long-lasting attenuation of the motor cortex rhythm, indicating a prolonged activation of the motor cortex in association with acute pain. In line with these findings, significantly altered reactivity of the motor cortex has been shown in patients suffering from chronic pain: in CRPS patients, rebound of the mu rhythm was diminished, suggesting that inhibition of the motor cortex may be defective in chronic pain (Juottonen et al., 2002). This view is in line with recent transcranial magnetic stimulation studies showing signs of disinhibition or hyperexcitability of the motor cortex in CRPS patients (Schwenkreis et al., 2003), and also agrees with the clinically frequently observed deficits of motor functions in chronic pain patients. The close interaction between the pain and motor systems may explain beneficial effects of mirror therapy and motor imagery in rehabilitation of CRPS (McCabe et al.., 2003; Moseley, 2004).

References

Akhtari, M., Mcnay, D., Mandelkern, M., Teeter, B., Cline, H. E., Mallick, J., et al. (1994). Somatosensory evoked response source localization using actual cortical surface as the spatial constraint. *Brain Topogr, 7,* 63–69.

Allison, T., McCarthy, G., Wood, C. C., Williamson, P. D., & Spencer, D. D. (1989). Human cortical potentials evoked by stimulation of the median nerve. 1. Cytoarchitectonic areas generating short-latency activity. *J Neurophysiol, 62,* 694–710.

Arendt-Nielsen, L., Yamasaki, H., Nielsen, J., Naka, D., & Kakigi, R. (1999). Magnetoencephalographic responses to painful impact stimulation. *Brain Res, 839,* 203–208.

Baumgartner, C., Sutherling, W. W., Di, S., & Barth, D. S. (1991). Spatiotemporal modeling of cerebral evoked magnetic fields to median nerve stimulation. *Electroencephalogr Clin Neurophysiol*, *79*, 27–35.

Bernard, J. F., & Besson, J. M. (1990). The spino (trigemino) pontoamygdaloid pathway: electrophysiological evidence for an involvement in pain processes. *J Neurophysiol*, *63*, 473–490.

Biermann, K., Schmitz, F., Witte, O. W., Konczak, J., & Schnitzler, A. (1998). Interaction of finger representation in the human first somatosensory cortex: a neuromagnetic study. *Neurosci Lett*, *251*, 13–16.

Bornhövd, K., Quante, M., Glauche, V., Bromm, B., Weiller, C, & Büchel, C. (2002). Painful stimuli evoke different stimulus-response functions in the amygdala, prefrontal, insula and somatosensory cortex: a single-trial fMRI study. *Brain*, *125*, 1326–1336.

Bragard, D., ACN Chen, & Plaghki, L. (1996). Direct isolation of ultra-late (C-fibre) evoked brain potentials by CO_2 laser stimulation of tiny cutaneous surface areas in man. *Neurosci Lett*, *209*, 81–84.

Brenner, D., Lipton, J., Kaufman, L., & Williamson, S. J. (1978). Somatically evoked fields of the human brain. *Science*, *189*, 81–83.

Bromm B., Lorenz J., & Scharein E. (1996). Dipole source analysis of brain activity in the assessment of pain. In: J. Kimura and H. Shibasaki, eds. *Recent Advances in Clinical Neurophysiology.* Amsterdam: Elsevier, pp. 328–335.

Büchel, C., Morris, J., Dolan, R. J., & Friston, K. J. (1998). Brain systems mediating aversive conditioning: an event-related fMRI study. *Neuron*, *20*, 947–957.

Buchner, H., Fuchs, M., Wischmann, H-A., Dossel, O., Ludwig, I., Knepper, A., et al. (1994). Source analysis of median nerve and finger stimulated somatosensory evoked potentials: Multichannel simultaneous recording of electric and magnetic fields combined with 3D-MR tomography. *Brain Topogr*, *6*, 299–310.

Buchthal, F., & Rosenfalck, A. (1966). Evoked action potentials and conduction velocity in human sensory nerves. *Brain Res*, *3*, 1–122.

Chen R., Corwell B., & Hallett M. (1999) Modulation of motor cortex excitability by median nerve and digit stimulation. *Exp Brain Res.* *129*(1):77–86.

Cheyne, D., & Weinberg, H. (1989). Neuromagnetic fields accompanying unilateral finger movements: pre-movement and movement-evoked fields. *Exp Brain Res*, *78*, 604–612.

Coghill, R. C., Talbot, J. D., Evans, A. C., Meyer, E., Gjedde, A., Bushnell, M. C., et al. (1994). Distributed processing of pain and vibration by the human brain. *J Neurosci*, *14*, 4095–4108.

Curio, G., Mackert, B-M., Burghoff, M., Koetitz, R., Abraham-Fuchs, K., & Harer, W. (1994). Localization of evoked neuromagnetic 600 Hz activity in the cerebral somatosensory system. *Electroencephalogr Clin Neurophysiol*, *91*, 483–487.

Davis, K. D., Kwan, C. L., Crawley, A. P., & Miklis D. J. (1998). Functional, study of thalamic and cortical activations evoked by cutaneous heat, cold, and tactile stimuli. *J Neurophysiol*, *80*, 1533–1546.

Elbert, T., Flor, H., Birbaumer, N., Knecht, S., Hampson, S., Larbig, W., et al. (1994). Extensive reorganization of the somatosensory cortex in adult humans after nervous system injury. *Neuroreport*, *5*, 2593–2597.

Elbert, T., Junghofer, M., Scholz, B., & Schneider, S. (1995a). The separation of overlapping neuromagnetic sources in first and second somatosensory cortices. *Brain Topogr*, *7*, 275–282.

Elbert, T., Pantev, C., Wienbruch, C., Rockstroh, B., & Taub, E. (1995b). Increased cortical representation of the fingers of the left hand in string players. *Science, 270*, 305–307.

Elbert, T., Sterr A., Flor H., Rockstroh B., Knecht S., Pantev C., et al. (1997). Input-increase and input-decrease types of cortical reorganization after upper extremity amputation in humans. *Exp Brain Res, 117*, 161–164.

Endo, H., Kato, Y., Kizuka, T., Masuda, T., & Takeda, T. (2004). Bilateral cerebral activity for unilateral foot movement revealed by whole-head magnetoencephalography. *Somatosens Motor Res, 21*, 33–43.

Erdler M., Beisteiner R., Mayer D., Kaindl T., Edward, V., Windischberger, C., et al. (2000). Supplementary motor area activation preceding voluntary movement is detectable with a whole-scalp magnetoencephalography system. *Neuroimage, 11*, 697–707.

Erne, S. N., Curio, G., Trahms, L., Trontelj, Z., & Aust, P. (1988). Magnetic activity of a single peripheral nerve in man. In: K. Atsumi, M. Kotani, S. Ueno, T. Katila & S.J. Williamson, eds. *Biomagnetism*. Tokyo: Denki University Press, pp. 166–169.

Flor, H., Elbert, T., Knecht, S., Wienbruch, C., Pantev, C., Birbaumer, N., et al. (1995). Phantom-limb pain as a perceptual correlate of cortical reorganization following arm amputation. *Nature, 375*, 482–484.

Foerster, O. (1936). The motor cortex in man in the light of Hughlings Jackson's doctrines. *Brain, 56*, 135–159.

Forss, N., Hari, R., Salmelin, R., Ahonen, A., Hamalainen, M., Kajola, M., et al. (1994a). Activation of the human posterior parietal cortex by median nerve stimulation. *Exp Brain Res, 99*, 309–315.

Forss, N., Salmelin, R., & Hari R. (1994b). Comparison of somatosensory evoked fields to airpuff and electric stimuli. *Electroencephalogr Clin Neurophysiol, 92*, 510–517.

Forss, N., Jousmaki, V., & Hari, R. (1995). Interaction between afferent input from fingers in human somatosensory cortex. *Brain Res, 685*, 68–76.

Forss, N., & Jousmaki, V. (1998). Sensorimotor integration in human primary and secondary somatosensory cortices. *Brain Res, 781*, 259–267.

Gallen, C. C., Sobel, D. F., Waltz, T., Aung, M., Copeland, B., Schwartz, B. J., et al. (1993). Noninvasive presurgical neuromagnetic mapping of somatosensory cortex. *Neurosurgery, 33*, 260–268.

Gallen, C. C., Schwartz, B., Rieke, K., Pantev, C., Sobel, D., Hirschkoff, E., et al. (1994). Intrasubject reliability and validity of somatosensory source localization using a large array biomagnetometer. *Electroencephalogr Clin Neurophysiol, 90*, 145–156.

Gallien, P., Aghulon, C., Durufle, A., Petrilli, S., de Crouy, A. C., Carsin, M., et al. (2003). Magnetoencephalography in stroke: a 1-year follow-up study. *Eur J Neurol, 10*, 373–382.

Garcia-Larrea, L., Frot, L. M., & Valeriani, M. (2003). Brain generators of laser-evoked potentials: from dipoles to functional significance. *Neurophysiol Clin, 33*, 279–292.

Gunji A., Hoshiyama M., & Kakigi R. (2001). Auditory response following vocalization; magnetoencephalographic study. *Clin Neurophysiol, 111*, 214–219.

Gunji, A., Kakigi, R., & Hoshiyama, M. (2000). Spatiotemporal source analysis of vocalization-associated magnetic fields. *Brain Res Cogn Brain Res, 9*, 157–163.

Grimm, Ch., Schreiber, A., Kristeva-Feige, R., Mergner, Th., Henning, J., & Lucking, C. H. (1998). A comparison between electric source localisation and fMRI during somatosensory stimulation. *Electroencephalogr Clin Neurophysiol, 106*, 22–29.

Hamalainen, M. S. (1992). Magnetoencephalography: A tool for functional brain mapping. *Brain Topogr, 5*, 95–102.

Hari, R., Kaukoranta, E., Reinikainen, K., Huopaniemie, T., & Mauno, J. (1983). Neuromagnetic localization of cortical activity evoked by painful dental stimulation in man. *Neurosci Lett, 42*, 77–82.

Hari, R., Reinikainen, K., Kaukoranta, E., Hamalainen, M., Ilmoniemi, R., Penttinen, A., et al. (1984). Somatosensory evoked cerebral magnetic fields from S1 and S2 in man. *Electroencephalogr Clin Neurophysiol, 57*, 254–263.

Hari, R., & Kaukoranta, E. (1985). Neuromagneic studies of somatosensory system: principles and example. *Prog Neurobiol, 24*, 233–256.

Hari, R., Hallstrom, J., Tiihonen, J., & Joutsiniemi, S-L. (1989). Multichannel detection of magnetic compound action fields of median and ulnar nerve. *Electroencephalogr Clin Neurophysiol, 72*, 277–280.

Hari, R., Hamalainen, H., Hamalainen, M., Kekoni, J., Sams, M., & Tiihonen, J. (1990). Separate finger representations at the human second somatosensory cortex. *Neuroscience, 37*, 245–249.

Hari, R. (1991). On brain's magnetic responses to sensory stimuli. *Journal of Clin Neurophysiol, 8*, 157–169.

Hari, R., Karhu., J, Hamalainen, M., Knuutila, J., Salonen, O., Sams, M., et al. (1993). Functional organization of the human first and second somatosensory cortices: a neuromagneic study. *Eur J Neurosci, 5*, 724–734.

Hari, R., Nagamine, T., Nishitani, N., Mikuni, N., Sato, T., Tarkiainen, A., et al. (1996). Time-varying activation of different cytoarchitectonic areas of the human SI cortex after tibial nerve stimulation. *Neuroimage, 4*, 111–118.

Hari, R., Portin, K., Kettenmann, B., Jousmaki, V., & Kobal, G. (1997). Right-hemisphere preponderance of responses to painful CO_2 stimulation of the human nasal mucosa. *Pain, 72*, 145–151.

Hari R., & Salmelin R. (1997) i. Human cortical oscillations: a neuromagnetic view through the skull. *Trends Neurosc 20*(1):44–49. Review.

Hari R., Forss N., Avikainen S., Kirveskari E., Salenius S., & Rizzolatti G. (1998). Activation of human primary motor cortex during action observation: a neuromagnetic study. *Proc Natl Acad Sci U S A* Dec 8; *95*(25), 15061–15065.

Hashimoto, I. (1988). Trigeminal evoked potentials following brief air puff: enhanced signal-to-noise ratio. *Ann Neurol, 23*, 332–338.

Hashimoto, I., Okada, K., Gatayama, T., & Yokoyama, S. (1991). Multichannel measurements of magnetic compound action fields of the median nerve in man. *Electroencephalogr Clin Neurophysiol, 81*, 332–336.

Hashimoto, I., Mashiko, T., Mizuta, T., Imada, T., Iwase, K., & Okazaki, H. (1994). Visualization of a moving quadrupole with magnetic mesurements of peripheral nerve action fields. *Electroencephalogr Clin Neurophysiol, 93*, 459–467.

Hashimoto, I., Mashiko, T., & Imada, T. (1996). Somatic evoked high-frequency magnetic oscillations reflect activity of inhibitory interneurons in the human somatosensory cortex. *Electroencephalogr Clin Neurophysiol, 100*, 189–203.

Hoshiyama, M., Kakigi, R., Koyama, S., Kitamura, Y., Shimojo, M., & Watanabe, S. (1995). Somatosensory evoked magnetic fields after mechanical stimulation of the scalp in humans. *Neurosci Lett, 195*, 29–32.

Hoshiyama, M., Kakigi, R., Koyama, S., Kitamura, Y., Shimojo, M., & Watanabe, S. (1996). Somatosensory evoked magnetic fields following stimulation of the lip in humans. *Electroencephalogr Clin Neurophysiol, 100*, 96–104.

Hoshiyama, M., Koyama, S., Kitamura, Y., Watanabe, S., Shimojo, M., & Kakigi, R. (1997). Activity in pariental cortex following somatosensory stimulation in man:

Magnetoencephalographic study using spatio-temporal source analysis. *Brain Topogr, 10*, 23–30.

Hoshiyama, M., Kakigi, R., Berg, P., Koyama, S., Kitamura, Y., Shimojo, M., et al. (1997). Identification of motor and sensory brain activities during unilateral finger movement: spatiotemporal source analysis of movement-associated magnetic fields. *Exp Brain Res, 115*, 6–14.

Hoshiyama, M., & Kakigi R. (2000). After-effect of transcutancous electrical nerve stimulation (TENS) on pain-related evoked potentials and magnetic fields in normal subjects. *Clin Neurophysiol, 111*, 717–724.

Howland, E. W., Wakai, R. T., Mjaanes, B. A., Balog, J. P., & Cleeland, C. S. (1995). Whole head mapping of magnetic fields following painful electric finger shock. *Brain Res Cogn Brain Res, 2*, 165–172.

Huang, M. X., Harrington, D. L., Paulson, K. M., Weisend, M. P., & Lee, R. R. (2004). Temporal dynamics of ipsilateral and contralateral motor activity during voluntary finger movement. *Hum Brain Mapp, 23*, 26–39.

Huang, M., Davis, L. E., Aine, C., Weisend, M., Harrington, D., Christner, R., et al. (2004). MEG response to median nerve stimulation correlates with recovery of sensory and motor function after stroke. *Clin Neurophysiol, 115*, 820–833.

Huttunen, J., Kobal, G., Kaukoranta, E., & Hari, R. (1986). Cortical responses to painful CO_2 stimulation of nasal mucosa: a magnetoencephalographic study in man. *Electroencephalogr Clin Neurophysiol, 64*, 347–349.

Huttunen, J., Hari, R., & Leinonen, L. (1987). Cerebral magnetic responses to stimulation of ulnar and median nerves. *Electroencephalogr Clin Neurophysiol, 66*, 391–400.

Huttunen, J., Ahlfors, S., & Hari, R. (1992). Interaction of afferent impulses in the human primary sensorimotor cortex. *Electroencephalogr Clin Neurophysiol, 82*, 176–181.

Hyvarinen, J., & Poranen, A. (1974). Function of the parietal association area 7 as revealed from cellular discharges in alert monkeys. *Brain, 97*, 673–692.

Ikeda, A., Lueders, H. O., Burgess, R. C., & Shibasaki, H. (1992). Movement-related potentials recorded from supplementary motor area and primary motor area. Role of supplementary motor area in voluntary movements. *Brain, 115*, 1017–1043.

Inoue, K., Hashimoto, I., Shirai, T., Kawakami, H., Miyachi, T., Mimori, Y., et al. (2004). Disinhibition of the somatosensory cortex in cervical dystonia-decreased amplitudes of high-frequency oscillations. *Clin Neurophysiol, 115*, 1624–1630.

Inoue, K., Shirai, T., Nakanishi., K, Hashizume, A., Harada, T., Mimori, Y., et al. (2005). Difference in somatosensory evoked fields elicited by mechanical and electrical stimulations: Elucidation of the human homunculus by a noninvasive method. *Hum Brain Mapp, 24*, 274–283.

Inui, K., Tran, T. D., Hoshiyama, M., & Kakigi, R. (2002a). Preferential stimulation of A delta fibers by intra-epidermal needle electrode in humans. *Pain, 96*, 247–252.

Inui, K., Tran, D. T., Qiu, Y., Wang, X., Hoshiyama, M., & Kakigi, R. (2002b). Pain-related magnetic fields evoked by intra-epidermal electrical stimulation in humans. *Clin Neurophysiol, 113*, 298–304.

Inui, K., Tran, D. T., Qiu, Y., Wang, X., Hoshiyama, M., & Kakigi, R. (2003a). A comparative magnetoencephalographic study of cortical activations evoked by noxious and innocuous somatosensory stimulations. *Neuroscience, 120*, 235–248.

Inui, K., Wang, X., Qiu, Y., Nguyen, B. T., Ojima, S., Tamura, Y., et al. (2003b). Pain processing within the primary somatosensory cortex in humans. *Eur J Neurosci, 17*, 2859–2866.

Inui, K., Wang, X., Tamura, Y., Kaneoke, Y., & Kakigi, R. (2004). Serial processing in the human somatosensory system. *Cereb Cortex, 14*, 851–857.

Inui, K, Tsuji, T, & Kakigi, R. (2006). Temporal analysis of cortical mechanisms for pain relief by tactile stimuli in humans. *Cereb Cortex, 33*, 355-365.

Itomi, K., Kakigi, R., Maeda, K., & Hoshiyama, M. (2000a). Dermatome versus homunculus: Detailed topography of the primary somatosensory cortex following trunk stimulation. *Clin Neurophysiol, 111*, 405–412.

Itomi, K., Kakigi, R., Mukai, T., & Hoshiyama, M. (2000b). Magnetic responses to shoulder and posterior head stimulation in humans. *Brain Topogr, 14*, 15–23.

Iwamura, Y., Iriki, A., & Tanaka, M. (1994). Bilateral hand representation in the postcentral cortex. *Nature, 369*, 554–556.

Jones, E. G., & Powell, T. P. S. (1970). Anatomical study of converging sensory pathways within the cerebral cortex of the monkey. *Brain, 93*, 793–820.

Jones, S. J., Halonen, J-P., & Shawkat, F. (1989). Centrifugal and centripetal mechanisms involved in the "gating" of cortical SEPs during movement. Electroencephalogr *Clin Neurophysiol, 74*, 36–45.

Jousmaki, V. & Hari, R. (1999). Somatosensory evoked fields to large-area vibrotactile stimuli. *Clin Neurophysiol, 110*, 905–909.

Juottonen K., Gockel M., Silén T., Hurri H., Hari R., & Forss N. (2002) Altered central sensorimotor processing in patients with complex regional pain syndrome. *Pain* 98(3):315–23.

Kakigi, R., & Shibasaki, H. (1984). Scalp topography of mechanically and electrically evoked somatosensory potentials in man. *Electroencephalogr Clin Neurophysiol, 59*, 44–56.

Kakigi, R., & Jones, S. J. (1985). Effects on median nerve SEPs of tactile stimulation applied to adjacent and remote areas of the body surface. *Electroencephalogr Clin Neurophysiol, 62*, 252–265.

Kakigi, R. (1986). Ipsilateral and contralateral SEP components following median nerve stimulation: Effects of interfering stimuli applied to the contralateral hand. *Electroencephalogr Clin Neurophysiol, 64*, 246–259.

Kakigi, R., & Jones, S. J. (1986). Influence of concurrent tactile stimulation on somatosensory evoked potentials following posterior tibial nerve stimulation in man. *Electroencephalogr Clin Neurophysiol, 65*, 118–129.

Kakigi, R., & Shibasaki, H. (1987). Generator mechanisms of giant somatosensory evoked potentials in cortical reflex myoclonus. *Brain, 110*, 1359–1373.

Kakigi, R., & Shibasaki, H. (1991). Effects of age, gender and stimulus side on the scalp topography of somatosensory evoked potentials following median nerve stimulation. *J Clin Neurophysiol, 8*, 320–330.

Kakigi, R., & Shibasaki, H. (1992). Effects of age, gender and stimulus side on the scalp topography of somatosensory evoked potentials following posterior tibial nerve stimulation in man. *J Clin Neurophysiol, 9*, 431–440.

Kakigi, R. (1994). Somatosensory evoked magnetic fields following median nerve stimulation. *Neurosci Res, 20*, 165–174.

Kakigi, R., Koyama, S., Hoshiyama, M., Shimojo, M., Kitamura, Y., & Watanabe, S. (1995a). Topography of somatosensory evoked magnetic fields following posterior tibial nerve stimulation. *Electroencephalogr Clin Neurophysiol, 95*, 127–134.

Kakigi, R., Koyama, S., Hoshiyama, M., Kitamura, Y., Shimojo, M., & Watanabe, S. (1995b). Pain-related magnetic fields following painful CO_2 laser stimulation in man. *Neurosci Lett, 192*, 45–48.

Kakigi, R., Koyama, S., Hoshiyama, M., Kitamura, Y., Shimojo, M., Watanabe, S., et al. (1996a). Effects of tactile interference stimulation on somatosensory evoked magnetic fields. *Neuroreport, 7*, 405–408.

Kakigi, R., Koyama, S., Hoshiyama, M., Kitamura, Y., Shimojo, M., & Watanabe S. (1996) Pain-related brain responses following CO_2 laser stimulation: Magnetoencephalographic studies. In: I. Hashimoto, Y.C. Okada & S. Ogawa, eds. Visualization of information processing in the human brain. *Electroencephalogr Clin Neurophysiol (Suppl) 47*, 110–120.

Kakigi, R., Shimojo, M., Hoshiyama, M., Koyama, S., Watanabe, S., Naka, D., et al. (1997). Effects of movement and movement imagery on somatosensory evoked magnetic fields following posterior tibial nerve stimulation. *Brain Res Cogn Brain Res, 5*, 241–253.

Kakigi, R., Tran, T. D., Qiu, Y., Wang, X., Nguyen, T. B., Inui, K., et al. (2003). Cerebral responses following stimulation of unmyelinated C-fibers in humans: electro- and magneto-encephalographic study. *Neurosci Res, 45*, 255–275.

Kakigi, R., Inui, K., & Tamura, Y. (2005). Electrophysiological studies on human pain perception. *Clin Neurophysiol, 116*, 743–763.

Kamada, K., Takeuchi, F., Kuriki, S., Oshiro, O., Houkin, K., & Abe, H. (1993). Functional Neurosurgical simulation with brain surface magnetic resonance images and magnetoencephalography. *Neurosurgery, 33*, 269–273.

Kanda, M., Nagamine, T., Ikeda, A., Ohara, S., Kunieda, T., Fujiwara, N., et al. (2000). Primary somatosensory cortex is actively involved in pain processing in human. *Brain Res, 853*, 282–289.

Kanno, A., Nakasato, N., Hatanaka, K., & Yoshimoto, T. (2003). Ipsilateral area 3b responses to median nerve somatosensory stimulation. *Neuroimage, 18*, 169–177.

Karhu, J., Hari, R., Lu, S. T., Paetau, R., & Rif, J. (1991). Cerebral magnetic fields to lingual stimulation. *Electroencephalogr Clin Neurophysiol, 80*, 459–468.

Karhu, J., Hari, R., Makela, J. P., Huttunen, J., & Knuutila, J. (1992). Cortical somatosensory magnetic responses in multiple sclerosis. *Electroencephalogr Clin Neurophysiol, 83*, 192–200.

Karhu, J, Hari, R, Paetau, R, Kajala, M, & Mervaala, E. (1994). Cortical reactivity in progressive myoclonus epilepsy. *Electroencephalogr Clin Neurophysiol, 90*, 93–102.

Kaufman, L., Okada, Y., Brenner, D., & Williamson, S. J. (1981). On the relation between somatic evoked potentials and fields. *Int J Neurosci, 15*, 223–239.

Kaukolanta, E., Hari R., Hamalainen, M., & Huttunen, J. (1986). Cerebral magnetic fields evoked by peroneal nerve stimulation. *Somatosens Res, 3*, 309–321.

Kawamura, T., Nakasato, N., Seki, K., Kanno, A., Fujita, S., Fijiwara, S., et al. (1996). Neuromagnetic evidence of pre- and post-central cortical sources of somatosensory evoked responses. *Electroencephalogr Clin Neurophysiol, 100*, 44–50.

Kenshalo Jr., D. R., & Willis Jr., W. D. (1991). The role of cerebral cortex in pain perception. In: A. Peters and E. G. Jones, eds. *The Cerebral Cortex*. New York: Plenum, pp. 153–212.

Kitamura, Y., Kakigi, R., Hoshiyama, M., Koyama, S., Shimojo, M., & Watanabe, S. (1995). Pain-related somatosensory evoked magnetic fields. *Electroencephalogr Clin Neurophysiol, 95*, 463–474.

Kitamura, Y., Kakigi, R., Hoshiyama, M., Koyama, S., & Nakamura, A. (1996). Effects of sleep on somatosensory evoked responses in human. A magnetoencephalographic study. *Brain Res Cogn Brain Res, 4*, 275–279.

Kitamura, Y., Kakigi, R., Hoshiyama, M., Koyama, S., Shimojo, M., & Watanabe, S. (1997). Pain-related somatosensory evoked magnetic fields following lower limb stimulation. *J Neurol Sci*, *145*, 187–194.

Knecht, S., Henningsen, H., Elbert, T., Flor, H., Hohling, C., Pantev, C., et al. (1995). Cortical reorganization in human amputees and mislocalization of painful stimuli to the phantom limb. *Neurosci Lett*, *201*, 262–264.

Knecht, S., Henningsen, H., Elbert, T., Flor, H, Hohling, C., Pantev, C., et al. (1996). Reorganizational and perceptional changes after amputation. *Brain*, *119*, 1213–1219.

Knecht, S., Henningsen, H., Hohling, C., Elbert, T., Flor, H., Pantev, C., et al. (1998). Plasticity of plasticity? Changes in the pattern of perceptual correlates of reorganization after amputation. *Brain*, *121*, 717–724.

Kristeva, R., Cheyne, D., & Deecke, L. (1991). Neuromagnetic fields accompanying unilateral and bilateral voluntary movements: topography and analysis of cortical sources. *Electroencephalogr Clin Neurophysiol*, *81*, 284–298.

Kristeva-Feige, R., Walter, H., Lutkenhoner, B., Hampson, S., Ross, B., Knorr, U., et al. (1994). A neuromagnetic study of the functional organization of the sensorimotor cortex. *Eur J Neurosci*, *6*, 632–639.

Kruger, L., Sampogna, S. L., Rodin, B. E., Clague, J., Brecha, N., & Yeh, Y. (1985). Thin-fiber cutaneous innervation and its intraepidermal contribution studies by labeling methods and neurotoxin treatment in rats. *Somatosens Res*, *2*, 335–356.

Lam, K., Kakigi, R., Kaneoke, Y,. Naka, D., Maeda, K., & Suzuki, H. (1999). Effects of visual and auditory stimulation on somatosensory evoked magnetic fields. *Clin Neurophysiol*, *110*, 295–304.

Lenz, F. A, Rios, M., Zirh, A., Chau, D., Krauss, G., & Lesser, R, P. (1998). Painful stimuli evoke potentials recorded over the human anterior cingulate gyrus. *J Neurophysiol*, *79*, 2231–2234.

Loose, R., Hamdy, S., & Enck, P. (2001). Magnetoencephalographic response characteristics associated with tongue movement. *Dysphagia*, *16*, 183–185.

Maclin, E., Rose, D. F., Knight, J. E., Orrison, W. W., & Davis, L. E. (1994). Somatosensory evoked magnetic fields in patients with stroke. *Electroencephalogr Clin Neurophysiol*, *91*, 468–475.

Maeda, K., Kakigi, R., Hoshiyama, M., & Koyama, S. (1999). Topography of the secondary somatosensory cortex in humans: a magnetoencephalographic study. *Neuroreport*, *10*, 301–306.

McCabe C.S., Haigh R.C., Ring E.F., Halligan P.W., Wall P.D., & Blake D.R. (2003). A controlled pilot study of the utility of mirror visual feedback in the treatment of complex regional pain syndrome (type 1). Rheumatology (Oxford). *42*(1), 97–101.

Makela, J. P. & Hari, R. (1992). Neuromagnetic auditory evoked responses after a stroke in the right temporal lobe. *Neuroreport*, *3*, 94–96.

Mauguiere, F., Merlet, I., Forss, N., Vanni, S., Jousmaki, V., Adeleine, P., et al. (1997a). Activation of a distributed somatosensory cortical network in the human brain: a dipole modeling study of magnetic fields evoked by median nerve stimulation. Part 1: Location and activation timing of SEF sources. *Electroencephalogr Clin Neurophysiol*, *104*, 281–289.

Mauguiere, F., Merlet, I., Forss, N., Vanni, S., Jousmaki, V., Adeleine, P., et al. (1997b). Activation of a distributed somatosensory cortical network in the human brain: a dipole modeling study of magnetic fields evoked by median nerve stimulation. Part 2: Effects of stimulus rate, attention and stimulus detection. *Electroencephalogr Clin Neurophysiol*, *104*, 290–295.

Mayville, J. M., Fuchs, A., & Kelso, J. A. (2005). Neuromagnetic motor fields accompanying self-paced rhythmic finger movement at different rates. *Exp Brain Res, 166,* 190–199.

Mima, T., Ikeda, A., Nagamine, T., Yazawa, S., Kunieda, T., Mikuni, N., et al. (1997). Human second somatosensory area: Subdural and magnetoencephalographic recording of somatosensory evoked responses. *J Neurol Neurosurg Psychiatry, 63,* 501–505.

Mima, T., Nagamine, T., Nakamura, K., & Shibasaki, H. (1998a). Attention modulates both pimary and second somatosensory cortical activities in humans: A magnetoencephalographic study. *J Neurophysiol, 80,* 2215–2221.

Mima, T., Nagamine, T., Nishitani, N., Mikuni, N., Ikeda, A., Fukuyama, H., et al. (1998b). Cortical myoclonus. sensorimotor hyperexcitability. *Neurology, 50,* 933–942.

Mogilner, A., Grossman, J. A. I., Ribary, U., Joliot, M., Volkmann, J., Rapaport, D., et al. (1993). Somatosensory cortical plasticity in adult humans revealed by magnetoencephalography. *Proc Natl Acad Sci USA, 90,* 3593–3597.

Mogilner, A., Nomura, M., Ribary, U., Jagow, R., Lado, F., Rusinek, H., et al. (1994). Neuromagnetic studies of the lip area of primary somatosensory cortex in humans: evidence for an oscillotopic organization. *Exp Brain Res, 99,* 137–147.

Moseley G.L. (2004). Graded motor imagery is effective for long-standing complex regional pain syndrome: a randomised controlled trial. *Pain 108*(1-2), 192–198.

Munger, B. L., & Halata, Z. (1983). The sensory innervation of primate facial skin. I. Hairy skin. *Brain Res Rev, 5,* 45–80.

Nagamine, T., Toro, T., Balish, M., Deuschl, G., Wang, B., Sato, S., et al. (1994). Cortical magnetic and electric fields associated with voluntary finger movements. *Brain Topogr, 6,* 175–183.

Nagamine, T., Makela, J., Mima, T., Mikuni, N., Nishitani, N., Satoh, T., et al. (1998). Serial processing of the somesthetic information revealed by different effects of stimulus rate on the somatosensory-evoked potentials and magnetic fields. *Brain Res, 791,* 200–208.

Naka, D., Kakigi, R., Koyama, S., Xiang, J., & Suzuki, H. (1998). Effects of tactile interference stimulation on somatosensory evoked magnetic fields following tibial nerve stimulation. *Electroencephalogr Clin Neurophysiol, 109,* 168–177.

Nakagawa, H., Namima, T., Aizawa, M., Uchi, K., Kaiho, Y., Yoshikawa, K., et al. (1998). Somatosensory evoked magnetic fields elicited by dorsal penile, posterior tibial and median nerve stimulation. *Electroencephalogr Clin Neurophysiol, 108,* 57–61.

Nakamura, A., Yamada, T., Goto, A., Kato, T., Ito, K., Abe, Y., et al. (1998). Somatosensory homunculus as drawn by MEG. *Neuroimage, 7,* 377–386.

Nakasato, N., Seki, K., Kawamura, T., Ohtomo, S., Kanno, A., Fujita, S., et al. (1996). Cortical mapping using an MRI-linked whole head MEG system and presurgical decision making. In: Hashimoto, Y. C. Okada & S. Ogawa, eds. Visualization of Information Processing in the Human Brain. *Electroencephalogr Clin Neurophysiol Suppl 47,* 333–341.

Nakasato, N., Kanno, A., Hatanaka, K., Ohtomo, S., Inoue, T., Shimizu, H., et al. (1999). Preoperative MEG, fMRI and intraoperative cortical stimulation methods for neurosurgical brain mapping. In: T. Yoshimoto, M. Kotani, S. Kuriki, H. Karibe & N. Nakasato, eds. *Recent Advances in Biomagnetism.* Sendai: Tohoku University Press. pp. 821–824.

Nakasato, N., Itoh, H., Hatanaka, K., Nakahara, H., Kanno, A., & Yoshimoto, T. (2001). Movement-related magnetic fields to tongue protrusion. *Neuroimage, 14,* 924–935.

Nakata, H., Inui, K., Nishihira, Y., Hatta, A., Sakamoto, M., Kida, T., et al. (2004). Effects of a go/nogo task on event-related potentials following somatosensory stimulation. *Clin Neurophysiol, 115,* 361–368.

Narich, L., Madonna, I., Opsomer, R. J., Pizzella, V., Romani, G. L., Torrioli, G., et al. (1991). Neuromagnetic somatosensory homunculus: a non-invasive approach in humans. *Neurosci Lett, 121,* 51–54.

Neshige, R., Luders, H., & Shibasaki, H. (1988). Recording of movement-related potentials from scalp and cortex in man. *Brain, 111,* 719–736.

Nguyen, B. T., Tran T. D., Hoshiyama, M., Inui, K., & Kakigi R. (2004). Face representation in the human primary somatosensory cortex. *Neurosci Res, 50,* 227–232.

Nguyen, T. B., Inui, K., Hoshiyama, M., & Kakigi, R. (2005). Face representation in the human secondary somatosensory cortex. *Clin Neurophysiol, 116,* 1247–1253.

Nihashi, T., Kakigi, R., Kawakami, O., Hoshiyama, M., Itomi, K., Nakanishi, H., et al. (2001). Representation of the ear in human primary somatosensory cortex. *Neuroimage, 13,* 295–304.

Nihashi, T., Kakigi, R., Okada, T., Sadato, N., Kashikura, K., Kajita, Y., et al. (2002). Functional magnetic resonance imaging evidence for a representation of the ear in human primary somatosensory cortex: comparison with MEG study. *Neuroimage, 17,* 1217–1226.

Nihashi, T., Kakigi, R., Hoshiyama, M., Miki K., Kajita, Y., Yoshida, J., et al. (2003). Effect of tactile interference stimulation of the ear in human primary somatosensory cortex: a magnetoencephalographic study. *Clin Neurophysiol, 114,* 1866–1878.

Nihashi, T., Naganawa, S., Sato, C., Kawai, H., Nakamura, T., Fukatsu, H., et al. (2005). Contralateral and ipsilateral responses in primary somatosensory cortex following electrical median nerve stimulation-an fMRI study. *Clin Neurophysiol, 116,* 842–848.

Novotny, G. E. K., & Gommert-Novotny, E. (1988). Intraepidermal nerves in human digital skin. *Cell Tissue Res, 254,* 111–117.

Opsommer, E., Masquelier, E., & Plaghki, L. (1999). Study of nerve conduction velocity of C-fibers in humans from thermal thresholds to contact heat (thermode) and from evoked brain potentials to radiant heat (CO_2 laser). *Neurophysiol Clin, 29,* 411–422.

Opsommer, E., Weiss, T., Plaghki, L., & Miltner, W. H. R. (2001a). Dipole analysis of ultralate (C-fibers) evoked potentials after laser stimulation of tiny cutaneous surface areas in humans. *Neurosci Lett, 298,* 41–44.

Opsommer, E., Weiss, T., Miltner, W. H., & Plaghki, L. (2001b). Scalp topography of ultralate (C-fibres) evoked potentials following thulium YAG laser stimuli to tiny skin surface areas in humans. *Clin Neurophysiol, 112,* 1868–1874.

Pantev, C., Gallen, C., Hampson, S., Buchanan, S., & Sobel, D. (1991). Reproducibility and validity of neuromagnetic source localization using a large array biomagnetometer. *Am J EEG Tech, 31,* 83–101.

Penfield, W., & Boldray, E. (1937). Somatic motor and sensory representation in the cerebral cortex of man as studied by electrical stimulation. *Brain, 60,* 389–443.

Peyron, R., Frot, M., Schneider, F., Garcia-Larrea, L., Mertens, P., Barral, F.G., et al. (2002). Role of operculoinsular cortices in human pain processing: Covering evidence from PET, fMRI, dipole modeling, and intracerebral recordings of evoked potentials. *Neuroimage, 17,* 1336–1346.

Ploghaus, A., Tracey, I., Clare, S., Gati, J. S., Rawlins, J. N. P., & Matthews, P. M. (2000). Learning about pain: The neural substrate of the prediction error for aversive events. *Proc Natl Acad Sci U S A, 97*, 9281–9286.

Ploghaus, A., Narain, C., Beckmann, C. F., Clare, S., Bantick, S., Wise, R., et al. (2001). Exacerbation of pain by anxiety is associated with activity in a hippocampal network. *J Neurosci, 21*, 9896–9903.

Ploner, M., Schmitz, F., Freund, H. J., & Schnitzler, A. (1999). Parallel activation of primary and secondary somatosensory cortices in human pain processing. *J Neurophysiol, 81*, 3100–3104.

Ploner, M., Schmitz, F., Freund, H. J., & Schnitzler, A. (2000). Differential organization of touch and pain in human primary somatosensory cortex. *J Neurophysiol, 83*, 1770–1776.

Praamstra, P, Schmitz, F, Freund, H. J., & Schnitzler, A. (1999). Magneto-encephalographic correlates of the lateralized readiness potential. *Brain Res Cogn Brain Res, 8*, 77–85.

Qiu, Y., Inui, K., Wang, X., Tran, T. D., & Kakigi, R. (2001). Conduction velocity of the spinothalamic tract in humans as assessed by CO_2 laser stimulation of C-fibers in men. *Neurosci Lett, 311*, 181–184.

Qiu, Y., Inui, K., Wang, X., Tran, T. D., & Kakigi, R. (2002). Effects of attention, distraction and sleep on CO_2 laser evoked potentials related to C-fibers in human. *Clin Neurophysiol, 113*, 1579–1585.

Qiu, Y., Fu, Q., Wang, X., Tran, T. D., Inui, K., Iwase, S., et al. (2003). Microneurographic study of C fiber discharges induced by CO_2 laser stimulation in humans. *Neurosci Lett, 353*, 25–28.

Qiu, Y., Inui, K., Wang, X., Nguyen, B. T., Tran, T. D., & Kakigi, R. (2004). Effects of distration on MEG responses ascending through C-fibers in humans. *Clin Neurophysiol, 115*, 636–646.

Qiu, Y., Honda, M., Noguchi, Y., Nakata, H., Tamura, Y., Tanaka, S., et al. (2006). Brain processing of the signals ascending through unmyelinated C fibers in humans, an event-related fMRI study. *Cereb Cortex, 16*, 1289–1295.

Pons, T. P., Garraghty, P. E., Ommaya, A. K., Kaas, J. H., Taub, E., & Mishkin, M. (1991). Massive cortical reorganization after sensory deafferentation in adult macaques. *Science, 252*, 1857–1860.

Raij TT, Vartiainen NV, Jousmäki V, Hari R. (2003). Effects of interstimulus interval on cortical responses to painful laser stimulation. *J Clin Neurophysiol. 20*(1), 73–79.

Raij T.T., Forss N., Stancák A., & Hari R. (2004). Modulation of motor-cortex oscillatory activity by painful Adelta- and C-fiber stimuli. *Neuroimage 23*(2), 569–573.

Robinson, D. L. (1973). Electrophysiological analysis of interhemispheric relations on the second somatosensory cortex of the cat. *Exp Brain Res, 18*, 131–144.

Rogers, R. L., Basile, L. F. H, Taylor, S., Sutherling, W. W., & Papanicolaou, A. C. (1994). Somatosensory evoked fields and potentials following tibial nerve stimulation. *Neurology, 44*, 1283–1286.

Rossini, P. M., Narici, L., Romani, G. L., Peresson, M., Torrioli, G., & Traversa, R. (1989). Simultaneos motor output and sensory input: cortical interference site resolved in humans via neuromagnetic measurements. *Neurosci Lett, 96*, 300–305.

Rossini, P. M., Narici, L., Martino, G., Pasquarelli, A., Peresson, M., Pizzella, V., et al. (1994). Analysis of interhemispheric asymmetries of somatosensory evoked magnetic fields to right and left median nerve stimulation. *Electroencephalogr Clin Neurophysiol, 91*, 476–482.

Rossini, P. M., Caltagirone, C., Castriota-Scanderbeg, A., Cicinelli, P., Gratta, C. D., Demartin, M., et al. (1998a). Hand motor cortical area reorganization in stoke: A study with fMRI, MEG and TCS maps. *Neuroreport, 9*, 2141–2146.

Rossini, P. M., Tecchio, F., Pizzella, V., Lupoi, D., Cassetta, E., Pasqualetti, P., et al. (1998b). On the reorganization of sensory hand areas after mono-hemispheric lesion: a functional (MEG)/anatomical (MRI) integrative study. *Brain Res, 782*, 153–166.

Rossini, P. M., Tecchio, F., Pizzella, V., Lupoi, D., Cassetta, E., & Pasqualetti, P. (2001). Interhemispheric differences of sensory hand areas after monohemispheric stroke: MEG/MRI integrative study. *Neuroimage, 14*, 474–485.

Roth, B. J., Sepulveda, N. G., & Wikswo, J. P. (1989). Using a magnetometer to image a two-dimensional current distribution. *J Appl Physiol, 65*, 361–372.

Sakamoto, K., Nakata, H., & Kakigi, R. (2008a) Somatotopic representation of the tongue in human secondary somatosensory cortex. *Clin Neurophysiol, 119*, 1664–1673.

Sakamoto, K., Nakata, H., & Kakigi, R. (2008b). Somatotopic representation of the tongue in human secondary somatosensory cortex. *Clin Neurophysiol, 119*, 2125–2134.

Sakuma, K., & Hashimoto, I. (1999a). High-frequency magnetic oscillations evoked by posterior tibial nerve stimulation. *Neuroreport, 10*, 227–230.

Sakuma, K., Sekihara, K., & Hashimoto, I. (1999b). Neural source estimation from a time-frequency component of somatic evoked high-frequency magnetic oscillations to posterior tibial nerve stimulation. *Clin Neurophysiol, 110*, 1585–1588.

Salenius S., Schnitzler A., Salmelin R., Jousmäki V., & Hari R. (1997) Modulation of the human cortical rolandic rhythms during natural sensorimotor tasks. *Neuroimage* 5, 221–228.

Salmelin, R. & Hari R. (1994) Spatiotemporal characteristics of sensorimotor MEG rhythms related to thumb movement. *Neuroscience* 60, 537–550.

Sarvas, J. (1987). Basic mathematical and electromagnetic concepts of the biomagnetic inverse problem. *Phys Med Biol, 32*, 11–12.

Sawamoto, N., Honda, M., Okada, T., Hanakawa, T., Kanda, M., Fukuyama, H., et al. (2000). Expectation of pain enhances responses to nonpainful somatosensory stimulation in the anterior cingulate cortex and parietal operculum/posterior insula: an event-related functional magnetic resonance imaging study. *J Neurosci, 20*, 7438–7445.

Schmidt, R. F., Schaible, H. G., Messlinger, K., Heppelmann, B., Hanesch, U., & Pawlak, M. (1994). Silent and active nociceptors: structure, functions, and clinical implications. In: G. F. Gebhart, D. L. Hammond and T. S. Jensen, eds. *Proceedings of the 7th World Congress on Pain*, Seattle, WA: IASP Press, pp. 213–250.

Schnitzler, A., Salmelin, R., Salenius, S., Jousmaki, V., & Hari, R. (1995a). Tactile information from the human hand reaches the ipsilateral primary somatosensory cortex. *Neurosci Lett, 200*, 25–28.

Schnitzler, A., Wittem, O. W., Cheyne, D., Haid, D., Vrba, J., & Freund, H. J. (1995b). Modulation of somatosensory evoked magnetic fields by sensory and motor interference. *Neuroreport, 6*, 1653–1658.

Schnitzler A., Salenius S., Salmelin R., Jousmäki V., & Hari R. (1997) Involvement of primary motor cortex in motor imagery: a neuromagnetic study. *Neuroimage*. 6(3):201–208.

Schnitzler, A., & Ploner, M. (2000). Neurophysiology and functional neuroanatomy of pain perception. *J Clin Neurophysiol, 17*, 592–603.

Seeck, M., Lazeyras, F., Michel, C. M., Blanke, O., Gericke, C. A., Ives, J., et al. (1998). Non-invasive epileptic focus localization using EEG-triggered functional MRI and electromagnetic tomography. *Electroencephalogr Clin Neurophysiol, 106*, 508–512.

Servos, P., Engel, S. A., Gati, J., & Menon, R. (1999). FMRI evidence for an inverted face representation in human somatosensory cortex. *Neuroreport, 10*, 1393–1395.

Shibasaki, H., Barrett, G., Halliday, E., & Halliday, A. M. (1980). Components of the movement-related cortical potential and their scalp topography. *Electroencephalogr Clin Neurophysiol, 49*, 213–26.

Shimizu, H., Nakasato, N., Mizoi, K., & Yoshimoto, T. (1997). Localizing the central sulcus by functional magnetic resonance imaging and magnetoencephalography. *Clin Neurol Neurosurg, 99*, 235–238.

Shimojo, M., Kakigi, R., Hoshiyama, M., Koyama, S., Kitamura, Y., & Watanabe, S. (1996a). Intracerebral interactions caused by bilateral median nerve stimulation in man. A magnetoencephalographyic study. *Neurosci Res, 24*, 175–181.

Shimojo, M., Kakigi, R., Hoshiyama, M., Koyama, S., Kitamura, Y., & Watanabe, S. (1996b), Differentiation of receptive fields in the sensory cortex following stimulation of various nerves of the lower limb in man. Magnetoencephalographic study. *J Neurosurg, 5*, 255–262.

Shimojo, M., Kakigi, R., Hoshiyama, M., Koyama, S., & Watanabe, S. (1997). Magnetoencephalographic study of intracerebral interactions caused by bilateral posterior tibial nerve stimulation in man. *Neurosci Res, 28*, 41–47.

Silén T., Forss N., Jensen O., & Hari R. (2000) Abnormal reactivity of the approximately 20-Hz motor cortex rhythm in Unverricht Lundborg type progressive myoclonus epilepsy. *Neuroimage* 12, 707–712.

Sobel, D. F., Gallen, C. C., Schwartz, B. J., Waltz, T. A., Copeland, B., Yamada, S., et al. (1993). Locating the central sulcus: Comparison of MR anatomic and magnetoencephalographic functional methods. *Am J Neuroradiol, 14*, 915–925.

Stancak, A., Raij, T. T., Pohja, M., Forss, N., & Hari, R. (2005). Oscillatory motor cortex-muscle coupling during painful laser and nonpainful tactile stimulation. *Neuroimage, 26*, 793–800.

Sterr, A., Muller, M. M., Elbert, T., Rockstroh, B., Pantev, C., & Taub, E. (1998a). Perceptual correlates of changes in cortical representation of fingers in blind multifinger Braille readers. *J Neurosci, 18*, 4417–4423.

Sterr, A., Muller, M. M., Elbert, T., Rockstroh, B., Pantev, C., & Taub, E. (1998b). Changed perception in Braille-readers. *Nature, 391*, 134–135.

Stippich, C., Freitag, P., Kassubek, J., Soros, P., Kamada, K., Kober, H., et al. (1998). Motor, somatosensory and auditory cortex localization by fMRI and MEG. *Neuroreport, 9*, 1953–1957.

Suk, J., Ribary, U., Cappell, J., Yamamoto, T., & Llinas, R. (1991). Anatomical localization revealed by MEG recordings of the human somatosensory system. *Electroencephalogr Clin Neurophysiol, 78*, 85–196.

Sutherling, W., Crandall, P., Darcey, T., Becker, D., Levesque, M., & Barth, D. (1988). The magnetic and electric fields agree with intracranial localizations of somatosensory cortex. *Neurology, 38*, 1705–1714.

Svensson, P., Minoshima, S., Beydoun, A., Morrow, T. J., & Casey, K. L. (1997). Cerebral processing of acute skin and muscle pain in humans. *J Neurophysiol, 78*, 450–460.

Tanosaki, M., Kimura, T., Takino, R., Iguchi, Y., Suzuki, A., Kurobe, Y., et al. (2002). Movement interference attenuates somatosensory high-frequency oscillations: contribution of local axon collaterals of 3b pyramidal neurons. *Clin Neurophysiol, 113*, 993–1000.

Tecchio, F., Rossini, P. M., Pizzella, V., Cassetta, E., Pasqualetti, P., & Romani, G. L. (1998). A neuromagnetic normative data set for hemispheric sensory hand cortical representations and their interhemispheric differences. *Brain Res Protoc, 2*, 306–314.

Tiihonen, J., Hari, R., & Hamalainen, M. (1989). Early deflections of cerebral magnetic responses to median nerve stimulation. *Electroencephalogr Clin Neurophysiol, 74*, 290–296.

Trahms, L., Erne, S. N., Trontel, Z., Curio, G., & Aust, P. (1989). Biomagnetic functional localization of a peripheral nerve in man. *Biophys J, 55*, 1145–1153.

Tran, T. D., Lam, K., Hoshiyama, M., & Kakigi, R. (2001). A new method for measuring the conduction velocities of A-β, Aδ- and C-fibers following electric and CO_2 laser stimulation in humans. *Neurosci Lett, 301*, 187–190.

Tran, T. D., Inui, K., Hoshiyama, M., Lam, K., & Kakigi, R. (2002a). Conduction velocity of the spinothalamic tract following CO_2 laser stimulation of C-fiber in humans. *Pain, 95*, 125–131.

Tran, T. D., Inui, K., Hoshiyama, M., Lam, K., Qiu, Y., & Kakigi, R. (2002b). Cerebral activation by the signals ascending through unmyelinated C-fibers in humans: a magnetoencephalographic study. *Neuroscience, 113*, 375–386.

Treede, R. D., Meyer, R. A., & Lesser, R. P. (1994). Similarity of threshold temperatures for first pain sensation, laser-evoked potentials, and nociceptor activation. In: G.F. Gebhart, D.L. Hammond and T.S. Jensen, eds. *Proceedings of the 7th world congress on pain*. Seattle: IASP Press, pp. 857–865.

Treede, R. D., Kenshalo, D. R., Gracely, R.H., & Jones, A. K. (1999). The cortical representation of pain. *Pain, 79*, 105–111.

Uesaka, Y., Ugawa, Y., Yumoto, M., Sakuta, M., & Kanazawa, I. (1993). Giant somatosensory evoked magnetic field in patients with myoclonus epilepsy. *Electroencephalogr Clin Neurophysiol, 87*, 300–305.

Uesaka, Y., Terao, Y., Ugawa, Y., Yumoto, M., Hanajima, R., & Kanazawa, I. (1996). Magnetoencephalographic analysis of cortical myoclonic jerks. *Electroencephalogr Clin Neurophysiol, 99*, 141–148.

Wang, X., Inui, K., Qiu, Y., & Kakigi, R. (2004). Cortical responses to noxious stimuli during sleep. *Neuroscience, 128*, 177–186.

Wasaka, T., Hoshiyama, M., Nakata, H., Nishihira, Y., & Kakigi, R. (2003). Gating of somatosensory evoked magnetic fields during the preparatory period of self-initiated finger movement. *Neuroimage, 20*, 1830–1838.

Wasaka, T., Nakata, H., Akatsuka, K., Kida, T., Inui, K., & Kakigi, R (2005). Differential modulation in human primary and secondary somatosensory cortices during the preparatory period of self-initiated finger movement. *Eur J Neurosci, 22*, 1239–1247.

Watanabe, S., Kakigi, R., Koyama, S., Hoshiyama, M., & Kaneoke, Y. (1998). Pain processing traced by magnetoencephalography in the human brain. *Brain Topogr, 10*, 255–264.

Weiss, T., Miltner, W. H. R., Dillmann, J., Meissner, W., Huonker, R., & Nowak, H. (1998). Reorganization of the somatosensory cortex after amputation of the index finger. *Neuroreport, 9*, 213–216.

Whitzel, B. L., Perrucelli, L., & Werner, G. (1969). Symmetry and connectivity in the body surface in somatosensory cortex: identification by combined magnetic and potential recordings. *J Physiol (Lond), 32*, 218–223.

Wikstrom, H., Huttunen, J., Korvenoja, A., Virtanen, J., Salonen, O., Aronen, H., et al. (1996). Effects of interstimulus interval on somatosensory evoked magnetic fields (SEFs): A hypothesis concerning SEF generation at the primary sensorimotor cortex. *Clin Neurophys* 1999 May; *110*(5):916–23.

Wikswo, J. P., & Freeman, J. A. (1980). Magnetic field of a nerve impulse: first measurements. *Science, 208*, 53–55.

Wikswo, J. P., Friedman, R. M., Kilroy, A. W., Van Wgeraat, J. M., & Buchanan, D. S. (1985). Preliminary measurements with micro SQUID. In: S. J. Williamson, M. Hoke, G. Stroink & M. Kotani, eds. *Advances in Biomagnetism.* New York: Plenum, pp. 681–684.

Wikswo, J. P. (1990). Biomagnetic sources and their models. In: S. J. Williamson, M. Hoke, G. Stroink & M. Kotani, eds. *Advances in Biomagnetism.* New York: Plenum, pp. 1–18.

Wood, C. C., Cohen, D., Cuffin, B. N., Yarita, M., & Allison, T. (1985). Electrical sources in human somatosensory cortex: identification by combined magnetic and potential recordings. *Science, 227*, 1051–1053.

Xu, X., Fujiwara, H., Shindo, K., Nagamine, T., & Shibasaki, H. (1997). Functional localization of pain perception in the human brain studied by PET. *Neuroreport, 8*, 555–559.

Xiang, J., Hoshiyama, M., Koyama, S., Kaneoke, Y., Suzuki, H., Watanabe, S., et al. (1997a). Somatosensory evoked magnetic fields following passive finger movement. *Brain Res Cogn Brain Res, 6*, 73–82.

Xiang, J., Kakigi, R., Hoshiyama, M., Kaneoke, Y., Naka, D., Takeshima, Y., et al. (1997b) Somatosensory evoked magnetic fields and potentials following passive toe movement in humans. *Electroencephalogr Clin Neurophysiol, 104*, 393–401.

Yang, T. T., Gallen, C. C., Schwartz, B.J., & Bloom, F. E. (1993). Noninvasive somatosensory homunculus mapping in humans by using a large-array biomagnetometer. *Proc Natl Acad Sci USA, 90*, 3098–3102.

Yang, T. T., Gallen, C. C., Ramachandran, V. S., Cobb, S., Schwartz, B.J., & Bloom, F. E. (1994). Noninvasive detection of cerebral plasticity in adult human somatosensory cortex. *Neuroreport, 5*, 701–704.

Yamasaki, H., Kakigi, R., & Naka, D. (1999). Effects of distraction on pain perception: Magneto- and electro-encephalographic studies. *Brain Res Cogn Brain Res, 8*, 73–76.

Yamasaki, H., Kakigi, R., Watanabe, S., & Hoshiyama, M. (2000). Effects of distraction on pain-related somatosensory evoked magnetic fields and potentials following painful electrical stimulation. *Brain Res Cogn Brain Res, 9*, 165–175.

13

MEG and Reading: From Perception to Linguistic Analysis

Riitta Salmelin

- Both timing and location of activation are essential in language research
- MEG reveals the spatiotemporal sequence of cortical activation in silent reading, with clear functional roles for activations
- Dyslexic vs. fluently reading adults: similar areas but abnormally weak or absent letter-string activation, delay in the stage of reading comprehension
- Children vs. adults: similar areas, functionally similar sequence of activation but everything delayed in time

Introduction

It is usually assumed that when we see a familiar word, like 'brain', the visual features must be processed first before the analysis can proceed to the content, apparently first at the level of single letters and then as a whole word, which further activates the word's meaning and its sound form. How much these later processing stages interact, and whether they occur sequentially or in parallel, as a single interactive process, is an issue currently under debate (Coltheart et al., 1993; Plaut et al., 1996). These theoretical models of reading are based largely on analysis of behavioral reaction times and error types in acquired and developmental reading disorders.

When seeking to describe the organization of normal reading at the level of the brain, it would seem reasonable to use the theoretical models as a conceptual framework rather than as a strict guideline of specific processes and their relationships. First, it is not certain that models derived from language disorders fully correspond to the normal function; second, the computations performed by the brain may not be divisible into the blocks suggested by the model; third, current theoretical models tend not to make quantitative predictions of measures that may be extracted with neuroimaging (timing, activation strength, localization).

For data-driven characterization of cerebral implementation of reading, knowledge of both location and timing of the activation is essential. This chapter focuses on the use of MEG in studying neural processes of fluent and impaired reading (for a review of MEG research into other aspects of language processing, see Salmelin, 2007). We will first track the cortical sequence of activation when reading familiar words and, thereafter, consider the case of unfamiliar words. After contrasting the sequence of activation in reading with that in speech perception, we will focus on cortical correlates of dyslexia. A comparison of reports on neurophysiological and hemodynamic signatures of reading then follows. We will close the chapter with a glimpse into recent advances and possible future directions.

Cortical Dynamics of Reading Familiar Words

Pre-lexical Analysis

Figure 13–1 depicts a paradigm used to tease apart early pre-lexical processes in reading (Tarkiainen et al., 1999). The subjects were shown (Finnish) words,

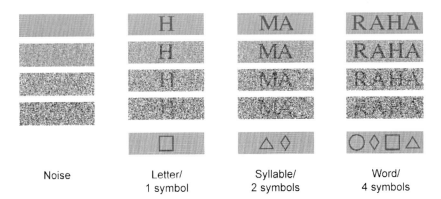

Noise   Letter/ 1 symbol   Syllable/ 2 symbols   Word/ 4 symbols

Figure 13–1. Paradigm for focusing on prelexical processes in reading. The amount of features to analyze (four levels of noise) and word-likeness of the stimuli (symbols; letters, syllables, words) were varied parametrically. Modified from Tarkiainen et al. (1999).

syllables, and single letters, imbedded in a noisy background, at four different noise levels. For control, the sequences also contained symbol strings. One sequence was composed of plain noise stimuli. The stimuli were thus varied along two major dimensions: The amount of features to process increased with noise and with the number of items in the string, letters or symbols. On the other hand, word-likeness was highest for clearly visible, complete words, and lowest for symbols and noise.

Figure 13–2 shows MEG data recorded from one subject. Time runs from 50 ms before stimulus onset to 250 ms after it. Within this time interval, there were two strong magnetic field patterns. The signal first concentrated over the right occipital cortex about 130 ms after stimulus onset (Type I). Here, the response was strongest to the highest noise level and smallest for words and symbols with no noise. It was followed by a prominent left-hemisphere activation at about 150 ms after word onset (Type II) which showed the opposite behavior: it was strongest and earliest for words with no noise, somewhat smaller and later for symbol strings, and nonexistent for the very noisy words. These types of responses were observed in almost every subject.

As illustrated in Figure 13–3, the data showed a clear dissociation between two processes within the first 200 ms: Visual feature analysis occurred at about 100 ms after stimulus presentation (detected in 9 of 12 subjects), with the active areas around the occipital midline, along the ventral visual stream. This signal increased with increasing noise and with the number of items in

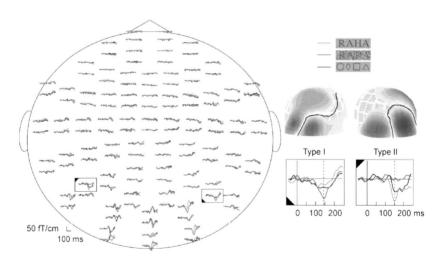

Figure 13–2. MEG responses to letter and symbol strings in one subject. The orange curves show responses to words with no noise, the green curves to words at the highest noise level, and black curves to symbol strings. A clear response particularly to noisy words (Type I) was followed by a left-hemisphere response that was strongest to the noiseless words (Type II). Modified from Tarkiainen et al. (1999).

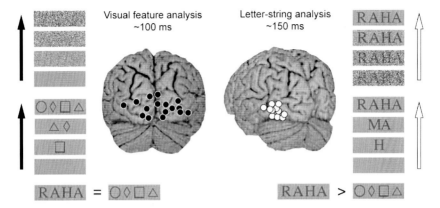

Figure 13–3. Dissociation of basic visual feature and letter-string analysis within 200 ms post-stimulus. Dots represent centers of active cortical patches collected from the individual subjects. Arrows indicate increasing strength of activation. Amount of features to analyze is the relevant variable at the first stage (~100 ms) and content at the next stage (~150 ms). From Salmelin (2007).

the string, similarly for letters and symbols. Only 50 ms later, at about 150 ms post-stimulus, the left inferior occipitotemporal cortex showed letter-string sensitive activation (10 of 12 subjects). This signal increased with the visibility of the letter strings. It was strongest for words, weaker for syllables, and still weaker for single letters. Crucially, the activation was significantly stronger for letter than symbol strings of equal length.

One may ask how specific these processes are to reading, or whether they reflect a more general transformation from visual to cognitive analysis. Category-specific occipitotemporal responses within the first 200 ms have been reported not only for letter-strings but, for example, also for numbers and faces—that is, for particularly important types of objects in our visual world (e.g., Allison et al., 1994). Tarkiainen and colleagues chose faces as test stimuli. The faces were masked the same way as the letter-strings, and the subjects' task was to identify the expressions on the faces (Tarkiainen et al., 2002). Here, the control stimuli were pictures of objects. Figure 13–4 compares early processing of letter-strings and faces in the same individuals. The stage of visual feature processing at about 100 ms was the same for both stimulus types. The timing, activated areas, and increase of activation with noise were indistinguishable. Thereafter, the processing routes diverged. The timing of the category-specific processing stage at about 150 ms was exactly the same for letter-strings and faces, and the activated areas showed large spatial overlap. However, the hemispheric balance was different. While both left and right occipitotemporal cortex respond to these stimuli (Cornelissen et al., 2003; Salmelin et al., 1996), letter-string-sensitive differentiation was detected essentially in the left hemisphere, whereas face-sensitive processing was more bilateral, with slight right-hemisphere predominance (Tarkiainen et al., 2002).

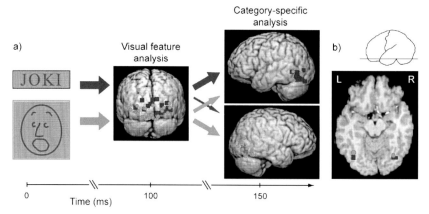

Figure 13–4. Letter-string and face analysis within 200 ms after stimulus presentation. (a) Cortical sequence of activation collected from individual subjects. Red indicates processing of letter-string stimuli and orange processing of face stimuli. (b) Mean (± SEM) location of category-specific activation at the base of the occipitotemporal cortex.
Modified from Tarkiainen et al. (2002).

What type of process does the activation at ~100 ms actually reflect? In order to obtain a simple estimate of the visual complexity of the stimulus images, Tarkiainen and colleagues computed the standard deviation of the gray values along each column, and then their mean value across the whole image (Tarkiainen et al., 2002). Equally well, one could compute the standard deviations along the rows. This measure of visual complexity is shown on the vertical axis in Figure 13–5. The horizontal axis depicts the cortical activation strength, normalized to the condition with highest noise, when this type of activation was strongest. The dots give the mean values for each stimulus category, averaged across subjects. The activation strength increased linearly with this very simple measure of visual complexity of the images, independent of the stimulus type. Accordingly, this processing stage seems to be determined directly by basic visual properties of the stimulus.

The content of the stimulus starts to matter in the subsequent category-specific processing stage, where the activation reaches the maximum at about 150 ms. In addition to the difference in hemispheric balance, there was a small but significant difference in location, with the face-sensitive activation centered about 6 mm anterior to the sources of the letter-string-specific response (Tarkiainen et al., 2002). The MEG data are in fairly good agreement with intracranial data, both with respect to the timing and location of letter-string-specific activation (Nobre et al., 1994), and the slightly more anterior center of activation for faces than for letter-strings (Nobre et al., 1994; Puce et al., 1996). The inferior occipitotemporal activation at ~150 ms apparently reflects pre-lexical analysis, as the response does not differentiate

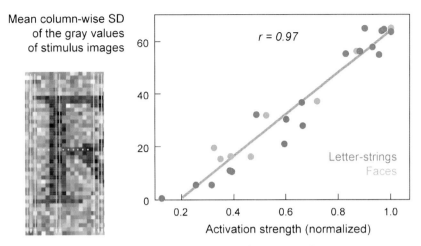

Figure 13–5. Effect of visual complexity on the occipital 100-ms response. Data from letter-string experiment in red and data from face experiment in orange. Strength of activation in this area was driven directly by basic visual properties, regardless of stimulus content.
Modified from Tarkiainen et al. (2002).

between words, nonwords, or consonant strings (Cornelissen et al., 2003; Salmelin et al., 1996; Wydell et al., 2003), again in agreement with intracranial recordings (Nobre et al., 1994).

Lexical–Semantic Analysis

The subsequent stage of reading comprehension may be characterized with the help of a well-established paradigm (Connolly & Phillips, 1994; Kutas & Hillyard, 1980), which uses sentences that create a very high expectation for a certain final word, and the researcher then varies the appropriateness of that word in the sentence context. Helenius and colleagues used four types of (Finnish) sentences: the final word was either the expected one (*e.g., The piano was out of tune*); rare, but semantically possible, (*e.g., When the power went out the house became quiet*, instead of *dark*); semantically wrong, but sharing the first letters with the expected word, referred to as the 'phonological' condition (*e.g., The gambler had a streak of bad luggage*, instead of *luck*); or totally anomalous (*e.g., The pizza was too hot to sing*). The sentences were shown one word at a time, and the responses were averaged with respect to the onset of the final word.

As illustrated in Figure 13–6, systematic stimulus-dependent variation was observed particularly in and around the left superior temporal cortex. The two types of semantically wrong sentence-ending words (phonological, anomalous) resulted in a prominent activation, reaching the maximum at about 400 ms after word onset. The signal was significantly weaker and short er-lasting (maximum at ~350 ms) for the rare but semantically possible final

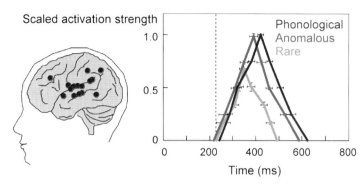

Figure 13–6. Lexical-semantic processing in the left hemisphere. *Left*: Source areas sensitive to semantic manipulation, collected from 10 subjects. *Right*: Mean (± SEM) time course of activation in the left superior temporal cluster. Colors indicate three different types of sentence-ending words (presented at time 0). The expected words did not evoke activation that would have exceeded the noise level.
Modified from Helenius et al. (1998).

words, and essentially non-existent for the expected words. This response is usually referred to as the N400 in EEG literature (N400m in MEG) and its behavior is generally considered as a signature of lexical-semantic processing (Kutas & Hillyard, 1980; Osterhout & Holcomb, 1995). In the right hemisphere, only about half of the subjects showed a qualitatively similar N400-type response (Helenius et al., 1998). In reading, lexical-semantic processing thus seems to be fairly strongly lateralized to the left hemisphere.

In fact, the complete suppression of the N400m response to the expected final words is far more remarkable than generation of the strong response to the semantically wrong words. Isolated words and the first words of sentences all elicit a strong N400/N400m response. When one proceeds along the sentence the response is gradually reduced to each word (Van Petten, 1995) until the expectation built by the context (semantic priming) is strong enough to entirely suppress the response to the expected word.

The onset of the N400m response, characterized by the latency at half the maximum response on the ascending slope, was positively correlated with the reaction time for recognizing real words in a lexical decision task (Helenius et al., 1998). In a series of MEG studies, Marantz, Pylkkänen and colleagues have demonstrated that the onset latency of the N400m activation (referred to as M350 in their studies) reflects lexical frequency. By varying both phonotactic probability and neighborhood density, these authors concluded that the response is related to lexical access rather than postlexical processing (Embick et al., 2001; Pylkkänen & Marantz, 2003; Pylkkänen et al., 2002).

When the active areas are modeled as Equivalent Current Dipoles (ECDs; cf. Chapter 6), sources of the N400m response are consistently localized to the superior temporal cortex (Halgren et al., 2002; Helenius et al., 1998; Pylkkänen

& Marantz, 2003; Salmelin et al., 1996; Simos et al., 1997), in the immediate vicinity of the auditory cortex (Helenius et al., 1998). Distributed models (cf. Chapter 8) suggest further spreading of activation to the anterior temporal and inferior frontal cortex (Halgren et al., 2002; Marinkovic et al., 2003). Involvement of the left temporal pole in semantic processing would agree with previous intracranial recordings (Halgren et al., 1994; Nobre & McCarthy, 1995) which did not, however, probe the superior temporal cortex.

Figure 13–7 summarizes the cortical dynamics of silent reading, as revealed by these MEG studies. First, there is basic visual feature analysis around the occipital midline, at about 100 ms; then, 50 ms later, lateralization to the left occipitotemporal cortex for letter-string analysis. Reading comprehension is reflected in the subsequent activation of the left superior temporal cortex at 200 to 600 ms.

The strong left-hemisphere lateralization of lexical-semantic processing in reading, at least in Finnish-speaking subjects, could possibly serve as a diagnostic tool. It has been used to evaluate cerebral implementation of reading comprehension in an aphasic patient with deep dyslexia (Laine et al., 2000). The central features of deep dyslexia are the abolishment of nonword reading, and semantic errors in reading: the patient may, for example, read the word "moon" as "crescent" (Coltheart, 1980). It has been suggested that

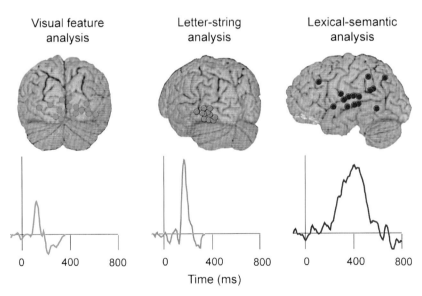

Figure 13–7. Cortical dynamics of silent reading in fluently reading subjects. Activation advanced from visual feature analysis in the occipital cortex (~100 ms) to letter-string analysis in the left occipitotemporal cortex (~150 ms) and further to activation of the left superior temporal cortex reflecting lexical-semantic analysis.
Modified from Salmelin et al. (2000).

in deep dyslexia, where extensive left-hemisphere damage leads to severely impaired reading, language processing is no longer subserved by the damaged left hemisphere but by the intact right hemisphere. The strange semantic errors would then reflect the limited capacity for word recognition in the right hemisphere (Weekes et al., 1997). The deep dyslexic patient studied by Laine and colleagues had a massive lesion in the left hemisphere, extending from the parietal and temporal to medial frontal areas (Laine et al., 2000). Nevertheless, when the patient was tested with the sentences ending with a congruent or incongruent word (Helenius et al., 1998), the remaining strip of the left superior temporal cortex still generated a sustained response that was graded by semantic relatedness, similar to the N400m identified in controls (cf. Figure 13–6). A simultaneous, weaker activation of the right superior temporal cortex did not vary with semantic congruity. Even in deep dyslexia, lexical-semantic processing thus seems to be subserved by the damaged left hemisphere like in normal subjects.

Cortical Dynamics of Reading Unfamiliar Words

When we encounter an unfamiliar word or a nonword the influential dual-route model of reading (Figure 13–9; Coltheart et al., 1993) states that we cannot use the lexical route because there is no representation for these letter-strings in our mental lexicon. Instead, we are supposed to process the letter-strings letter-by-letter and convert each letter to its corresponding sound in order to obtain a sound form for the letter-string, which again may lead to some type of semantic association.

The dual-route model predicts that for real words the lexical route dominates and, in that case, the word length has little effect. Processing of nonwords, on the other hand, would rely on the letter-level grapheme-to-phoneme conversion, and subsequent phonological processing. Nonword length should thus have a strong effect on the amount of phonological processing required.

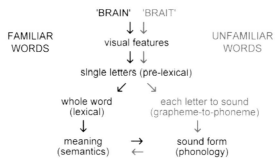

Figure 13–8. Outline of the dual-route model of reading. Modified from Coltheart et al. (1993).

Behaviorally, it has been found that naming latencies are shorter for short than long words, and that this length effect is markedly enhanced when naming non-words (Weekes, 1997). The use of the phonological route, and thus the length effect, is thought to be particularly pronounced in a regular orthography.

The Finnish language has an exceptionally regular one-to-one correspondence between graphemes and phonemes and should, therefore, be well suited for cortical evaluation of the potential lexical-semantic vs. phonological routes of reading. Wydell and colleagues varied the letter-string length and lexicality by presenting short and long real Finnish words (4 and 8 letters) and short and long pronounceable nonwords in a randomized order (Wydell et al., 2003). The subjects were occasionally prompted to read the string aloud, in an unpredictable fashion, thus emphasizing full phonological encoding of the letter-strings.

There were only two areas and time windows where the activation showed systematic dependence on stimulus lexicality or length (Figure 13–9; cf. Chapter 6 where this data set was used as an example in demonstrating source analysis of complex cognitive data). An early length effect was evident in the occipital midline at about 100 ms after stimulus onset. The long letter-strings grouped together and evoked a stronger response than the short letter-strings, regardless of letter-string type (lexicality). Based on previous knowledge about cortical dynamics of silent reading, reviewed above, this response is likely to reflect basic visual feature analysis. The subsequent activation in the left inferior occipitotemporal cortex, interpreted as letter-string-sensitive activation (cf. Figure 13–7), did not vary with length or lexicality, in agreement with existing MEG and intracranial data (Cornelissen et al., 2003; Nobre et al., 1994; Salmelin et al., 1996).

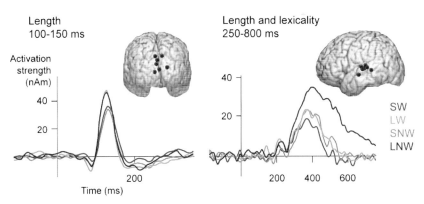

Figure 13–9. Cortical effects of letter-string length and lexicality. Colors denote short and long words (SW, LW) and short and long nonwords (SNW, LNW). A pure length effect (LW, LNW > SW, SNW) was observed in the occipital cortex at 100–150 ms. Interaction between length and lexicality (LNW >> SNW, LW ≥ SW) was detected in the left superior temporal cortex at 250–800 ms.
Modified from Wydell et al. (2003).

Lexicality affected the activation pattern from about 250 ms onwards, in line with previous MEG observations (Salmelin et al., 1996). The effect was found most consistently in the left superior temporal cortex. For short and long real words, the response was remarkably similar. However, the long nonwords evoked an activation that was significantly stronger and lasted twice as long as that for the short nonwords. The cortical differentiation thus seemed to agree with the behavioral pattern that letter-string length has a particularly strong effect on nonword naming.

The cortical area and time window displaying the lexicality-by-length interaction is very similar to that of the N400m activation that was evident in the sentence reading task, and clearly sensitive to semantic manipulation (cf. Figure 13–6; Helenius et al., 1998). But here the picture is more intricate, because the stimulus length also influences the activation. If we accept the dual-route model then the length effect should be interpreted as reflecting phonological processing.

In fact, when one considers the sentence-reading task in more detail, it turns out that the responses to the two different types of semantically wrong sentence-ending words were not identical. When the word had the wrong meaning but the same initial letters as the expected word, referred to as the phonological condition, the response lasted about 50 ms longer than for the completely wrong word (Helenius et al., 1998). Sublexical information thus affected the response at this late stage, from ~350 ms onwards. Accordingly, these data sets on Finnish-speaking subjects seem to suggest that there is both semantic and phonological influence at 250 to 600 ms after stimulus onset in the left superior temporal cortex, which shows in activation strength and duration when reading words and nonwords (Salmelin et al., 1996; Wydell et al., 2003), and in duration in the sentence-reading task (Helenius et al., 1998).

English language has a highly irregular correspondence between graphemes and phonemes, which allows generation of stimuli that are expected to require specifically lexical-semantic processing (exception words) or phonological encoding (pseudohomophones, pseudowords). Using this type of stimuli in their MEG study, Simos and colleagues (Simos et al., 2002a) reported activation of the left superior temporal gyrus for all word types, and involvement of the middle temporal gyrus and mesial temporal lobe in semantic analysis. This pattern could be specific to the type of processing required in reading English, or it might reflect the data analysis approach chosen by the authors, where dipolar sources are sought every 4 ms and comparisons are based on the number of dipolar sources identified within each region of interest (instead of, for example, dipole source amplitudes or their time courses of activation). However, a recent study using that same analysis approach for characterizing cortical dynamics of word and pseudoword reading in English-speaking subjects, found identical areas of activation for both word types (Wilson et al., 2005). Differences between word types only emerged in the left superior temporal cortex, in activation strength (pseudowords>words) and timing (words<pseudowords), thus essentially agreeing with the pattern observed in Finnish-speaking subjects (Salmelin et al., 1996; Wydell et al., 2003).

Perception of Written vs. Spoken Language

The N400m activation reflecting lexical-semantic processing in reading is generated remarkably close to the auditory cortex (1–2 cm; Helenius et al., 1998). An intuitive and tempting interpretation would be to suggest that the development of language comprehension is driven by speech perception, hence the spatial nearness, and that this process develops into a supramodal mechanism (Marinkovic et al., 2003) that eventually serves all (language) comprehension, independent of input modality. Nevertheless, a reading-evoked N400m response in the left superior temporal cortex, influenced by semantic priming, has been detected also in a congenitally deaf subject (unpublished data) which speaks against auditorily driven development of the semantic N400m activation during language acquisition – but obviously does not preclude possible auditorily driven predisposition to semantic processing in the superior temporal cortex that could have developed over the course of human evolution.

When subjects listen to sentences with semantically congruent or incongruent endings (Helenius et al., 2002b) or perform semantic judgment on spoken words (Marinkovic et al., 2003) MEG data show an N400m response graded by semantic relatedness, very similar in timing and location to that observed in reading (Figure 13–10a). As illustrated in Figure 13–10b, simple tones and synthetic single vowels and consonant–vowel syllables typically evoke only a prominent response at about 100 ms post-stimulus (e.g., Hari, 1990; Parviainen et al., 2005; Salmelin et al., 1999). When listening to natural speech, words and sentences, the N100m response is followed by a pronounced N400m response (e.g., Biermann-Ruben et al., 2005; Helenius et al., 2002b; Marinkovic et al., 2003), with a brief reduction of activity in between, at about 200 ms.

The speech signals arrive as sound waves (acoustic features), and from these signals the brain extracts speech sounds (phonetic features) and speech sound sequences (phonology), which further activate the meaning of the word. MEG studies have shown that processing of acoustic-phonetic features of speech is reflected in the N100m response (Parviainen et al., 2005; Poeppel et al., 1996). Categorical perception of phonemes occurs by ~150 ms (Phillips et al., 2000; Vihla et al., 2000).

Qualitatively, the sequence is thus relatively similar in reading and speech perception, with language-specific activation emerging by 100–150 ms and evidence for lexical-semantic processing from 200–300 ms onwards. In both modalities, brief reduction of time-locked activity is detected at about 200 ms. The specific process(es) within the time window approximately from 150 to 300 ms post-stimulus remain poorly understood in both reading and speech perception.

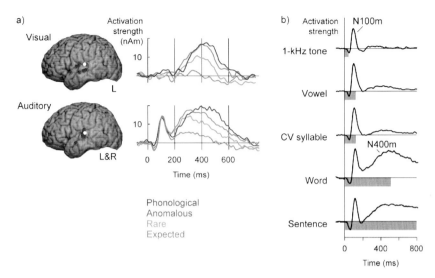

Figure 13–10. Time course of activation in the superior temporal cortex. (a) Lexical-semantic processing in visual *vs.* auditory perception, as indicated by a graded response to semantically congruent and incongruent sentence-ending words. The white dot indicates location of the auditory cortex, as determined from the N100m response to simple 1-kHz tones. (b) Activation evoked by different types of auditory stimuli. Note the emergence of the N400m response when advancing from artificial consonant-vowel (CV) syllables to natural spoken words.

Cortical Correlates of Developmental Dyslexia

Dyslexia is characterized by a difficulty in learning to read and write in the absence of any obvious deficit in general intelligence, or in the ability to acquire new information. Problems in phonological processing are also typically reported in dyslexia, and they are often thought to be the underlying cause of this disorder (Bradley & Bryant, 1983). What is the neurophysiological basis of impaired reading in dyslexia?

The first MEG study on reading in dyslexia compared passive viewing of 7- to 8-letter Finnish words and nonwords in fluently reading and dyslexic adults matched for age and level of education (Salmelin et al., 1996). In control subjects, activation proceeded from occipital to inferior occipitotemporal cortex bilaterally, and further to the left superior temporal cortex and the sensorimotor cortex in both hemispheres (cf. Figure 13–7). Systematic differences between control and dyslexic subjects were observed only in the left hemisphere (Figure 13–11). The dyslexic subjects did not activate the left occipitotemporal and superior temporal cortex but showed, instead, activation of the left inferior frontal cortex at about 300 ms post-stimulus. Shaywitz and colleagues, in their functional magnetic resonance imaging (fMRI) study

0 – 200 ms   200 – 400 ms

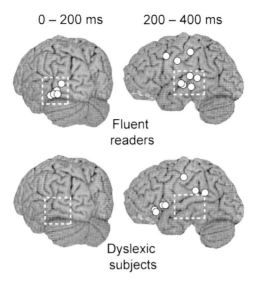

Fluent
readers

Dyslexic
subjects

Figure 13–11. Differences in cortical activation between dyslexic and control subjects in silent reading of isolated words and nonwords. The white rectangles denote cortical areas and time windows in which a salient response was detected in fluently reading subjects but not in dyslexic individuals. Modified from Salmelin et al. (1996).

(Shaywitz et al., 1998), reported a qualitatively similar combination of posterior underactivation with anterior overactivation in dyslexia.

Early cortical processes of reading in dyslexia were targeted in a follow-up study that employed words masked by various levels of noise and symbol strings, as illustrated in Figure 13–1 (Helenius et al., 1999b). The data demonstrated that the response at ~100 ms reflecting low-level visual feature analysis was intact in dyslexia, but that the subsequent activation of the left occipito-temporal cortex associated with letter-string analysis at ~150 ms was nondetectable or abnormally weak in dyslexic subjects (Figure 13–12). When lexical-semantic processing was probed using sentences that ended with semantically congruent or incongruent words, the onset of the N400m response was found to be delayed by about 100 ms in dyslexic subjects as compared with controls (Helenius et al., 1999a).

These findings point to disruption of the reading process at the stage of letter-string analysis, at about 150 ms after seeing a word. In fluent readers, this activation is likely to be the gateway from visual to linguistic analysis, a fast route that automatically sets letter-strings apart from other visual objects and facilitates fast reading. The lack of this fast route for written language is most probably the immediate reason for the slow and inaccurate reading performance that is characteristic to dyslexia.

However, this result is clearly no final answer. It raises further questions: are the problems limited to words, or does the abnormally weak activation

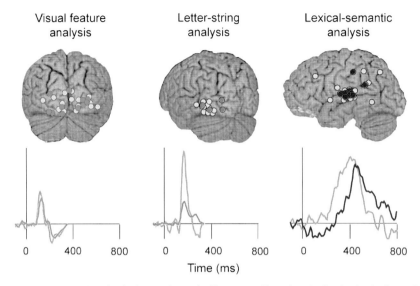

Figure 13–12. Cortical dynamics of silent reading in dyslexic (color) and fluently reading subjects (gray). In dyslexic subjects, there was a marked lack of activation in the left occipitotemporal cortex at ~150 ms and delay in activation of the left superior temporal cortex at ~400ms.
Modified from Salmelin et al. (2000).

reflect a more general deficit in the left occipitotemporal cortex—or, possibly, in the time window of category-specific processing when we start to deal with entities? Tarkiainen and colleagues tested these options by using face stimuli that were masked the same way as the letter-strings (cf. Figure 13–1). Occipital activation reflecting basic visual feature analysis was again found to be intact. The subsequent category-specific activation to faces in the inferior occipito-temporal cortex was normal as well, with timing and hemispheric balance similar to that in controls (Tarkiainen et al., 2003). Presence of a salient face-sensitive response at ~150 ms in the left inferior occipitotemporal cortex speaks against a general functional deficit in this cortical area or time window. The left occipitotemporal underactivation thus seems to be fairly specific to letter-strings. Abnormally weak activation in the left occipitotemporal cortex in dyslexic subjects is a consistent finding in hemodynamic imaging studies of reading as well (Brunswick et al., 1999; Paulesu et al., 2001; Shaywitz et al., 1998).

It should be noted, however, that in a series of MEG experiments on word and nonword reading in English-speaking children with dyslexia, Simos and colleagues did not find differences between participants with dyslexia and control participants in an early (less than 200 ms) activation that they identi-fied at the base of the temporal cortex (Simos et al., 2000a; Simos et al., 2000b; Simos et al., 2002b). At present, it remains unclear if this apparent discrep-ancy is due to the participants' age, their native language, or the applied MEG analysis technique.

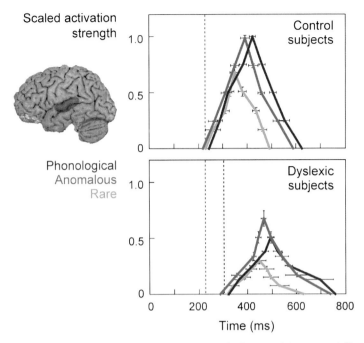

Figure 13–13. Lexical-semantic activation in dyslexic subjects and fluently reading controls. Note the 100-ms delay at the onset in the dyslexic group. The diminished activation to the phonological word type (wrong meaning but initial letters the same as in the expected word) as compared with the anomalous sentence-ending words suggests a sublexical influence in dyslexic reading.
Modified from Helenius et al. (1999a).

Figure 13–13 displays the time course of lexical-semantic activation in dyslexic and control subjects to different types of unexpected sentence-ending words (Helenius et al., 1999a). Apart from the striking 100-ms delay at the onset, the pattern in the dyslexic subjects differed from that in controls in other ways as well. In fluent readers, the responses to completely anomalous words and to the wrong words beginning with the expected letters ('phonological') were equally strong, suggesting that these subjects read a word as a whole, and detected immediately if it was wrong. In dyslexic subjects, however, the response to the phonological words was significantly weaker than to the anomalous words. This difference suggests either that the responses to the phonological word type were quite variable in latency or, which is more likely, that the dyslexic subjects occasionally mistook the phonological word for the expected one, which resulted in reduction of the averaged response. In any case, it seems that the dyslexic subjects did not take a word in as a whole, but rather advanced in smaller units. The signals were overall smaller in dyslexic than control subjects, indicating involvement of a smaller or less synchronous neuronal population.

In dyslexia, cortical abnormalities in reading apparently start in letter-string-sensitive analysis at ~150 ms, with further effects in later processing stages. Recent MEG studies on speech perception in dyslexia have shown a qualitatively similar pattern, with differences between dyslexic and control groups emerging within the first 200 ms (Helenius et al., 2002a; Nagarajan et al., 1999; Parviainen et al., 2005), and a delay (~50 ms) in the onset of the subsequent stage of semantic processing (Helenius et al., 2002b). It thus seems that in dyslexia there are abnormalities in both auditory and visual language perception, but the discrepancies are particularly pronounced in the visual domain. Indeed, the relationship between audition and vision would seem reasonable from a developmental point of view. Cortical specificity to letter strings must certainly arise with experience. Children first learn to listen to spoken words and only much later make the connection between the symbolic written words and the original phonological code. Efficient integration of written and spoken language is clearly a prerequisite for learning to read. Problems in cerebral implementation of speech perception could certainly impede and be further amplified in neural organization of reading.

Neurophysiological vs. Hemodynamic View Of Reading

Pre-Lexical Analysis

Both neurophysiological and hemodynamic imaging studies indicate that in the left inferior occipitotemporal cortex, there are neurons that are particularly interested in letter-strings (Cohen et al., 2000; Nobre et al., 1994; Tarkiainen et al., 1999) and that this activation is abnormally weak in dyslexic individuals who have difficulties in learning to read and write (Helenius et al., 1999b; Paulesu et al., 2001). This is apparently quite an amazing correspondence between fundamentally different techniques, and it seems very attractive. Because of that, it is all the more important to consider whether the neurophysiological and hemodynamic signatures reflect the same, unitary process.

There seems to be a small difference in the mean location of the letter-string-sensitive activation as determined with MEG, or with fMRI and positron emission tomography (PET). Based on anatomical landmarks, the source area in MEG falls on Brodmann area 19 (Tarkiainen et al., 2002) whereas fMRI/PET studies report activation of area 37 (Cohen et al., 2000; Cohen et al., 2002). When the MEG coordinates are converted into Talairach space the source area is found to be centered 1–2 cm posterior and about 0.5 cm medial to the center of the hemodynamically determined maximum (Tarkiainen et al., 2002).

Functionally, there are also potentially important differences. The MEG, EEG, or intracranial response does not differentiate between real words, pseudowords or even consonant strings (Allison et al., 1994; Cornelissen et al., 2003; Nobre et al., 1994; Salmelin et al., 1996; Wydell et al., 2003).

It appears to be interested in letter-like strings, potential language. Hemodynamic studies, on the other hand, have often reported a significantly stronger response in this area to real words than consonant strings (Brunswick et al., 1999; Paulesu et al., 2000). BA 37 has, in fact, been recently dubbed a Visual Word Form Area, where neurons would become attuned to the orthographic system of the language during reading acquisition (Cohen et al., 2000; Cohen et al., 2002); this interpretation has been challenged (Price & Devlin, 2003).

One plausible way to reconcile the findings is to assume that MEG detects the onset of letter-string-sensitive analysis which is not detected in, or does not dominate, the hemodynamic signal. fMRI/PET would detect subsequent activation along the ventral stream, where neurons would be increasingly sensitive to the word-likeness of the letter-strings but show weaker synchronization, or be less rigorously time-locked to stimulus presentation, and might thus go undetected in MEG, at least with the usual analysis techniques (Cornelissen et al., 2003; Salmelin and Helenius, 2004).

Semantic and Phonological Analysis

As for the subsequent stages of semantic and phonological analysis, the MEG data reviewed above suggest that the left superior temporal activation at 200 to 600 ms reflects both of those processes (Figure 13–14a). The response is reduced by semantic priming, and there is stronger activation to pseudowords than real words.

During the past few years, the representation of semantic and phonological processes in reading has been addressed in a number of fMRI/PET studies. Jobard and others, based on a meta-analysis of 35 reports (Jobard et al., 2003), suggest the pattern sketched in Figure 13–14b. Semantic processing was most consistently associated with activation of the triangular part of the inferior frontal gyrus, posterior middle temporal gyrus, and basal temporal cortex, whereas phonological processing was reflected in activation of the superior temporal cortex, supramarginal gyrus, and opercular part of the inferior frontal gyrus.

There is some agreement between neurophysiological and hemodynamic methods for phonological processing, but apparently none for semantic analysis. The left superior temporal cortex is implicated in phonology both by MEG and hemodynamic measures, but only MEG assigns it a role in semantics. For this particular pattern, one could consider a rather simplistic account: In fMRI/PET studies the active brain areas are determined by specific subtractions. Based on the dual-route model of reading, areas involved in phonological analysis are thought to be revealed by subtracting activations to real words from those to pseudowords. Areas involved in semantic processing, on the other hand, would be sought by the inverse subtraction. Based on the MEG data, and assuming that both semantic and phonological manipulation affects essentially the same neuronal population, such subtractions would

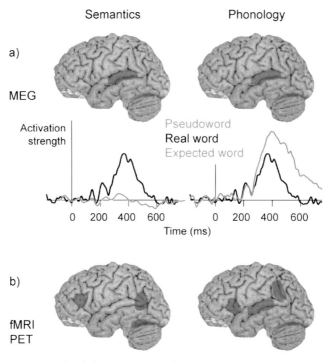

Figure 13–14. Cerebral loci associated with semantic and phonological analysis of written words using (a) MEG and (b) fMRI/PET. For MEG, time course of activation in the left superior temporal cortex is shown as well. From Salmelin and Kujala (2006).

indeed show activation of the left superior temporal cortex for the comparison pseudowords > words (phonology) but none for the comparison words > pseudowords (semantics).

On the other hand, one may also ask whether the differences might be due to the choice of language. Most of the MEG studies were performed using Finnish, whereas English has been the prevalent language in fMRI/PET studies. A recent fMRI study used Japanese language, which has a highly regular orthography, like Finnish (Ischebeck et al., 2004). One of the tasks—silent articulation of visually familiar and unfamiliar words and pseudowords—was very similar to that used in the MEG study of word and pseudoword reading described above (Wydell et al., 2003). Nevertheless, in the fMRI pattern, there was again a striking lack of left superior temporal activation, now also for phonological processing. Clearly, it will be essential to establish the similarities and differences between hemodynamic and MEG measures, what they tell about the processes involved in reading, and how these processes are organized in the brain.

Recent Advances and Future Directions

Cortical Sequence of Activation in Children Learning To Read

In developmental dyslexia, irregularities in the cortical sequence of reading (and speech perception) are most obvious from about 150 ms until 300–350 ms after word presentation. Disturbingly, this is the time window that remains rather poorly understood in cortical dynamics of fluent reading as well. What happens after the initial letter-string-specific activation in the left occipitotemporal cortex, and before lexical-semantic processing reflected in activation of the left superior temporal cortex? Does the former directly drive the latter?

The possible interdependence between the early occipitotemporal and subsequent superior temporal activation, is difficult to establish in adult subjects with relatively little interindividual variability in response timing, and rigid neuronal implementation of language function. Children at the verge of becoming fluent readers are an interesting subject population in this respect, as one would expect clearly more interindividual variability in (timing of) activation sequences in children than adults. Even more importantly, one should be able to establish whether the strength or timing of the occipitotemporal letter-string activation is correlated with the developing reading skills or, possibly, if this activation rapidly appears at a specific point in functional and/or anatomical maturation.

A recent MEG study mapped neural correlates of letter-string perception in 7–8-year-old children who were in the first grade of elementary school (Parviainen et al., 2006). Based on a set of standardized behavioral tests, these children were expected to become fluent readers. Figure 13–15 depicts the cortical sequence of silent reading in children and in adults (cf. Figure 13–7). The sequence of activation was functionally quite similar in the two groups, with visual feature analysis in the occipital cortex, subsequent letter-string-sensitive activation in the left occipitotemporal cortex and, finally, sustained activation in the left superior temporal cortex. However, in children the activation was delayed in time as compared with the adults, by about 50 ms at the stage of visual feature analysis, and by about 100 ms at the stage of letter-string analysis. Importantly, there was a significant correlation in both timing and strength of activation between the occipital and left occipitotemporal responses, on the one hand, and between the occipitotemporal and left temporal responses, on the other hand, thus implying a causal sequence of activation from occipital via left occipitotemporal to left superior temporal cortex.

A letter-string-sensitive response in the left occipitotemporal cortex was detected in about half of the children, which is clearly a smaller percentage than in fluently reading adult subjects (detected in almost every individual). In those children who did show a salient letter-string response, the cortical activation strength was strongly correlated with the child's ability to analyze speech sounds. The cortical activation strength was decreased with better phonological skills, thus approaching the adult level of activation, which

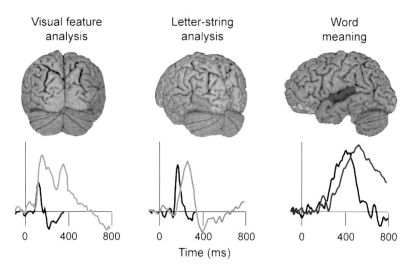

Figure 13–15. Cortical dynamics of silent reading in children (color) and in fluently reading adults (black). In children, the sequence of activation was qualitatively similar to that in adults but delayed in time.
Modified from Parviainen et al. (2006).

is generally much lower than in children. Since the ability to analyze speech sounds is considered a prerequisite for reading acquisition (Bradley & Bryant, 1983), this intriguing correlation again points to an important role for the left inferior occipitotemporal cortex in reading acquisition and fluent reading.

Studies on children learning to read are likely to prove essential also for understanding the relationship between perception of spoken and written language. Cortical activation patterns in dyslexic adults seem to point to impaired integration of auditory and visual information that may be specific to language, or possibly reflects a more general difficulty in multisensory integration. This type of interactions between input modalities, particularly in the interesting early time windows (< 300 ms), are quite difficult to assess in the relatively rigid adult brain. The developing brain of a child could provide a clearer view into such processes.

Extracting Information from Rhythmic Background Activity

The different components of reading are typically probed with rather artificial experimental setups that allow good control of the task and the stimulus properties. While this is a well-argumented and necessary approach, the brain correlates of language processing may appear quite different in more natural contexts that the brain is tuned for. For example, how important is the occipitotemporal letter-string area when we are reading continuously, in more realistic conditions?

    In order to move from stimulus-driven to increasingly realistic language tasks, one needs to find new ways to analyze the MEG data. Because no external trigger signals are available, the activation sequence must be determined directly from brain activity. Although, theoretically, MEG is well suited for identifying brain areas with correlated time courses of activation, it is a conceptually, mathematically, and computationally challenging problem. Dynamic Imaging of Coherent Sources (DICS; see Chapter 9) is a tool for performing connectivity analysis on non-averaged MEG data (Gross et al., 2001) that was initially applied for characterization of the motor system where muscle activity provides an external, non-brain reference signal (Gross et al., 2001; Gross et al., 2002).

    Recently, this method was further developed for use on cognitive tasks, in which there are typically no external reference signals available (Kujala et al., 2007; Salmelin and Kujala, 2006). Subjects were reading stories that were shown to them word by word, in rapid serial visual presentation that simulates natural reading but without need for making saccades (Kujala et al., 2007). Words were shown at three rates that were selected individually for each subject according to their cognitive performance. At the fast rate the subject could not understand the story, at the medium rate the subject was able to understand part of the text, with effort, and at the slowest rate the story was easy to follow.

    Coupling between brain areas (Figure 13–16) was detected at a frequency of about 10 Hz, which seems to represent an inherent carrier frequency in the brain, as it was not affected by the rate at which the words were presented. The nodes of the left-hemisphere network formed an interesting compilation

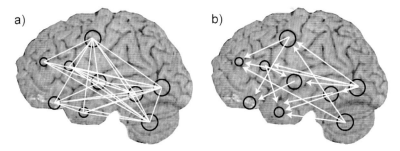

Figure 13–16. Coupling between brain areas during a continuous reading task. The network included the occipito-temporal cortex, superior, anterior and medial temporal cortex, face motor cortex, insula, cerebellum, and prefrontal and orbitofrontal cortex (indicated by black circles; surface projection). (a) The nodes formed a strongly interconnected network; the larger the black circle the more connections between that node and the other nodes. (b) Connections were mostly bidirectional, but for part of the connections there was a dominant direction of information flow, indicated by the arrowheads.
Modified from Kujala et al. (2007).

of brain areas that have been identified in activation studies on various aspects of language function, using either MEG, fMRI or PET, or intracranial recordings: The occipitotemporal node corresponds approximately to the letter-string area, and the superior, anterior and medial temporal areas have been suggested to be involved in semantic and phonological analysis. Face motor cortex, insula and the cerebellum are typically reported in language production, thus suggesting a connection between sensory and motor processes even in silent reading. The prefrontal and orbitofrontal cortex have been associated especially with visual recognition and working memory.

The entire network was strongly interconnected (Figure 13–16a). The connections were mostly bidirectional, but for part of the connections there was a dominant direction of information flow, as evaluated with Granger causality (Figure 13–16b). Intriguingly, the left inferior occipitotemporal cortex, together with the cerebellum, turned out to be the main forward-driving node of the network, again emphasizing the significance of this area in reading. Indeed, in the light of this network structure it is not surprising that impaired neural processing in this area in dyslexia may seriously affect the ability to read fluently.

Rhythmic cortical activity also shows event-related modulation that is not as tightly time-locked to the stimulus or task onset/offset as the strictly phase-locked evoked responses, and may offer important complementary information of brain function (see Chapters 6–9). Localization of rhythmic activity, and especially of those areas in which rhythmic activity is reduced, is not straightforward. Recently, methods have been developed that allow visualization and localization of brain areas where the level of rhythmic activity within a specific frequency range is suppressed below a predefined base level; DICS, mentioned above, is one of those methods. Within the domain of MEG as a measure of brain function, it will be essential to understand the relationship between evoked responses, event-related modulation of cortical rhythms and connectivity patterns, as regards their location, timing and functional dependence on parametric variation of stimuli and tasks. Furthermore, the relationship of these MEG signatures with hemodynamic measures, such as the fMRI BOLD signal, will need to be established for efficient use of neuroimaging methods in unraveling the principles of neural processing.

Interaction and Labeling of Linguistic Processes at the Neural Level

A relevant issue in reading that will need to be clarified in detail is the spatiotemporal representation of semantic and phonological processing, and their possible interaction. The brain may well turn out to be uninterested in such divisions but, for the time being, such labels serve as a reasonable conceptual framework for clarifying the neural basis of language function. An additional concept to consider is syntax and its interplay with semantics, in time and space (Service et al., 2007). Furthermore, the modality-specific vs. supramodal nature of semantic, phonological, and syntactic processing, and the nearness of both visually and auditorily evoked N400m response to the primary auditory cortex, deserve careful investigation.

Perhaps the time is now ripe for starting to let the brain inform us about the ways in which it prefers to cope with written language, and the types of processes implemented at the neuronal level. Combined spatial and temporal information will be essential in that endeavor.

References

Allison, T., McCarthy, G., Nobre, A., Puce, A., & Belger, A. (1994). Human extrastriate visual cortex and the perception of faces, words, numbers, and colors. *Cerebral Cortex, 5*, 544–554.

Biermann-Ruben, K., Salmelin, R., & Schnitzler, A. (2005). Right rolandic activation during speech perception in stutterers: an MEG study. *Neuroimage, 25*, 793–801.

Bradley, L., & Bryant, P. E. (1983). Categorizing sounds and learning to read – a causal connection. *Nature, 301*, 419–421.

Brunswick, N., McCrory, E., Price, C. J., Frith, C. D., & Frith, U. (1999). Explicit and implicit processing of words and pseudowords by adult developmental dyslexics – A search for Wernicke's Wortschatz? *Brain, 122*, 1901–1917.

Cohen, L., Dehaene, S., Naccache, L., Lehericy, S., DehaeneLambertz, G., Henaff M., et al. (2000). The visual word form area – Spatial and temporal characterization of an initial stage of reading in normal subjects and posterior split-brain patients. *Brain, 123*, 291–307.

Cohen, L., Lehericy, S., Chochon, F., Lemer, C., Rivaud, S., & Dehaene, S. (2002). Language-specific tuning of visual cortex functional properties of the Visual Word Form Area. *Brain, 125*, 1054–1069.

Coltheart, M. (1980). Deep dyslexia: A right-hemisphere hypothesis. In: K. Patterson & J. C. Marshall (eds.). *Deep dyslexia*. London: Routledge & Kegan Paul. pp. 326–380.

Coltheart, M., Curtis, B., Atkins, P., & Haller, M. (1993). Models of reading aloud: dual-route and parallel-distributed-processing approaches. *Psychological Review, 100*, 589–608.

Connolly, J. F., and Phillips, N. A. (1994). Event-related potential components reflect phological and semantic processing of the terminal word of spoken sentences. *Journal of Cognitive Neuroscience, 6*, 256–266.

Cornelissen, P., Tarkiainen, A., Helenius, P., & Salmelin, R. (2003). Cortical effects of shifting letter-position in letter-strings of varying length. *Journal of Cognitive Neuroscience, 15*, 731–746.

Embick, D., Hackl, M., Schaeffer, J., Kelepir, M, & Marantz, A. (2001). A magnetoencephalographic component whose latency reflects lexical frequency. *Cognitive Brain Research 10*, 345–348.

Gross, J., Kujala, J., Hämäläinen, M., Timmermann, L., Schnitzler, A, & Salmelin, R. (2001). Dynamic imaging of coherent sources: Studying neural interactions in the human brain. *Proceedings of the National Academy of Sciences of USA, 98*, 694–699.

Gross, J., Timmermann, J., Kujala, J., Dirks, M., Schmitz, F., Salmelin, R., et al. (2002). The neural basis of intermittent motor control in humans. *Proceedings of the National Academy of Sciences of USA, 99*, 2299–2302.

Halgren, E., Baudena, P., Heit, G., Clarke, M., & Marinkovic, K. (1994). Spatio-temporal stages in face and word processing. 1. Depth-recorded potentials in the human occipital, temporal and parietal lobes. *Journal of Physiology* (Paris) *88*, 1–50.

Halgren, E., Dhond, R. P., Christensen, N., Van Petten, C., Marinkovic, K., Lewine, J. D., et al. (2002). N400-like magnetoencephalography responses modulated by semantic context, word frequency, and lexical class in sentences. *Neuroimage, 17*, 1101–1116.

Hari, R. (1990). The neuromagnetic method in the study of the human auditory cortex. In: F. Grandori, M. Hoke, and G. L. Romani (eds.). *Auditory Evoked Magnetic Fields and Electric Potentials.* Vol 6. Basel: S. Karger, pp. 222–282.

Helenius, P., Salmelin, R., Richardson, U., Leinonen, S., & Lyytinen, H. (2002a). Abnormal auditory cortical activation in dyslexia 100 msec after speech onset. *Journal of Cognitive Neuroscience, 14*, 603–617.

Helenius, P., Salmelin, R., Service, E., & Connolly, J. F. (1998). Distinct time courses of word and sentence comprehension in the left temporal cortex. *Brain, 121*, 1133–1142.

Helenius, P., Salmelin, R., Service, E., & Connolly, J. F. (1999a). Semantic cortical activation in dyslexic readers. *Journal of Cognitive Neuroscience, 11*, 535–550.

Helenius, P., Salmelin, R., Service, E., Connolly, J. F., Leinonen, S., & Lyytinen, H. (2002b). Cortical activation during spoken-word segmentation in nonreading-impaired and dyslexic adults. *Journal of Neuroscience, 22*, 2936–2944.

Helenius, P., Tarkiainen, A., Cornelissen, P., Hansen, P.C., & Salmelin, R. (1999b). Dissociation of normal feature analysis and deficient processing of letter-strings in dyslexic adults. *Cerebral Cortex, 9*, 476–483.

Ischebeck, A., Indefrey, P., Usui, N., Nose, I., Hellwig, F., & Taira, M. (2004). Reading in a regular orthography: An fMRI study investigating the role of visual familiarity. *Journal of Cognitive Neuroscience, 16*, 727–741.

Jobard, G., Crivello, F., & TzourioMazoyer, N. (2003). Evaluation of the dual route theory of reading: a metanalysis of 35 neuroimaging studies. *Neuroimage, 20*, 693–712.

Kujala, J., Pammer, K., Cornelissen, P., Roebroeck, A., Formisano, E., & Salmelin R. (2007). Phase coupling in a cerebro-cerebellar network at 8-13 Hz during reading. *Cerebral Cortex, 17*, 1476–1485.

Kutas, M., and Hillyard, S. A. (1980). Reading senseless sentences: brain potentials reflect semantic incongruity. *Science, 207*, 203–205.

Laine, B., Salmelin, R., Helenius, P., & Marttila R. (2000). Brain activation during reading in deep dyslexia: An MEG study. *Journal of Cognitive Neuroscience, 12*, 622–634.

Marinkovic, K., Dhond, R. P., Dale, A. M, Glessner, M., Carr, V., & Halgren, E. (2003). Spatiotemporal dynamics of modality-specific and supramodal word processing. *Neuron, 38*, 487–497.

Nagarajan, S., Mahncke, H., Salz, T., Tallal, P., Roberts, T., & Merzenich, M. M. (1999). Cortical auditory signal processing in poor readers. *Proceedings of the National Academy of Sciences of USA, 96*, 6483–6488.

Nobre, A. C., Allison, T., & McCarthy, G. (1994). Word recognition in the human inferior temporal lobe. *Nature, 372*, 260–263.

Nobre, A. C., and McCarthy, G. (1995). Language-related field potentials in the anterior-medial temporal lobe: II. Effects of word type and semantic priming. *Journal of Neuroscience, 15*, 1090–1098.

Osterhout, L., & Holcomb, PJ. (1995). Event-related potentials and language comprehension. In: M. D. Rugg M. G. H. Coles (eds.). *Electrophysiology of mind*. Oxford:
Oxford University Press. pp, 171–215.

Parviainen, T., Helenius, P., Poskiparta, E., Niemi, P., & Salmelin, R. (2006). Cortical sequence of word perception in beginning readers. *Journal of Neuroscience, 26*,
6052–6061.

Parviainen, T., Helenius, P., & Salmelin, R. (2005). Cortical differentiation of speech and
nonspeech sounds at 100 ms: implications for dyslexia. *Cerebral Cortex, 15*, 1054–1063.

Paulesu, E., Demonet, J. F., Fazio, F., McCrory, E., Chanoine, V., Brunswick, N., et al.
(2001). Dyslexia: Cultural diversity and biological unity. *Science, 291*, 2165–2167.

Paulesu, E., McCrory, E., Fazio, F., Menoncello, L., Brunswick, N., Cappa, S. F., et al.
(2000). A cultural effect on brain function. *Nature Neuroscience, 3*, 91–96.

Phillips, C., Pellathy, T., Marantz, A., Yellin, E., Wexler, K., Poeppel, D., et al. (2000).
Auditory cortex accesses phonological categories: An MEG mismatch study. *Journal of Cognitive Neuroscience, 12*, 1038–1055.

Plaut, D., McClelland, J., Seidenberg, M., & Patterson, K. (1996). Understanding
normal and impaired word reading: computational principles in quasi-regular
domains. *Psychological Review, 103*, 56–115.

Poeppel, D., Yellin, E., Phillips, C., Roberts, T. P. L., Rowley, H. A, Wexler, K.,
et al. (1996). Task-induced asymmetry of the auditory evoked M100 neuromagnetic field elicited by speech sounds. *Cognitive Brain Research, 4*, 231–242.

Price, C. J., & Devlin, J. T. (2003). The myth of the visual word form area. *Neuroimage,
19*, 473–481.

Puce, A., Allison, T., Asgari, M., Gore, J. C., & McCarthy, G. (1996). Differential
sensitivity of human visual cortex to faces, letterstrings, and textures: a functional
magnetic resonance imaging study. *Journal of Neuroscience, 16*, 5205–5215.

Pylkkänen, L., & Marantz, A. (2003). Tracking the time course of word recognition
with MEG. *Trends in Cognitive Sciences, 7*, 187–189.

Pylkkänen, L., Stringfellow, A., & Marantz, A.(2002). Neuromagnetic evidence for the
timing of lexical activation: an MEG component sensitive to phonotactic probability but not to neighborhood density. *Brain and Language, 81*, 666–678.

Salmelin, R. (2007). Clinical neurophysiology of language: The MEG approach. *Clinical
Neurophysiology, 118*, 237–254.

Salmelin, R., & Helenius, P. (2004). Functional neuroanatomy of impaired reading in
dyslexia. *Scientific Studies of Reading, 8*, 257–272.

Salmelin, R., Helenius, P., & Service, E.(2000). Neurophysiology of fluent and impaired reading: a magnetoencephalographic approach. *Journal of Clinical Neurophysiology, 17*, 163–174.

Salmelin, R., & Kujala, J. (2006). Neural representation of language: activation versus
long-range connectivity. *Trends in Cognitive Sciences, 10*, 519–525.

Salmelin, R., Schnitzler, A., Parkkonen, L., Biermann, K., Helenius, P., Kiviniemi, K.,
et al.(1996). Native language, gender, and functional organization of the auditory
cortex. *Proceedings of the National Academy of Sciences of USA, 96*, 10460–10465.

Salmelin, R., Service, E., Kiesilä, P., Uutela, K., & Salonen O. (1996). Impaired visual
word processing in dyslexia revealed with magnetoencephalography. *Annals of
Neurology, 40*, 157–162.

Service, E., Helenius, P., Maury, S., & Salmelin, R. (2007). Localization of syntactic
and semantic brain responses using magnetoencephalography. *Journal of Cognitive
Neuroscience 19*, 1193–1205.

Shaywitz, S. E., Shaywitz, B. A., Pugh, K. R., Fulbright, R. K., Constable, R. T., Mencl, W. E., et al. (1998). Functional disruption in the organization of the brain for reading in dyslexia. *Proceedings of the National Academy of Sciences of USA, 95,* 2636–2641.

Simos, P. G., Basile, L. F., & Papanicolaou, A. C. (1997). Source localization of the N400 response in a sentence-reading paradigm using evoked magnetic fields and magnetic resonance imaging. *Brain Research, 762,* 29–39.

Simos, P. G., Breier, J. I., Fletcher, J. M., Bergman, E., & Papanicolaou, A. C. (2000a) Cerebral mechanisms involved in word reading in dyslexic children: A magnetic source imaging approach. *Cerebral Cortex, 10,* 809–816.

Simos, P. G., Breier, J. I., Fletcher, J. M., Foorman, B. R., Bergman, E., Fishbeck, K., et al. (2000b). Brain activation profiles in dyslexic children during non-word reading: a magnetic source imaging study. *Neuroscience Letters, 290,* 61–65.

Simos, P. G., Breier, J. I., Fletcher, J. M., Foorman, B. R., Castillo, E. M., & Papanicolaou, A. C. (2002a). Brain mechanisms for reading words and pseudowords: an integrated approach. *Cerebral Cortex, 12,* 297–305.

Simos, P. G., Fletcher, J. M., Bergman, E., Breier, J. I., Foorman, B. R., Castillo, E. M., et al. (2002b). Dyslexia-specific brain activation profile becomes normal following successful remedial training. *Neurology, 58,* 1203–1213.

Tarkiainen, A., Cornelissen, P. L., & Salmelin, R. (2002). Dynamics of visual feature analysis and object-level processing in face versus letter-string perception. *Brain, 125,* 1125–1136.

Tarkiainen, A., Helenius, P., Hansen, P. C., Cornelissen, P. L., & Salmelin, R. (1999). Dynamics of letter string perception in the human occipitotemporal cortex. *Brain, 122,* 2119–2131.

Tarkiainen, A., Helenius, P., & Salmelin, R. (2003). Category-specific occipitotemporal activation during face perception in dyslexic individuals: an MEG study. *Neuroimage, 19,* 1194–1204.

Van Petten, C. (1995). Words and sentences: event-related brain potential measures. *Psychophysiology, 32,* 511–525.

Vihla, M., Lounasmaa, O. V., & Salmelin, R. (2000). Cortical processing of change detection: Dissociation between natural vowels and two-frequency complex tones. *Proceedings of the National Academy of Sciences of USA, 97,* 10590–10594.

Weekes, B., Coltheart, M., & Gordon, E. (1997). Deep dyslexia and right hemisphere reading – a regional cerebral blood flow study. *Aphasiology, 11,* 1139–1158.

Weekes, B. S. (1997). Differential effects of number of letters on word and nonword latency. *Quarterly Journal of Experimental Psychology, 50A,* 439–456.

Wilson, T. W., Leuthold, A. C., Lewis, S. M., Georgopoulos, A. P., & Pardo, P. J. (2005). The time and space of lexicality: a neuromagnetic view. *Experimental Brain Research, 162,* 1–13.

Wydell, T. N., Vuorinen, T., Helenius, P., & Salmelin, R. (2003). Neural correlates of letter-string length and lexicality during reading in a regular orthography. *Journal of Cognitive Neuroscience, 15,* 1052–1062.

14

The Use of MEG in Clinical Settings

Jyrki P. Mäkelä

- Clinical MEG measurements need to provide useful information for diagnostics or treatment in individual patients
- At present, this condition is realized in patients with medically intractable epilepsy going through workup for epilepsy surgery, or in patients going to the surgery of tumors in the vicinity of eloquent cortical regions
- As errors in data interpretation may produce harmful effects on the patients, particular care for measurement accuracy and artifact rejection, and close collaboration with the team responsible for the treatment are needed in clinical MEG measurements
- Search for diagnostic MEG markers in several neurodegenerative diseases and in traumatic brain injury patients will probably provide the new clinical applications of MEG in the future

Introduction

Search for clinical applications has paralleled the development of MEG from its early phases in the seventies (Hughes et al., 1977). The possibilities of MEG in clinical use were first demonstrated by studies of patients with several types of epilepsy (Barth et al., 1982; Modena et al., 1982; Barth et al., 1984). At the time, data were obtained sequentially by moving the one-sensor instrument, using simultaneously-measured EEG signal as a trigger for averaging, to detect epileptic spikes in the MEG signal from measurements at different sites (Barth et al., 1984). Already these early efforts demonstrated that MEG is able to identify source locations of epileptiform spikes and their spread to the opposite hemisphere 20 ms later (Barth et al., 1982), and multiple sources of epileptic activity in individual patients (Barth et al., 1984). Recordings of somatosensory evoked fields (SEFs) with small-coverage instruments were also able to locate the central sulcus accurately, as compared with intracranial recordings (Sutherling et al., 1988). The co-registration of the source localization of evoked responses with anatomical magnetic resonance imaging (MRI) paved the way for use of MEG in preoperative planning (Gallen et al., 1993; Kamada et al., 1993).

The need for multichannel detectors for clinical practice has been obvious since the very first clinical studies (Modena et al., 1982). The development has led to instruments covering the whole scalp (Ahonen et al., 1993; Vrba et al., 1993). These devices have considerably speeded up MEG recordings, and made large-scale utilization of MEG feasible in clinical patients. With these instruments, one can observe simultaneous magnetic activity from the entire scalp surface. Moreover, a possible inaccuracy caused by repetitive probe positioning is avoided. Functional landmarks in several sensory modalities can be created within a single measurement session, and the spread of epileptiform activity can be followed across the lateral cortical surfaces. Both spontaneous MEG and evoked responses can be used to depict active cortical areas, by superimposing the source locations of the spontaneous activity and evoked fields on the patient's MRIs. MEG provides accurate data on individual patients; averaging across patients, which would blur individual differences and diminish clinical applicability, is not needed. The noninvasiveness of MEG allows repeated recordings as often as desired. Despite impressive development of instruments, identification of epileptogenic cortical areas, and localization of eloquent cortices, have remained the mainstay of clinical MEG—although MEG teams are making an extensive search for individually useful MEG signals, e.g., in patients suffering from stroke, Parkinson's disease, chronic pain, or Alzheimer's disease.

General Aspects

The use of MEG in clinical settings requires an approach different from that in research. Typically, individual features in measurements are of crucial importance in clinical patient studies, whereas they are of minor interest or even confounding in research settings that aim to reveal general features of the brain function. Different approaches in the practical performance of measurements are also apparent. Healthy control subjects are often familiar with the recording environment, whereas patients seldom visit a MEG unit more than one or two times. However, high motivation for obtaining personally significant results from measurements often produces excellent cooperation by patients, despite the unfamiliar environment. Careful explanation of the recording procedures to the patient, as well as taking into account the functional problems caused by the patient's condition in planning and executing the measurements, improve the obtained results. It is useful to have a nurse with a patient in the shielded room to improve communication and explain the needed procedures. This can reduce the patient's anxiety, as well as serving the need to monitor the patient to prevent unexpected events, particularly when acute cases are studied.

Furthermore, the research questions in clinical patients need to reflect the needs of clinical practice, not the interests of the researcher. A close collaboration between the team performing MEG recordings, and the persons responsible for clinical decisions, is quintessential in obtaining the best results.

Technical Aspects Relevant in Clinical Settings

The high quality of the data is of prime importance in measurements influencing clinical decisions, e.g., on extent of surgery in the region of epileptogenic brain, or in the vicinity of irretrievable cortical areas. The effects of various artifact sources on the results need to be fully understood.

Data Quality

Epileptic discharges produce MEG activity with a signal-to-noise ratio sufficient to allow reliable analysis without signal averaging. When sensory responses or motor function are studied, signal averaging is needed; it is useful to average the responses alternately to two different bins for evaluation of their reproducibility. In patients with cortical lesions, interstimulus interval or stimulus intensity may need modification from those applied in healthy control subjects, to ensure that the responses are robust enough for analysis. The signal-to-noise ratio can be improved by signal processing; for example, by digital or spatial filtering. In studies of evoked responses, the averaged signals are often low-pass filtered digitally, to suppress the high-frequency noise. Spatial filters are based on an assumption that the distribution of the target signal differs from that of environmental noise, biological artifacts, or brain activity outside the function studied (Hämäläinen and Hari, 2002). These filters allow the removal or suppression of noise subspace—caused, e.g., by cardiac artifacts—from the data (Jousmäki and Hari, 1996). The filter types need to be selected on the basis of clinical details of the patient, and the loss of clinically useful information should not occur.

Magnetic Artifacts

MEG signals are extremely tiny, and the recordings are sensitive to artifacts produced by moving magnetic materials. Even hair dyes or cosmetics may contain magnetic particles. Naturally, any magnetic material worn by the patient needs to be removed. Use of nonmagnetic laboratory garments may be useful. As in basic research, eye movements, producing strong magnetic signals, need to be recorded to remove related artifacts from brain signals. It is essential to strive toward signals that are as artifact-free as possible, although new signal-processing methods for artifact removal make a more relaxed attitude tempting.

Unfortunately, in studies of patients, the possibilities for non-removable artifact sources abound. Dental materials, shunts needed to treat hydrocephalus, clips closing aneurysms, or lid springs needed in the treatment of the lid lag in facial paresis, may all be magnetic. Occasionally, ferromagnetic dust due to drilling in a previous neurosurgical operation may produce disturbances that lower signal quality. MR imaging may aggravate these artifacts; consequently, it is a useful policy to perform MRI *after* the MEG recordings, if possible. Use of demagnetization instruments may turn out to be helpful in some cases. Occasionally, the exclusion of the most affected channels may facilitate the data analysis. In studies of patients with epilepsy, magnetic electrodes—including sphenoidal electrodes, or magnetic leads—may produce severe disturbances. Vagus nerve stimulators or pacemakers may render MEG recordings useless. These problems can occasionally be prevented by selecting electrodes and instrumentation carefully. The magnetic artifacts sometimes consist of slow drifts, and can be removed if the signals of interest are in a higher frequency range. However, high-pass filtering may deform significantly the waveforms of fast signals, and thus it is often inefficient in artifact removal.

Recent developments may, fortunately, alleviate artifact-related problems. Computational removal of artifacts is developing quickly. The signal space separation algorithm allows the recognition of magnetic signals from different subspaces, e.g., from the head and its surroundings. The method utilizes Maxwell's equations, and exact information about the geometry and sensitivity of the sensor array, to decompose the multichannel MEG signals into a device-independent representation, separating contributions of sources internal and external to the sensor array. Further suppression of artifacts in the internal space is obtained by detecting signals with similar temporal patterns in the signals of both spaces that are emanating from strong artifact sources not completely suppressed by the basic geometrical separation. These common temporal patterns are then projected out of the signals originating in the internal space. This leaves the tiny brain signals intact (Taulu & Simola, 2006). This method suppresses artifacts generated, e.g., by eye blinks or by dental fillings. Even very strong artifacts generated by a vagus nerve stimulator (Tanaka et al. 2009), or electric stimulation of subthalamic nucleus in Parkinsonian patients, are suppressed—provided that the amplifiers of the MEG system do not drift completely out of the measurement range (Mäkelä et al., 2007). Similarly, signal processing that applies the beamformer method attenuates spatially correlated noise, and makes it feasible to obtain recordings from patients with magnetic dental fillings (Cheyne et al., 2007). One case report describes the use of beamformers in suppression of magnetic noise caused by a deep brain stimulator for treatment of chronic pain (Kringelbach et al., 2007).

Accuracy of MEG-MRI Overlay

In clinical applications, the MEG device coordinate system needs to be related to the anatomical coordinate system of the subject's head. This is usually accomplished by attaching head position indicator coils on scalp locations related to the fiducial points on the head, and by calculating the head position from magnetic signals produced by weak currents at the coils. Naturally, accuracy at this phase is crucial in preoperative measurements, because errors in the transformation of the coordinates are directly reflected as inaccuracy in the final results. It is useful to utilize signals from at least four indicator coils, and digitize tens of sites of the patient's scalp and face, in addition to fiducial points, for a fit with the MR images later on. Digital photographs of the fiducial points add confidence in locating them later from the MR images. Well-established physiological landmarks—such as sources of early median nerve SEFs and auditory evoked fields—provide confidence in the success of the MEG-MRI overlay, particularly when their source orientations match the gyral anatomy. These should be recorded, in addition to spontaneous activity recordings used in location of the epileptic cortical areas. As some diseases may alter brain anatomy relatively rapidly due to edema or rapid growth, the time lapse between MRI and MEG recordings should not be too long.

The detection of head movements during the MEG measurement is important for the accuracy of the MEG source localization. Whereas adult patients are usually highly motivated and remain motionless, with about 1 mm standard deviation of the measured head positions (Uutela et al., 2001), movements may increase inaccuracy in pediatric measurements, or, e.g., in epileptic seizures. Continuous head position monitoring has been developed to monitor the position of the patient's head during MEG recordings (Uutela et al., 2001; Medvedovsky et al., 2007), and appears to be useful in ictal epilepsy recordings (Vitikainen et al., 2009). The present compensation systems operate in a range of a few centimeters, and may strengthen noise signals (Uutela et al., 2001). Combined artifact suppression alleviates this problem (Medvedovsky et al., 2007). The accuracy of the source localization will increase further with these applications, particularly in pediatric neurology. If such solutions are not available, head fixation with cushions may turn out to be useful. The head can also be lined to one side of the helmet dewar to enhance the signal amplitude on the side of the interest.

Patient Safety

Unexpected events, such as epileptic seizures or drug-induced respiratory suppression, are more probable in studies of patients than in control subjects.

If studied supine, safety belts or railings may prevent the subject from falling off the bed in such instances. The examiners should be well versed on how to get the subject quickly out of the gantry if needed. Resuscitation equipment, oxygen system and, preferably, suction instrumentation need to be prepared for an emergency.

Routine Clinical Applications

MEG in Epilepsy

MEG recordings are a useful adjunct in planning epilepsy surgery. MEG appears to be particularly beneficial in the study of patients with non-lesional neocortical epilepsy, and in patients with large lesions, where it may provide unique information on the epileptogenic zone in relation to the lesion (for reviews, see Pataraia et al., 2002; Barkley & Baumgartner, 2003; Knowlton & Shih, 2004). Naturally, the preoperative localization of eloquent cortices can be made with the same methods in epileptic patients as in control subjects, and their relation to epileptic zone can be visualized (Figure 14–1). Sources of epileptic spikes can be integrated into neuronavigation systems (Iida et al., 2005). It has been suggested that MEG source localization, using a single-dipole model, can provide unique localization information not available with other noninvasive methods in patients with epilepsy (Mamelak et al., 2002). The clustering of the sources of individual interictal spikes (Figure 14–2) has demonstrated a high correlation with electrocorticography (ECoG) (Lamusuo et al., 1999; Mamelak et al., 2002). If source clusters are located in the nonresectable eloquent cortex, residual seizures remain probable (Iida et al., 2005), and a high correlation of the resection volume with the brain region containing MEG source clusters of epileptic spikes has been shown to predict favorable outcome in epilepsy surgery (Fischer et al., 2005). MEG can also encourage epilepsy surgery when displaying focal epileptiform activity, whereas traditional methods suggest multifocal activity or demonstrate bilateral, multifocal or diffuse ictal onset, indicating an unfavorable candidate for epilepsy surgery (Schwartz et al., 2008).

Temporal Dynamics of Epileptiform Activity

Excellent temporal resolution of MEG makes it possible to describe, in addition to interictal spike source locations, the temporal sequence of spike propagation by using multidipole models. In some patients, it is possible to follow the spread of epileptic activity from one hemisphere to another (Figure 14-1), or within a hemisphere. The identification of the earliest source of epileptic activity naturally makes the localization of the epileptogenic zone more reliable (Hari et al., 1993; Paetau et al., 1999; Lin et al., 2003; Yu et al., 2004; Hara et al., 2007). The analysis of epileptiform MEG by using multidipole models is more demanding and time-consuming than applying a single dipole model

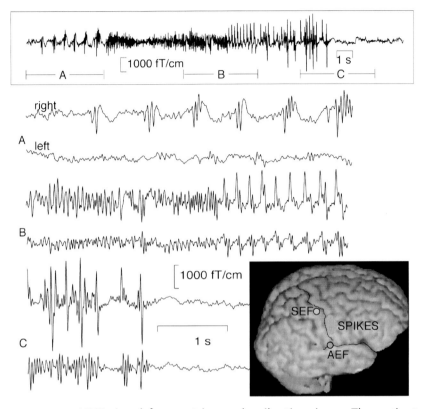

Figure 14–1. MEG signal from a triggered epileptic seizure. The patient has partial epilepsy with seizures triggered by touching of the left gum or corner of the mouth, including left facial jerking. The whole seizure from the channel showing the maximum signal in the right hemisphere is depicted in the box above. Below, the sections A, B and C show the development of the seizure, as well as activity in the corresponding region in the left hemisphere, in enlarged form. Before the seizure onset, spikes emerge more frequently and become polyphasic in the right frontoparietal region. No notable activity over the left hemisphere is seen during the first 6 s; afterwards, the spike discharge spreads to the left side as well. After the seizure, interictal spikes are absent. The sources of epileptic activity (spikes) cluster to the face motor cortex representation. Sources of median nerve SEFs and AEFs are shown to indicate irretrievable areas. Modified from Forss et al. (1995).

into each spike and calculating the clusters of sources—but should be attempted, as the obtained additional data may significantly aid in the clinical decision-making. Application of minimum norm estimate and dynamic statistical parametric mapping may be used to study the temporal development of epileptiform activity as well (Hara et al., 2007).

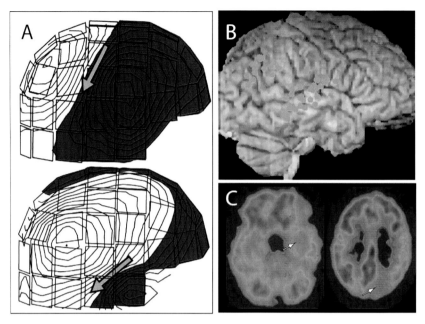

Figure 14–2. (A) Dipolar field patterns from two different epileptiform spike types in the right parietal and temporal lobe in a patient with intractable epilepsy, going through epilepsy surgery evaluation. (B) Clusters of spike sources superimposed on the patient's 3D MRI. (C) PET data demonstrating hypometabolism in right temporal and parietal lobe (arrows). SEEG demonstrated right temporal and parieto-occipital epileptiform activity. MRI showed a small region of atrophy in the right parietal region. Right parietal region was operated, resulting in worthwhile reduction of seizures (Engel's classification IIIa).
Modified from (Lamusuo et al. 1999).

Sensitivity of MEG in Epilepsy

Although methodological properties limit feasible recording times in epileptic patients, the average sensitivity of MEG for epileptiform activity has been found to be 70% in a series of 455 patients going through presurgical epilepsy evaluation (Stefan et al., 2003). Similar general sensitivity of 73%, with the yield of 92% in patients with extratemporal, and 50% in patients with medial temporal lobe epilepsy, has been described (Knowlton et al., 1997). Information crucial for final decision making has been obtained by MEG in about 10% of the studied patients (Stefan et al., 2003; Sutherling et al. 2008). Abnormal slow-wave activity may also occur in the vicinity of the epileptogenic area. The MEG sources of this activity were concordant with the consensus finding, based on other evaluation methods, concerning the presumed epileptiform region in 48% of the patients—as often as ictal noninvasive video EEG monitoring (Gallen et al., 1997). Combining source localization of the abnormal slow-wave activity with interictal epileptiform spikes enhanced localization of the affected hemisphere in patients with temporal epilepsy (Fernandez et al., 2004), and should be included in the analysis of epileptiform activity when available. In intracranial EEG recordings, high-frequency oscillations in the 60–100 Hz range appear to be highly localized in the seizure onset zone, in patients with nonlesional neocortical epilepsy (Worrell et al., 2004). Time will tell if these signals can be reliably picked up and analyzed by MEG as well.

Enhancing the Gain of MEG in Studies of Epileptic Patients

One factor diminishing the yield of MEG in patients with epilepsy is the lack of epileptiform activity in the limited time window of the recording. Usually, a recording of at least 30 minutes of spontaneous activity, including periods of drowsiness, is needed. Hyperventilation for 3 minutes is a practical way to enhance the appearance of spikes in MEG measurements. MEG artifacts often abound during hyperventilation, but the study of the post-hyperventilation period may turn out to be useful. Photostimulation, routinely used in EEG recordings, is more inconvenient to use effectively in the MEG setup. Sleep deprivation during the night preceding the recording will increase the probability of the detection of the epileptic activity, although the quality of evoked fields may decrease due to the lowered vigilance. Monitoring occipital MEG signals to detect alpha rhythm changes may be useful to guarantee good quality of the evoked fields.

Tapering of antiepileptic medication may provoke epileptiform activity; follow-up on the hospital ward is needed for this procedure. Some epileptiform activity can be detected only during sleep; consequently, recording during the night may prove useful. The yield of MEG recordings has been claimed to approach 100% when patients with temporal lobe epilepsy were on subtherapeutic anticonvulsant levels, and sleep was encouraged (Assaf et al., 2004). Video recording may provide useful clues of the epilepsy syndrome and signal interpretation, if seizures occur during the MEG measurement.

Anesthesia may be needed when studying children between ages 6 months–5 years; an anesthetic regimen using propofol appears not to reduce the occurrence of epileptiform activity, and has caused no problems in association with MEG recordings (Balakrisnan et al., 2007; Szmuk et al., 2003), although it may produce seizures in rare cases (e.g., Mäkelä et al., 1993). Appearance of epileptiform activity is enhanced by clonidine (Kettenmann et al., 2005), and by some anesthetic agents and, consequently, recordings under anesthesia may even enhance detection of the epileptic spikes. Naturally, particularly careful monitoring of the patient by oximetry and heart rate detection is required if anesthesia or sedation is used. Administration of anxiolytic drugs may also be necessary in some cases (e.g. Schwartz et al., 2008).

Interictal vs. Ictal MEG

Ictal measurements are possible in several types of epilepsy (Figure 14–1), although body movements may render the signal non-analyzable. However, the initiation of the epileptiform discharges may be detected before the onset of body movements even in these cases. Sources of interictal spikes were found to be in the same area as the sources of ictal spikes (Shiraishi et al., 2001; Tilz et al., 2002; Tang et al., 2003); thus interpretation of interictal spikes in MEG appears to be a useful and effective noninvasive method for localizing primary seizure foci (Tang et al., 2003). However, ictal MEG produced localizing information superior to interictal MEG in three out of six patients (Eliashiv et al., 2002); our experience also indicates that ictal recordings should be done when they are logistically feasible. New, more comfortable gantries and continuous head position localization make this type of experiment more feasible (Vitikainen et al., 2009).

Comparison of MEG with Electrocorticography

Invasive video EEG monitoring has been a gold standard for defining the epileptogenic cortex prior to surgery. However, it is quite demanding for the patient and may cause bleeding or infections (Hamer et al., 2002). As epilepsy surgery is usually elective, such events should be prevented if possible. Furthermore, a rough estimate concerning the epileptogenic cortical areas is required before the insertion of the intracranial electrodes. MEG source localization aids in selecting sites for grids to be used in subdural EEG recordings (Mamelak et al., 2002; Vitikainen et al. 2009; Knowlton et al. 2009; Sutherling et al. 2008). It has been suggested as particularly useful in the detection of epileptic activity after lesionectomy, or unsuccessful removal of the epileptic zone, because dural adhesions may hamper the insertion of subdural electrode grids in these patients (Kirchberger et al., 1998).

Comparisons of preoperative MEG findings with ECoG have occasionally found almost complete matches (Lamusuo et al., 1999; Otsubo et al., 2001), whereas some others report lower values (Mamelak et al., 2002). The patient populations have been quite variable, and the location of the seizure focus probably affects the degree of correlation between MEG and invasive EEG recordings.

Combination of MEG with ictal SPECT may replace invasive EEG monitoring (Knowlton, 2006). Combining MEG with navigated transcranial magnetic stimulation may also turn out to be useful in diminishing invasive EEG measurements (Vitikainen et al., 2009). MEG appears to be as accurate as interictal and ictal invasive video-EEG (Papanicolaou et al., 2005)—and ictal MEG recordings produced localization equivalent or superior to invasive EEG in five out of six patients (Eliashiv et al., 2002). Nevertheless, although MEG predicted 82% of findings in invasive recordings of 49 patients, epileptogenic cortex remained nonlocalized in 7 of them by MEG, whereas invasive recordings were diagnostic (Knowlton et al., 2006).

Complementary Properties of MEG and EEG in Clinical Settings

MEG and EEG signals look similar, and the knowledge of different visual patterns of epileptiform phenomena, collected since the 1920s, can be applied in MEG analysis. Nevertheless, MEG source modeling provides information not available in EEG. In simultaneous recordings of epileptiform activity by MEG and subdural ECoG it has been estimated that at least 4 cm^2 of synchronously active cortex is needed to produce a detectable MEG spike (Mikuni et al., 1997). However, even cortical spikes associated with 6–10 cm^2 of synchronous activity in ECoG rarely generate scalp-recordable EEG interictal spikes; an area exceeding 10 cm^2 is required for recognizable scalp potentials (Tao et al., 2005). Indeed, in a cohort of 70 candidates for epilepsy surgery, whole-head MEG detected epileptiform activity in 72%, and simultaneous 70-channel EEG in 61% of the patients. MEG revealed epileptiform activity in one third of the EEG-negative patients, particularly in patients having lateral neocortical epilepsy or cortical dysplasia (Knake et al., 2006). Furthermore, a higher ratio of spikes unique to MEG (8/12 patients) compared with EEG (2/12 patients) is detected when the signals are overlapped by sleep changes; this has been attributed to stronger contribution of radial sources of sleep spindles and vertex waves on EEG (Ramantani et al., 2006). MEG may be useful in detecting epileptic activity deep in the sulci, masked in EEG by more superficial radial activity in the gyri (Merlet et al., 1997)—e.g., in Landau-Kleffner syndrome, in which the spike activity typically resides deep in the Sylvian fissure (Paetau et al., 1999; Iwasaki et al., 2003). Consequently, MEG can be applied also in patients with suspected epilepsy but with a normal EEG, and in epilepsy patients whose epilepsy type remains unclassified on the basis of the EEG.

The simultaneous recording of MEG and EEG, and the use of both methods in modeling the epileptiform activity, is crucial for a complete view of the epileptogenic zone. Combined MEG and EEG can identify the source areas and their activation sequences in more detail, thereby helping to select patients with a single pacemaker area and prospects for good outcome after surgery (Lewine et al., 1999; Paetau et al., 1999), and should at least be included into analysis of particularly difficult cases of intractable epilepsy. Strategies for a unified model of brain electric activity as recorded both by MEG and EEG have been delineated (Huang et al., 2007); however, they have not yet been utilized in the analysis of epileptiform activity.

Detection of Mesial Epileptiform Activity by MEG?

Direct detection by MEG of epileptic activity in the mesial temporal cortex and deep orbitofrontal cortices is difficult because gradiometers are relatively insensitive to deep sources (Mikuni et al., 1997). It has been proposed that source current orientations in the temporal region separate between mesial and lateral neocortical epileptiform activity (Assaf et al., 2004), but the finding appears not to extend to all patients (Lamusuo et al., 1999). However, new

MEG instruments contain magnetometers, which are more sensitive to deep sources (and to noise). The "brain noise" in magnetic measurements is clearly stronger in the low- than high-frequency range; consequently the relative signal-to-noise ratio in magnetometers is better for signals having high-frequency components (Parkkonen and Curio, personal communication). Accordingly, magnetic auditory brainstem responses have been detected by magnetometers after applying intense averaging (Parkkonen et al., 2009). This indicates that magnetometers may pick up deep fast-frequency epileptiform activity in a data-driven manner, and should be used when study of deep sources is necessary. Indeed, such activity has recently been observed in magnetometer signals of patients with temporal lobe epilepsy (Enatsu et al., 2008). Consequently, magnetometer signals should be analyzed particularly carefully when, e.g., mesial or insular epileptiform activity is implicated by clinical semiology.

Localization of Eloquent Areas in Patients with Brain Tumors

Tumors or vascular malformations may distort brain anatomical landmarks, making it impossible to identify, e.g., motor areas on the basis of anatomy. Functional landmarks depicting eloquent brain areas have been suggested as a valuable planning adjunct before brain tumor surgery (e.g., Gallen et al., 1995; Bittar et al., 1999; Lehericy et al., 2000; Kober et al., 2001b; Mäkelä et al., 2006). MEG landmarks may encourage surgery in cases where key cortical areas are displaced but unaffected by tumor masses, and may facilitate maximal resection in tumors abutting the eloquent cortex. In patients with tumor invasion into eloquent cortical regions, they suggest the selection of alternative treatment strategies (Ganslandt et al., 2004). Several types of functional landmarks—produced, e.g., by sources of somatosensory, auditory, visual or speech-related evoked fields—enable presurgical mapping tailored to individual patient needs. The distance between these landmarks and the area needing operation has been shown to predict the risk of complications (Hund et al., 1997). In 119 patients with gliomas, 46% were not considered for surgery because MEG source localization indicated tumor invasion of eloquent cortex; 54% of the patients were operated, and 6% suffered from neurological deterioration. This compared favorably with functionally significant deficits reported previously in 17-20% of the operated patients (Ganslandt et al., 2004).

The identification of MEG sources, superimposed on 3-dimensional MRI surface rendering, helps presurgical planning to find the optimal "surgical corridor" to the lesion (Kamada et al., 1993; Gallen et al., 1995). Preoperative discussion with the patient about surgical alternatives—e.g., the trade-offs involved between the amount of resection and the possible functional deficit—is also made more accurate with this approach, and it should be made available when clinical symptoms suggest close proximity of eloquent areas and brain pathology.

During surgery, the orientation to the brain in a limited field of view is facilitated by 3-D reconstructions of brain anatomy including cortical veins, and with superimposed functional landmarks (Figure 14–3). If intraoperative stimulation or recordings are required, the selection of stimulation sites, or the adequate grid position for monitoring of evoked potentials during craniotomies, is made easier by functional landmarks, which serve as "intraoperative road maps" for the most efficient sites (Mäkelä et al., 2001; Schiffbauer et al., 2002).

The most common application of functional mapping is the localization of the central sulcus (Figure 14–3). The sources of the somatosensory evoked fields (SEFs) to median nerve stimuli are located in the posterior wall of the central sulcus (Sutherling et al., 1988). Preoperative functional localization with MEG generally agrees with direct intraoperative mapping of the somatosensory cortical areas. About 200 cases of SEF source localizations and intraoperative cortical mapping have been published, with a satisfactory concordance (for references, see Mäkelä et al., 2006), suggesting that handling of the inverse problem in dipole modeling matches the neurophysiological reality. The reported mean difference of about 10 mm between the pre- and intraoperative localizations (Mäkelä et al., 2001, Rezai et al., 1996,

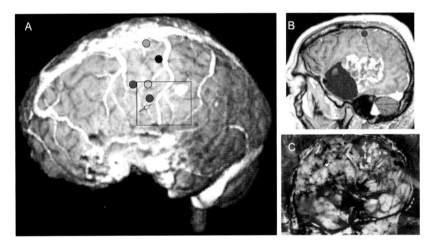

Figure 14–3. A 3D MR surface rendering (including veins) of a patient with a recurring GIII glioma in the left temporal lobe.(A) Dots indicate SEF sources of tibial (red), median nerve (light blue) and lip (dark blue) stimulation, and coherence maxima to wrist (purple) and ankle (yellow) extensions. (B) A sagittal MR section demonstrates that the source of responses to lip stimuli is in the close vicinity of the tumor. (C) Intraoperative view from the tumor region. Dural adhesions from the previous operation blur the anatomy, but the vein bifurcation (arrow) close to the source of lip SEFs, and tumor, Is readily identifiable and enables estimation of the tumor location and its relation to the somatosensory cortex.

Schiffbauer et al., 2002) needs to be related to methodological factors. For example, SEF sources are typically located within sulci, and cortical stimulation and recordings are performed from the visible gyral surface. No clear information exists about the spread of the stimulation current within the cortex. Schiffbauer et al. (2002) observed that the same response to cortical stimulation was obtained from sites with spatial variation of 11 ± 1 mm. Moreover, the 1-cm separation of electrode centers in the grids used to record intraoperative cortical SEPs, does not allow millimeter-scale comparisons between pre- and intraoperative recordings.

Motor evoked fields, recorded by time-locking of MEG signal with movements, identify the motor cortex in the anterior wall of the central sulcus, but are complex to interpret because of concomitant somatosensory activity (Rezai et al., 1996); they have been deemed not particularly useful in clinical settings (Lin et al., 2007). Correlograms between electromyography (EMG) and cortical spontaneous MEG during, e.g., wrist or ankle extension (Salenius et al., 1997) yield fast and selective localization of the motor cortex in most patients. Statistically significant MEG–EMG coherence can be recorded in about two out of three patients, and it independently confirms the SEF localization of the central sulcus. With proper signal analysis, the applicability of the coherence method approaches 100% (Kim & Chung, 2007). The combined use of several functional landmarks makes the localization of the central sulcus more accurate, increases the detection of possible methodological errors (Mäkelä et al., 2001), and should be used routinely.

Functional Localization in Planning Radiotherapy

Stereotactic radiation therapy with high single doses is suitable for lesions with sharp boundaries, such as cortical meningioma, and for high-grade glioma recidives. When applying high doses, it is important to avoid radiation to the surrounding intact brain areas. MEG source locations may provide useful information for the dose planning if the lesion is located close to eloquent brain areas (Aoyama et al., 2003).

Fusion of MEG Localizations with Neuronavigation Systems

MEG landmarks (Rezai et al., 1996; Ganslandt et al., 1997; Schiffbauer et al., 2002), and sources of epileptiform activity (Iwasaki et al. 2003) can be incorporated into image-guided stereotactic methods for a more precise navigation during operation. However it has been shown that the cortical surface shifts 5–10 mm after dural opening during the surgery (Roberts et al., 1998). The largest shift sometimes occurs near the center of the craniotomy, which is usually the brain region of the greatest interest (Hill et al., 2000). These shifts may introduce problems for pre- and intraoperative site comparison. Depicting surface veins in combination with 3-D brain structures and functional landmarks can be used for visual feedback in intraoperative navigation (e.g. Mäkelä et al., 2001).

Comparison of MEG with fMRI in Localization of the Central Sulcus

Functional MRI (fMRI) provides information about the location of the sensorimotor cortex in about 90-95% of the studied patients (Krings et al., 2001; Pujol et al., 2008). Although the method is not applicable in patients with a complete hand paralysis, it is needed in about 7% of patients harboring an intracranial mass (Pujol et al., 2008). Differences in central sulcus localization by MEG and fMRI have been reported; a 15±5 mm mean difference of the SEF source location, and the somatosensory elicited activation in fMRI in the same patients (Kober et al., 2001b) may exceed the gyral width. In patients with tumors in the vicinity of the central sulcus, the fMRI and MEG localization of the central sulcus were discordant in about 20% of the affected hemispheres; MEG localizations matched with the intraoperative mapping (Inoue et al., 1999; Korvenoja et al., 2006). As fMRI integrates brain activity over a period of several seconds, it reveals the whole cortical network participating in the processing of external stimuli or a task. Limited resolution in the time domain may consequently result in difficulties in separating the primary areas from secondary processing areas. Strong fMRI activations in nonprimary areas may, therefore, confound the interpretation of activation maps (Korvenoja et al., 2006). This drawback is avoided in MEG measurements detecting cortical activity with millisecond temporal accuracy, which separates the primary somatosensory cortex response from secondary activations (Hari & Forss, 1999); MEG should be used when detailed central sulcus localization is needed.

Approaching MEG Applications in Clinical Settings

Combination of MEG with Subcortical Pathway Mapping

Subcortical pathway mapping with intraoperative electrical stimulation of the white matter fibers related to sensorimotor and language areas have been suggested to optimize the risk-benefit ratio in the surgery of low-grade gliomas invading eloquent regions (Duffay et al., 2003). The combination of MEG source localization with 3D anisotropy contrast imaging allows such optimization preoperatively. The eloquent motor system including pyramidal tracts (Kamada et al., 2003), the anatomy of the optic radiation, and the functional localization of the primary visual cortex (Inoue et al., 2004), as well as the arcuate fasciculus joining the posterotemporal auditory MEG sources to the frontal cortex (Kamada et al. 2007), have been visualized for optimal preoperative planning of the tumor surgery. Evidently, in the near future this approach will be useful for highly detailed surgical planning. Integration of

MEG and diffusion tensor imaging is also suggested to be more sensitive than conventional imaging methods in detecting subtle neuronal lesions in mild traumatic brain injury (Huang et al., 2009).

Language Lateralization by MEG

The detection of language lateralization is important for the presurgical evaluation of some neurosurgical patients. Hemispheric language dominance is assessed by the "Wada test," injection of amobarbital into internal carotid artery to stop the function of one hemisphere at a time. Concomitantly, the language and memory functions of the non-anesthetized hemisphere are tested. However, because the procedure involves a risk of complications, is sensitive to the cross-flow of amobarbital to the other hemisphere, poses difficulties in interpretation especially when verbal memory is tested, and can be replicated extremely seldomly (Klöppel and Büchel, 2005), a reliable noninvasive test for language dominance would be desirable.

Search for language lateralization with MEG has often been based on calculations of sequential single dipole sources accounting for auditory evoked fields (AEFs) 50–700 ms after the stimulus onset, elicited by recognition memory task for spoken words. In a series of 100 patients, these AEFs were not applicable to laterality analysis in 15% of the patients; complete agreement with Wada test was obtained in 87% of the remaining patients. Although the sequential single dipole model probably does not capture the complex speech-related processes, the activity in the perisylvian auditory areas detected by this method has been considered useful for preoperative planning (Papanicolaou et al., 2004; Merrified et al. 2007). The method combines speech lateralization and activation of short-term memory processes; both provide useful information in planning of temporal lobe surgery. Listening to synthetized vowel sounds produced late AEFs with dipole sources lateralized to the left hemisphere in 85% of the patients in whom intraoperative cortical stimulation found left-hemisphere sites essential for language, and demonstrated right-sided lateralization in two patients with right-hemisphere predominance in the Wada test (Szymanski et al., 2001). More simple tests, based on stronger 100-ms AEF in the dominant auditory cortex for speech than nonspeech stimuli, have been developed (Gootjes et al., 1999; Parviainen et al., 2005; Kirveskari et al., 2006), but the results have not yet been compared with the Wada test. Silent naming of visually presented pictures suppresses spontaneous MEG activity in the 8–100 Hz range; the laterality of stronger suppression in the inferior frontal gyrus region was congruent with the result of the Wada test in 95% of the patients (Hirata et al., 2004). Similarly, the speech laterality estimation from 13–25 Hz activity-decrease in the inferior frontal regions during responses to deviant stimuli in an auditory oddball task comprised from short words agrees with results of the Wada Test in 95% of the cases (Kim & Chung, 2008). These promising approaches to language lateralization require further studies.

MEG Localization of Speech-Related Activity Within Hemispheres

The preoperative localization of speech-related areas within the hemispheres would also be beneficial in planning surgical approaches in some neurosurgical patients. The functional localization of the auditory cortex by using sources of N100m AEFs is useful for planning surgery in the left temporal lobe, because the left auditory cortex is often surrounded by the language-related cortex (Nakasato et al., 1997). Current MEG techniques cannot identify the whole set of speech-related cortical areas directly, and it is not obvious which aspect of language should be mapped for clinical purposes. The study could be guided, e.g., by an identification of disease-induced problems in specific aspects of language. A targeted stimulus design could then be used for functional localization of brain areas involved in the affected processing stage, for example, by studying activations related to naming objects, or elicited by visually presented words (Salmelin, 2007).

Visually presented words forming sentences elicit MEG responses in the vicinity of the left auditory cortex at about 400 ms after the word onset (Helenius et al., 1998). Anomalous words ending sentences activate the left perisylvian cortex more strongly than the words producing expected endings. Although the source modeling of the widespread activity related to language tasks requires expertise, it may produce useful information as functional landmarks (Figure 14–4). It is probable, however, that modeling of the speech-related brain activity by current dipoles shows only some parts of the cortical network related to reading, speech production, and perception. Minimum-norm or minimum-current estimates may turn out to be useful in analyzing widespread activation patterns related to speech perception or reading (Kober et al., 2001a; Hirata et al. 2004).

Surgery of tumors or epileptic foci near eloquent areas is occasionally performed during awake craniotomy, which allows the patient to report sensations elicited by cortical stimulation. This approach is exciting in studies of speech-related activity, and allows comparison of pre- and intraoperative functional localization. However, the access to cortical areas is limited by the size of the craniotomy, and the number of tasks that can be done to a waking patient during surgery is restricted. Consequently, these studies require careful planning. Testing multiple aspects of speech perception and production, in a time scale sensible for study of a clinical patient, is particularly demanding. Standardized series of activation paradigms have been suggested to be desirable in fMRI studies of language lateralization and representation in the brain (Klöppel & Büchel, 2005). This is true for MEG studies of language as well.

Future Applications of MEG in Clinical Settings

To add regular clinical MEG indications (see, e.g., recommendations of American Academy of Neurology 2009), extensive search for new ways to use

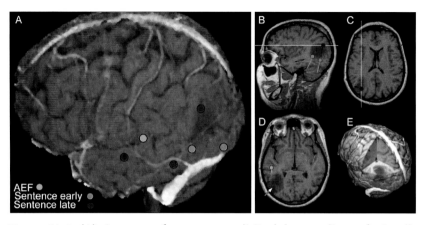

Figure 14–4. (A) Sources of responses elicited by reading of visually presented words forming sentences, which had potentially abnormal endings. Last words produce clear responses; the source locations are superimposed on patient's 3D MRI surface rendering. The yellow dots display the sources of early activations and the red ones are sources activated later on. Green dot indicates the source of the N100m AEF. (B) and (C) Sagittal and horizontal MR sections show that the activations elicited by reading are in close vicinity of the tumor. (D) The arrow points to the "surgical corridor" selected by the neurosurgeon. (E) 3D MRI reconstruction with digital section in the parietal lobe illustrates the 3D extent of the tumor. During awake craniotomy, stimulation of the cortex in the posterior margin of the tumor produced difficulties in seeing the written words, whereas the stimulation of lower and upper margin disturbed the understanding of the sentence meaning. The surgeon approached the tumor exactly from its center and carefully extended the resection to the margins of the tumor. No clear defects in speech production or understanding were observed after the operation.

MEG in clinics is underway. Most promising approaches include detection of plastic changes elicited by different types of brain or peripheral nervous system pathology. Modification of spontaneous MEG signals, detected by various signal analysis methods in patients with stroke, head trauma or degenerative brain diseases, may also provide clinically useful information in the future.

For interpretation of MEG results in terms of clinical research, it is useful to obtain as much information as possible about the studied patients by combining clinical data from various directions—such as genetic properties, clinical details, anatomic and functional MR imaging, neuropsychology, physiotherapy, etc. Occasionally, joining a study of a clinical patient group already collected for another research purpose, with a MEG examination, may turn out to be useful. If the study is prospective, careful planning of patient selection criteria is mandatory, and usually not as easy as expected.

Strict criteria prolong the research project, whereas too loose a patient selection makes interpretation of the results difficult.

Cortical Reorganization

Objective means to predict potential for rehabilitation and to follow its course would be useful in the follow-up of neurological patients. It has been suggested that extensive practice, or lack of use, of a certain body part may change the somatotopic organization of the primary sensory cortex. Cortical representations of fingers, as depicted by SEF sources elicited by tactile finger stimulation, have been shown to differentiate after the treatment of syndactyly (Mogilner et al., 1993). Moreover, the amputation of the arm modifies SEF source structure in a manner suggesting plastic changes in the primary sensory cortex (Flor et al., 1995). MEG studies have recently shown that modifications of SEF source locations occur in association with chronic pain without nerve deafferentation (Juottonen et al., 2002; Maihöfner et al., 2003). Furthermore, abnormal ipsilateral SEFs developed in association with the mirror-like spread of chronic regional pain from one upper limb to another, during a 3-year follow-up of one patient (Forss et al., 2005). Such changes might be useful as objective correlates of perceived pain. The changes in SEF source organization are, at least to some extent, reversible, suggesting that rehabilitation should be targeted for regaining the orderly somatotopic arrangement at the primary sensory cortex (Maihöfner et al., 2004). An objective follow-up of such changes is an intriguing new possibility for clinical applications.

Experiments related with a possible cerebral plasticity underlying recovery after stroke, have searched for changes in SEF source organization. Narrowed cortical area harboring the sources of SEFs in patients with first-ever monohemispheric stroke have been described (Rossini et al., 2003), but so far, except for some source displacement possibly due to perilesional edema, no unusual source structure has been demonstrated. Instead, source strengths and response latencies appear to be correlated with the severity of the clinical picture (Wikström et al. 1999; Gallien et al. 2003; Oliviero et al. 2005). Enhanced excitability of the affected hemisphere and spared posterior parietal responses have been linked with high functionality of the affected hand, whereas the enhanced excitability in the unaffected hemisphere has been linked with large cortical lesions in the affected hemisphere (Oliviero et al., 2004).

Use of a single dipole model in analyzing possible plastic changes may not be as straightforward as it seems. For example, the orderly tonotopic organization of AEF N100m sources has formed a basis for the investigation of such phenomena as reorganization of auditory cortex in tinnitus subjects, or possible anomalies of auditory cortex in schizophrenic patients. However, a recent carefully executed study has shown that organization of AEF sources demonstrated no significant frequency dependence at all in most healthy subjects, causing concern about the conclusions in clinical studies based on orderly tonotopic organization in control subjects (Lütkenhöner et al., 2003). The quantitative differences of source locations derived from single dipole modeling pertinent in these studies require large normative data bases to fully realize the significance of these changes.

Low-grade gliomas frequently invade eloquent structures, but may produce little or no neurological deficit at the phase they present with seizures. It has been suggested that functional tissue may persist within the tumor, that eloquent areas may be redistributed around the tumor, or that the function disturbed by the tumor is compensated with activity in remote areas within the same or opposite hemisphere The type of reorganization naturally affects directly the presurgical planning (Duffay, 2005). Arteriovenous malformations reaching central sulcus region have been suggested to modify SEF sources in about 30% of the patients; in 10%, the shifts of sources to the opposite hemisphere were observed (Vates et al., 2002). However, the clearest shifts to the opposite hemisphere occurred in sources of SEFs to lip stimulation, known to have bilateral representation in healthy subjects as well. Occasionally, incomplete tumor resections may induce reshaping of functional cortex, and a total removal of the tumor may be feasible after a few years (Duffay, 2005). Follow-up of such development obviously provides new vistas for functional mapping by MEG.

Modifications of Spontaneous MEG by Neurological Diseases

Pathological, low-frequency spontaneous brain electric activity, surrounding focal ischemic brain lesions, has been described in MEG recordings, and it has been associated with preserved and metabolically active but acidotic cortical tissue, contributing to salvageable tissue surrounding stroke (Kamada et al., 1997). Some studies (e.g., Mäkelä et al., 1998b; Tecchio et al., 2005) have shown modifications of the spontaneous activity in the non-stroke hemisphere as well. The functional significance of slow wave activity in the affected and unaffected hemispheres remains to be elucidated (Butz et al., 2004). However, synchronous low-frequency activity has been suggested to form a part of brain plasticity and anatomical reorganization within the adult brain, since it is strongly correlated with axonal sprouting in the animal model of ischemic brain lesions (Charmichael & Chesselet, 2002). It is well known that ischemic injury to one brain area changes function in numerous connected brain regions (Cramer, 2004). Tracking such changes and correlating them with clinical recovery of the patients is an exciting direction for future MEG studies in patients; new signal processing tools may ease the analysis of the rich patterns of activity displayed in spontaneous MEG.

Abnormalities of spectral content of the spontaneous MEG have been associated with memory disorders in patients after herpes simplex encephalitis (Mäkelä et al., 1998a), thalamic strokes (Mäkelä et al., 1998b), in patients with mild head trauma having cognitive problems (Lewine et al., 2007;

Huang et al.,2009), and in Alzheimer's disease (Fernandez et al., 2006a,b; Osipova et al., 2005). Although patients suffering from these disorders display differences from age-matched control subjects on the group level, no clear factors separating individual patients from control subjects have emerged. Furthermore, no robust correlations between the spectral abnormalities and neuropsychological findings have been reported. Time will tell, whether new analysis methods searching for cortico-cortical spatial (Schnitzler and Gross, 2005), phase-related (Palva et al., 2005), and temporal correlations (Linkenkaer-Hansen et al., 2005) of spontaneous MEG activity will produce more robust differences in individual patients.

The vistas produced by new artifact-rejection methods to study effects of electric stimulation of central brain and peripheral nervous system, are promising completely new research possibilities by mapping the effects of this causal intervention in different patient groups with MEG. Pathophysiology of, e.g., Parkinson's disease, chronic pain, depression, obsessive-compulsive disorders, or minimal cognitive state, can be studied in a controlled manner, as neurostimulators appear to be useful in these conditions. The stimulation effects are reversible, unlike those of lesions, and even blinded methods are possible after artifact removal (Kringelbach et al., 2007).

As demands for evidence-based treatments are increasing, there is, in addition to figuring out better and better ways to study patients, also a need to show the benefit of the MEG measurements by well-designed, prospective, randomized studies of large patient groups by, hopefully, demonstrating improved results (see, e.g., Sutherling et al., 2008, Knowlton et al. 2009), and shortened treatment times. Obviously, these studies would benefit from joint efforts of several laboratories involved in clinical applications of MEG. Although this type of research may not appeal to neuroscientists, the MEG community should direct energy towards these studies as well, as the future availability of clinical MEG may be influenced by lack of such studies.

Conclusions

MEG is a valuable tool to use in clinical settings. Nevertheless, it is clear that it is only a part of a multifaceted clinical evaluation deriving information from all available sources for the benefit of the patient. The relative weight of MEG in this evaluation depends on individual clinical details of each patient. The emerging applications are highly exciting, and will provide new opportunities for MEG studies in clinical settings.

Acknowledgments

Supported by the Academy of Finland. E. Kirveskari made valuable comments on the manuscript.

References

Ahonen, A., Hämäläinen, M., Kajola, M., Knuutila, J., Laine, P., Lounasmaa, O., et al. (1993). 122-channel SQUID instrument for investigating the magnetic signals from human brain. *Physica Scripta*, *T49*, 198–205.

American Academy of Neurology Professional Association (AANPA). (2009). *Magnetoencephalography (MEG) Policy. Recommended by the AANPA Medical Economics and Management Committee. Approved by the AANPA Board of Directors on May 8, 2009.* St. Paul, MN: AANPA.

Aoyama, H., Kamada, K., Shirato, H., Takeuchi, F., Kuriki, S., Iwasaki, Y., et al. (2003). Visualization of the corticospinal tract pathway using magnetic resonance axonography and magnetoencephalography for stereotactic irradiation planning of arteriovenous malformations. *Radiother Oncol*, *68*, 27–32.

Assaf B., Karkar K., Laxer K., Garcia P., Austin E., Barbaro N., et al. (2004). Magnetoencephalography source localization and surgical outcome in temporal lobe epilepsy. *Clin Neurophysiol*, *115*, 2066–2076.

Balakrishnan, G., Grover, K. M., Mason, K., Smith, B., Barkley, G., Tepley, N., et al. (2007). A retrospective analysis of the effect of general anesthetics on the successful detection of interictal epileptiform activity in magnetoencephalography. *(2007) Anesth Analg*, *104*, 1493–1497.

Barkley, G., & Baumgartner, C. (2003). MEG and EEG in epilepsy. *J Clin Neurophysiol*, *20*, 163–178.

Barth, D., Sutherling, W., Engel Jr., J., & Beatty, J. (1982). Neuromagnetic localization of epileptiform spike activity in the human brain. *Science*, *218*, 891–894.

Barth, D., Sutherling, W., Engel Jr., J., & Beatty, J. (1984). Neuromagnetic evidence of spatially distributred sources underlying epileptiform spikes in the human brain. *Science*, *223*, 293–296.

Bittar, R., Olivier, A., Sadikot, A., Andermann, F., Comeau, R., Cyr, M., et al. (1999) Localization of somatosensory function by using positron emission tomography scanning; a comparison with intraoperative cortical stimulation. *J Neurosurg*, *90*, 478–483.

Butz, M., Gross, J., Timmermann, L., Moll, M., Freund, H. & Witte, O. (2004). Perilesional pathological oscillatory activity in the magnetoencepohalogram of patients with cortical brain lesions. *Neurosci Lett*, *355*, 93–96.

Charmichael, S., & Chesselet, M. (2002). Synchronous neuronal activity is a signal for axonal sprouting after cortical lesions in the adult. *J Neurosci*, *22*, 6062–6070.

Cheyne, D., Bostan, A., Gaetz, W., & Pang E. W. (2007). Event-related beamforming: A robust method for presurgical functional mapping using MEG. *Clin Neurophysiol*, *118*, 1691–1704.

Cramer, S. (2004). Functional Imaging in stroke recovery. *Stroke*, *35*(Suppl. I), 2695–2698.

Duffay, H. (2005). Lessons from brain mapping in surgery for low-grade glioma: insights into associations between tumour and brain plasticity. *Lancet Neurol*, *4*, 476–485.

Duffay, H., Capelle, L., Denvil, D., Sichez, N., Gaticnol, P., Taillandier, L., et al. (2003). Usefulness of intraoperative electrical subcortical mapping during surgery for low-grade gliomas located within eloquent brain regions: functional results in a consecutive series of 103 patients. *J Neurosurg*, *98*, 764–778.

Ebersole, J. (1999). Non-invasive pre-surgical evaluation with EEG/MEG source analysis. *Electroenceph Clin Neurophysiol, Suppl. 50,* 167–174.

Enatsu, R., Mikuni, N., Usui, K., Matsubayashi, J., Taki, J., Begum, T., et al. (2008). Usefulness of MEG magnetometer for spike detection in patients with mesial temporal epileptic focus. *NeuroImage 41,* 1206–1219.

Fernandez, A., Hornero, R., Mayo, A., Poza, J., Gil-Gregorio, P. & Ortiz, T. (2006a). MEG spectral profile in Alzheimer's disease and mild cognitive impairment. *Clin Neurophysiol, 117,* 306–314.

Fernandez, A., Turrero, A., Zuluaga, P., Gil, P., Maestu, F., Campo, P., et al. (2006b) Magnetoencephalographic parietal delta dipole density in mild cognitive impairment:preliminary results of a method to estimate the risk of developing Alzheimer disease. *Arch Neurol, 63,* 427–430.

Fischer, M., Scheler, G., & Stefan, H. (2005). Utilization of magnetoencephalography results to obtain favourable results in epilepsy surgery. *Brain, 128,* 153–157.

Flor, H., Elbert, T., Knecht, S., Wienbruch, C., Pantev, C., Birbaumer, N., et al. (1995). Phantom-limb pain as a perceptual correlate of cortical reorganization following arm amputation. *Nature, 375,* 482–484.

Forss, N., Kirveskari, E., & Gockel, M. (2005). Mirror-like spread of chronic pain. *Neurology, 65,* 748–750.

Forss, N., Mäkelä, J., Keränen, T., & Hari, R. (1995). Trigeminally triggered epileptic hemifacial convulsions. *NeuroReport, 6,* 918–920.

Gallen, C., Schwartz, B., & Bucholz, R. (1995). Presurgical localization of functional cortex using magnetic source imaging. *J Neurosurg, 82,* 988–994.

Gallen, C., Sobel, D., Waltz, T., Aung, M., Copeland, B., Schwartz, B., et al. (1993). Noninvasive presurgical mapping of somatosensory cortex. *Neurosurgery, 33,* 260–268.

Gallen, C., Tecoma, E., Iragui, V., Sobel, D., Schwartz, B., & Bloom, F. (1997) Magnetic source imaging of abnormal low-frequency magnetic activity in presurgical evaluatios of epilepsy. *Epilepsia, 38,* 452–460.

Ganslandt, O., Buchfelder, M., Hastreiter, P., Grummich, P., Fahlbusch, R., & Nimsky, C. (2004). Magnetic source imaging supports clinical decision making in glioma patients. *Clin Neurol Neurosurg, 107,* 20–26.

Ganslandt, O., Steinmeier, R., Kober, H., Vieth, J., Kassubeck, J., Romstöck, J., et al. (1997). Magnetic source imaging combined with image-guided frameless stereotaxy: a new method in surgery around the motor strip. *Neurosurgery, 41,* 621–628.

Gootjes, L., Raij, T., Salmelin, R., & Hari, R. (1999). Left-hemisphere dominance for processing of vowels: a whole-scalp neuromagnetic study. *NeuroReport, 10,* 2987–2991.

Hamer, H. M., Morris, H. H., Mascha, E. J., Karafa, M. T., Bingaman, W. E., Bej, M. D., et al. (2002). Complications of invasive video-EEG monitoring with subdural grid electrodes. *Neurology, 58,* 97–103.

Hara, K., Lin, F.-H., Camposano, S., Foxe, D. M., Grant P. E., Bourgeois, B. F., et al. (2007). Magnetoencephalographic mapping of interictal spike propagation:a technical and clinical report. *AJNR, 28,* 1486–1488.

Hari, R., Ahonen, A., Forss, N., Granström, M.-L., Hämäläinen, M., Kajola, M., et al. (1993). Parietal epileptic mirror focus detected with a whole-head neuromagnetometer. *NeuroReport, 5,* 45–48.

Hari, R., & Forss, N. (1999). Magnetoencephalography in the study of human somatosensory cortical processing. *Phil Trans R Soc Lond B, 354*, 1145–1154.

Helenius, P., Salmelin, R., Service, E., & Connolly, J. (1998). Distinct time courses of word and context comprehension in the left temporal cortex. *Brain, 112*, 1133–1142.

Hill, D., Castellano Smith, A., Simmons, A., Maurer, C., Cox, T., Elwes, R., et al. (2000). Sources of error in comparing functional magnetic resonance imaging and invasive electrophysiological recordings. *J Neurosurg, 93*, 214–223.

Hirata, M., Kato, A., Taniguchi, M., Saitoh, Y., Ninomiya, H., Ihara, A., et al. (2004). Determination of language dominance with synthetic aperture magnetometer: comparison with the Wada test. *NeuroImage, 23*, 46–53.

Huang, M-X., Song, T., Hagler D. J., Podgorny, I., Jousmäki, V., Cui, L., et al. (2007). A novel integrated MEG and EEG analysis method for dipolar sources. *Neuro-Image, 37*, 731–748.

Huang, M-X, Theilmann, R., Robb, A., Angeles, A., Nichols, S., Drake, A., et al. (2009). Integrated imaging approach with MEG and DTI to detect mild traumatic brain injury in military and civilian patients. *J Neurotrauma, 26*, 1213–1226.

Hughes, J., Cohen, J., Mayman, C., Scholl, M., & Hendrix, D. (1977). Relationship of the magnetoencephalogram to abnormal activity in the electroencephalogram. *J Neurol, 217*, 79–93.

Hund, M., Rezai, A., Kronberg, E., Cappell, J., Zoneshayn, M., Ribary, U., et al. (1997). Magnetoencephalographic mapping: basis of new functional risk pro-file in the selection of patients with cortical brain lesions. *Neurosurgery, 40*, 936–943.

Hämäläinen, M., & Hari, R. (2002). Magnetoencephalographic characterization of dynamic brain activation: basic principles and methods of data collection and source analysis. In: J. Mazziotta (ed.). *Brain Mapping: the methods.* (pp. 227–253) London, New York: Elsevier.

Iida, K., Otsubo, H., Matsumoto, Y., Ochi, A., Oishi, M., Holowka, S., et al. (2005). Characterizing magnetic spike sources by using magnetoencephalography-guided neuronavigation in epilepsy surgery in pediatric patients. *J Neurosurg, (Pediatrics 2), 102*, 187–196.

Inoue, T., Fujimura, M., Kumabe, T., Nakasato, N., Higano, S., & Tominaga, T. (2004). Combined three-dimensional anisotropy contrast imaging and magnetoencepha-lography guidance to preserve visual function in a patient with an occipital lobe tumor. *Minim Invas Neurosurg, 47*, 249–252.

Inoue, T., Shimizu. H., Nakasato, N., Kumabe, T., & Yoshimoto, T. (1999). Accuracy and limitation of functional magnetic resonance imaging for identification of the central sulcus: comparison with magnetoencephalography in patients with brain tumors. *NeuroImage, 10*, 738–748.

Iwasaki, M., Nakasato, N., Shamoto, H. & Yoshimoto, T. (2003). Focal magnetoence-phalographic spikes in the superior temporal plane undetected by scalp EEG. *J Clin Neurosci, 10*, 236–238.

Jousmäki, V., & Hari, R. (1996). Cardiac artifacts in magnetoencephalogram. *J Clin Neurophysiol, 13*, 172–176.

Juottonen, K., Gockel, M., Silen, T., Hurri, H., Hari, R., & Forss, N. (2002). Altered central sensorimotor processing in patients with complex regional pain syndrome. *Pain, 98*, 315–323.

Kamada, K., Todo, T., Masutani, Y., Aoki, S., Ino, K., Morita, A., et al. (2007). Visualization of the frontotemporal language fibers by tractography combined with functional magnetic resonance imaging and magnetoencephalography. *J Neurosurg, 106*, 90–98.

Kamada, K., Houkin, K., Takeuchi, F., Ishii. N., Ikeda, J., Sawamura, Y., et al. (2003). Visualization of the eloquent motor system by integration of MEG, functional, and anisotropic diffusion-weighted MRI in functional neuronavigation. *Surg Neurol, 59*, 353–362.

Kamada, K., Saguer, M., Möler, M., Wichlow, K., Katenhauser, M., Kober, H. et al. (1997). Functional and metabolic analysis of cerebral ischemia using magnetoencephalography and proton magnetic resonance spectroscopy. *Ann Neurol, 42*, 554–563.

Kamada, K., Takeuchi, F., Kuriki, S., Oshiro, O., Houkin, K., & Abe, H. (1993). Functional neurosurgical simulation with brain surface magnetic resonance images and magnetoencephalography. *Neurosurgery, 33*, 269–273.

Kettenmann, B., Feichtinger, M., Tilz, C., Kaltenhäuser, M., Hummel, C., & Stefan, H. (2005). Comparison of clonidine to sleep deprivation in the potential to induce spike or sharp wave activity. *Clin Neurophysiol, 116*, 905–912.

Kim, J. S., & Chung, C. K. (2007). Robust source analysis of oscillatory motor cortex activity with inherently variable phase delay. *NeuroImage, 37*, 518–529.

Kim, J. S., & Chung, C. K. (2008). Language lateralization using MEG beta frequency desynchronization during auditory oddball stimulation with one-syllable words. *NeuroImage, 42*, 1499–1507.

Kirchberger, K., Hummel, C., & Stefan, H. (1998). Postoperative multichannel magnetoencephalography in patients with recurrent seizures after epilepsy surgery. *Acta Neurol Scand, 98*, 1–7.

Kirveskari, E., Salmelin, R., & Hari, R. (2006). Neuromagnetic responses to vowels vs. tones reveal hemispheric lateralization. *Clin Neurophysiol,117*, 643–648.

Klöppel, S., & Büchel, C. (2005). Alternatives to the Wada test: a critical view of functional magnetic resonance imaging in preoperative use. *Curr Opin Neurol, 18*, 418–423.

Knowlton, R. (2006). The role of FDG-PET, ictal SPECT and MEG in the epilepsy surgery evaluation. *Epilepsy & Behav, 8*, 91–101.

Knowlton, R., Laxer, K., Aminoff, M., Roberts, T., Wong, S., & Rowley, H. (1997). Magnetoencephalography in partial epilepsy: clinical yield and localization accuracy. *Ann Neurol, 42*, 622–631.

Knowlton, R., & Shih, J. (2004). Magnetoencephalography in epilepsy. *Epilepsia, 45*(Suppl. 4), 61–71.

Knowlton R., Elgavish R., Howell J., Blount J., Burneo J., Faught E., et al. (2006). Magnetic source imaging versus intracranial electroencephalogram in epilepsy surgery: a prospective study. *Ann Neurol, 59*, 835–842.

Knowlton, R., Radzan, S., Limdi, N., Elgavish, R., Kkillen, J., Blount, J., et al. (2009). Effect of epilepsy magnetic source imaging on intracranial electrode placement. *Ann Neurol 65*: 716–723.

Kober, H., Möller, M., Nimsky, C., Vieth, J., Fahlbusch, R., & Ganslandt, O. (2001a). New approach to localize speech-relevant brain areas and hemispheric dominance using spatially filtered magnetoencephalography. *Hum Brain Mapp, 14*, 236–250.

Kober, H., Nimsky, C., Moller, M., Hastreiter, P., Fahlbusch, R., & Ganslandt, O. (2001b). Correlation of sensorimotor activation with functional magnetic resonance imaging and magnetoencephalography in presurgical functional imaging: a spatial analysis. *NeuroImage, 14*, 1214–1228.

Korvenoja, A., Kirveskari, E., Aronen, H., Avikainen, S., Brander, A., Huttunen, J., et al. (2006). Localization of primary sensorimotor cortex:comparison of magnetoencephalography, functional MR imaging and intraoperative cortical mapping. *Radiology, 241*, 213–222.

Kringelbach, M., Jenkinson, N., Owen, S. L. F., & Aziz, T. Z. (2007). Translational principles of deep brain stimulation. *Nature Rev Neurosci, 8*, 623–635.

Kringelbach, M., Jenkinson, N., Greren A. L., Owen, S. L. F., Hansen, P. C., Cornelissen, P. L., et al. (2007). Deep brain stimulation for chronic pain investigated with magnetoencephalography. *NeuroReport,18*, 223–228.

Krings, T., Reiniges, M., Erberich, S., Kemeny, S., Rohde, V., Spetzger, U., et al. (2001). Functional MRI for presurgical planning: problems, artefacts and solution strategies. *J Neurol Neurosurg Psych, 70*, 749–760.

Lamusuo, S., Forss, N., Ruottinen, H.-M., Bergman, J., Mäkelä, J., Mervaala, E., et al. (1999). 18-F FDG PET and whole-scalp MEG localization of epileptogenic cortex. *Epilepsia, 40*, 921–930.

Lehericy, S., Duffay, H., Cornu, P., Capelle, L., Pidoux, B., Carpentier, A., et al. (2000). Correspondence between functional magnetic resonance imaging somatotopy and individual brain anatomy of the central region: comparison with intraoperative stimulation in patients with brain tumors. *J Neurosurg, 92*, 589–598.

Lewine, J., Andrews, R., Chez, M., Patil, A., Devinsky, O., Smith, M., et al. (1999) Magnetoencephalographic patterns of epileptiform activity in children with regressive autism spectrum disorders. *Pediatrics, 104*, 405–418.

Lewine, J., Davis, J. T., Bigler, ED., Thoma, R., Hill, D., Funke, M., et al. (2007). Objective documentation of traumatic brain injury subsequent to mild head trauma:Multimodal brain imaging with MEG, SPECT and MRI. *J Head Trauma Rehabil, 22*,141–155.

Lin, P. T., Berger, M. S., & Naragajan, S. S. (2006). Motor field sensitivity for preoperative localization of motor cortex. *J Neurosurg, 105*, 588–594.

Lin, Y.-Y., Chang, K.-P., Hsieh, J.-C., Yeh, T.-C., Hsiang, Y.-Y., Kwan, S.-Y., et al. (2003). Magnetoencephalographic analysis of bilaterally synchronous discharges in benign rolandic epilepsy of childhood. *Seizure, 12*, 448–455.

Linkenkaer-Hansen, K., Monto, S., Rytsälä, H., Suominen, K., Isometsä, E., & Kähkönen, S. (2005). Breakdown of long-range temporal correlations in theta oscillations in patients with major depressive disorder. *J Neurosci, 25*, 10131–10137.

Lütkenhöner, B., Krumbholz, K., & Seither-Preisler, A. (2003). Studies of tonotopy based on wave N100 of the auditory evoked field are problematic. *NeuroImage, 19*, 935–949.

Maihöfner, C., Handwerker, H., Neundorfer, B., & Birklein, F. (2004). Cortical reorganization during recovery from complex regional pain syndrome. *Neurology, 63*, 693–701.

Maihöfner, C., Handwerker, H., Neundörfer, B., & Birklein, F. (2003). Patterns of cortical reorganization in complex regional pain syndrome. *Neurology, 61*, 1707–1715.

Mamelak, A., Lopez, N., Akhtari, M., & Sutherling, W. (2002) Magnetoencepha-
lography-directed surgery in patients with neocortical epilepsy. *J Neurosurg, 97*,
865–873.

Merlet, I., Paetau, R., Garcia-Larrea, L., Uutela.K, Granström, M.-L., & Maguiere, F.
(1997) Apparent asynchrony between interictal electric and magnetic spikes. *NeuroReport, 8*, 1071–1076.

Merrified, W. S., Simos, P. G., Papanicolau, A. C., Philpott, LM., & Sutherling, W. W.
(2007). Hemispheric language dominance in magnetoencephalography: Sensitivity,
specificity and data reduction techniques. *Epilepsy Behav, 10*, 120–128.

Mikuni, N., Nagamine, T., Ikeda, A., Terada, K., Taki, W., Kimura, J., et al. (1997).
Simultaneous recording of epileptiform discharges by MEG and subdural electrodes in temporal lobe epilepsy. *NeuroImage, 5*, 298–306.

Modena, I., Ricci, G., Barbanera, S., Romani, G., & Carelli, P. (1982). Biomagnetic
measurements of spontaneous brain activity in epileptic patients. *Electroenceph clin
Neurophysiol, 54*, 622–628.

Mogilner, A., Grossman, A., Ribary, U., Joliot, M., Volkmann, J., Rapaport, D., et al.
(1993). Somatosensory cortical plasticity in adult humans revealed by magnetoencephalography. *Proc Natl Acad Sci USA, 90*, 3593–3597.

Mäkelä J.P., Forss N., Jääskeläinen J., Kirveskari E., Korvenoja A., & Paetau R. (2006).
Magnetoencephalography in neurosurgery. *Neurosurgery, 59*, 493–510.

Mäkelä, J.P., Kirveskari, E., Seppä, M., Hämäläinen, M., Forss, N., Avikainen, S.,
et al. (2001). Three-dimensional integration of brain anatomy and function to facilitate intraoperative navigation around the sensorimotor strip. *Hum Brain Mapp,
12*, 180–192.

Mäkelä, J. P., Salmelin, R., Hokkanen, L., Launes, J., & Hari, R. (1998a). Neuromagnetic sequelae of herpes simplex encephalitis. *Electroenceph clin Neurophysiol, 106*,
251–258.

Mäkelä, J. P., Salmelin, R., Kotila, M., Salonen, O., Laaksonen, R., Hokkanen, L., et al.
(1998b). Left thalamic infarctions modify neuromagnetic cortical signals. *Electroenceph clin Neurophysiol, 106*, 433–443.

Mäkelä, J.P., Taulu, S., Ahonen, A., Pohjola, J., & Pekkonen, E. (2007). Effects of
subthalamic nucleus stimulation on spontaneous sensorimotor MEG activity in a
Parkinsonian patient. *International Congress Series, 1300*, 345–348.

Mäkelä, J. P., Iivanainen, M., Pieninkeroinen, I. P., Waltimo, O., Lahdensuu, M.
(1993). Seizures associated with propofol anesthesia. *Epilepsia, 34*, 832–835.

Nakasato, N., Kumabe, T., Kanno, A., Ohtomo, S., Mizoi, K., & Yoshimoto, T. (1997).
Neuromagnetic evaluation of cortical auditory function in patients with temporal
lobe tumors. *J Neurosurg, 86*, 610–618.

Oliviero, A., Tecchio, F., Zappasodi, F., Pasqualetti, P., Salustri, C., Lupoi, D., et al.
(2004). Brain sensorimotor hand area functionality in acute stroke: insights from
magnetoencephalography. *NeuroImage, 23*, 542–550.

Osipova, D., Ahveninen, J., Jensen, O., Ylikoski, A., & Pekkonen, E. (2005). Altered
generation of spontaneous oscillations in Alzheimer's disease. *NeuroImage, 27*,
835–8411.

Otsubo H., Ochi A., & Elliot, I. (2001). MEG predicts epileptic zone in
lesional extrahippocampal epilepsy: 12 pediatric surgery cases. *Epilepsia, 42*,
1523–1530.

Paetau, R., Granström, M.-L., Blomstedt, G., Jousmäki, V., Korkman, M., & Liukko-nen, E. (1999). Magnetoencephalography in presurgical evaluation of children with the Landau-Kleffner syndrome. *Epilepsia, 40*, 326–335.

Palva, J., Palva, S., & Kaila, K. (2005). Phase synchrony among neuronal oscillations in the human cortex. *J Neurosci, 25*, 3962–3972.

Papanicolaou, A., Simos, P., Castillo, E., Breier, J., Sarkari, S., Pataraia, E., et al. (2004). Magnetoencephalography: a noninvasive alternative to the Wada procedure. *J Neurosurg, 100*, 867–876.

Papanicolau A., Pataraia E., Billingsley-Marshall R., Castillo E., Wheless J., Swank P., et al. (2005). Toward the substitution of invasive electroencephalography in epilepsy surgery. *J Clin Neurophysiol, 22*, 231–237.

Parkkonen, L., Fujiki, N., & Mäkelä, JP. (2009). Sources of auditory brainstem responses revisited: Contribution by magnetoencephalography. *Human Brain Mapping 30*, 1772–1782.

Parviainen, T., Helenius, P., & Salmelin, R. (2005). Cortical differentiation of speech and nonspeech sounds at 100 ms: implications for dyslexia. *Cerebral Cortex, 15*, 1054–1063.

Pataraia, E., Baumgartner, C., Lidinger, G., & Deecke, L. (2002) Magnetoencephalo-graphy in presurgical epilepsy evaluation. *Neurosurg, Rev. 25*, 141–159.

Pujol, J., Deus, J., Acebes, JJ., Villanueva, A., Aparicio, A., Soriano-Mas, C., et al. (2008). Identification of the sensorimotor cortex with functional MRI: frequency and actual contribution in a neurosurgical context. *J Neuroimaging, 18*, 28–33.

Ramantani, G., Boor, R., Paetau, R., Ille, N., Feneberg, R., Rupp, A., et al. (2006). MEG versus EEG: influence of background activity on interictal spike detection. *J Clin Neurophysiol, 23*, 498–508.

Rezai, A., Hund, M., Kronberg, E., Zoneshayn, M., Cappell, J., Ribary, U., et al. (1996). The interactive use of magnetoencephalography in stereotactic image-guided neurosurgery. *Neurosurgery, 39*, 92–102.

Roberts, D., Hartov, A., Kennedy, F., Miga, M., & Paulsen, K. (1998). Intraoperative brain shift and deformation: a quantitative analysis of cortical displacement in 28 cases. *Neurosurgery, 42*, 749–760.

Rossini, P., Calautti, C., Pauri, F., & Baron, J.-C. (2003) Post-stroke reorganization in the adult brain. *Lancet Neurol, 2*, 493–502.

Salenius, S., Portin, K., Kajola, M., Salmelin, R., & Hari, R. (1997). Cortical control of human motoneuron firing during isometric contractions. *J Neurophysiol, 77*, 3401–3405.

Salmelin, R., Hari, R., Lounasmaa, O. V., & Sams, M. (1994). Dynamics of brain activation during picture naming. *Nature, 368*, 463–465.

Salmelin, R. (2007). Clinical neurophysiology of language: the MEG approach. *Clin Neurophysiol, 118*, 237–254.

Schiffbauer, H., Berger, M., Ferrari, P., Freudenstein, D., Rowley, H., & Roberts, T. (2002). Preoperative magnetic source imaging for brain tumor surgery: a quantita-tive comparison with intraoperative sensory and motor mapping. *J Neurosurg, 97*, 1333–1342.

Schnitzler, A., & Gross, J. (2005). Normal and pathological oscillatory communication in the brain. *Nature Neurosci, 6*, 285–296.

Shiraishi, H., Watanabe, Y., Watanabe, M., Inoue, Y., Fujiwara, T., & Yagi K. (2001). Interictal and ictal magnetoencephalographic study in patients with medial frontal lobe epilepsy. *Epilepsia*, *42*, 875–882.

Stefan, H., Hummel, C., Scheler, G., Druschky, K., Tilz, C., Kaltenhäuser, M., et al. (2003). Magnetic brain source imaging of focal epileptic activity: a synopsis of 455 cases. *Brain*, *126*, 2396–2405.

Sutherling, W., Crandall, P., Darcey, T., Becker, D., Levesque, M., & Barth, D. (1988). The magnetic and electric fields agree with intracranial localizations of somatosensory cortex. *Neurology 38*, 1705–1714.

Sutherling, W., Mamelak, A., Thyerlei, D., Maleeva, T., Minazad, Y., Philpott, L., et al. (2008) Influence of magnetic source imaging for planning intracranial EEG in epilepsy. *Neurology 71*, 990–996.

Schwartz, E. S., Dlugos, D. L., Storm, P. B., Dell, J., Magee, R., Flynn, T. P., et al. (2008). Magnetoencephalography for pediatric epilepsy: how we do it. *Am J Neuroradiol 29*(5), 832–837.

Szmuk, P., Kee, S., Pivalizza, E. G., Warters, R., Abramson, D. C., & Ezri, T. (2003). Anaesthesia for magnetoencephalography in children with intractable seizures. *Paediatric Anaesth*, *13*, 811–817.

Szymanski, M., Perry, D., Cage, N. M., Rowley, H., Walker, J., Berger, M., et al. (2001). Magnetic source imaging of late evoked field responses to vowels: toward an assessment of hemispheric dominance for language. *J Neurosurg*, *94*, 445–453.

Tang, L., Mantle, M., Ferrari, P., Schiffbauer, H., Rowley, A. A., Barbaro, N. M., et al. (2003). Consistency of interictal and ictal onset localization using magnetoencephalography in patients with partial epilepsy. *J Neurosurg*, *98*, 837–845.

Tanaka, N., Thiele, E., Madsen, J., Bourgeois, B., & Stufflebeam, S. (2009). Magnetoencephalographic analysis in patients with vagus nerve stimulator. *Pediatr Neurol 41*, 383–387.

Tao, J. X., Ray, A., Hawes-Ebersole, S., & Ebersole, J. S. (2005) Intracranial EEG substrates of scalp EEG interictal spikes. *Epilepsia*, *46*, 669–676.

Taulu, S., Simola, J., & Kajola, M. (2005). Applications of the signal space separation method. *IEEE Trans Sign Proc*, *53*, 3359–3372.

Taulu, S., & Simola, J. (2006), Spatiotemporal signal space separation method for rejecting nearby interference in MEG measurements. *Phys Med Biol*, *51*, 1759–1768.

Tecchio, F., Zappasodi, F., Pasqualetti, P., Tombini, M., Salustri, C., Oliviero, A., et al. (2005). Rhythmic brain activity at rest from rolandic areas in acute monohemispheric stroke: a magnetoencephalographic study. *NeuroImage*, *28*, 72–83.

Tilz, C., Hummel, C., Kettenmann, B., & Stefan, H. (2002). Ictal onset localization of epileptic seizures by magnetoencephalography. *Acta Neurol Scand*, *106*, 190–195.

Uutela, K., Taulu, S., & Hämäläinen, M. (2001). Detecting and correcting for head movements in neuromagnetic measurements. *NeuroImage*, *14*, 1424–1431.

Vates, E., Lawton, M., Wilson, C., McDermott, M., Halbach, V., Roberts, T., et al. (2002). Magnetic source imaging demonstrates altered cortical distribution of function in patients with arteriovenous malformations. *Neurosurgery*, *51*, 614–622.

Vitikainen A-M., Lioumis P., Metsähonkala L., Salli E., Komssi S., Kicic D., et al. (2009). Combined use of non-invasive techniques for improved functional localization for a selected group of epilepsy surgery candidates. *NeuroImage 45*, 342–348.

Vrba, J., Betts, K., Burbank, M., Cheung, T., Fife, A., Haid, G., et al. (1993). Whole cortex 64 channel SQUID biomagnetometer system. *IEEE Trans Appl Sup. 3*, 1878–1882.

Worrell, G. A., Parish, L., Cranstoun, S. D., Jonas, R., Baltuch G., & Litt, B. (2004). High-frequency oscillations and seizure generation in neocortical epilepsy. *Brain, 127*, 1496–1506.

Yu, H., Nakasato, N., Iwasaki, M., Shamoto, H., Nagamatsu, K., & Yoshimoto, T. (2004) Neuromagnetic separation of secondarily bilateral synchronized spike foci: report of three cases. *J Clin Neurosci, 11*, 644–648.

15

Using Magnetoencephalography to Elucidate the Principles of Deep Brain Stimulation

Morten L. Kringelbach, Peter C. Hansen,
Alex L. Green, and Tipu Z. Aziz

- The correlational nature of neuroimaging makes it difficult to understand neural mechanisms
- However, deep brain stimulation (DBS) used together with magnetoencephalography (MEG) can provide a powerful causal tool for both elucidating the fundamental oscillatory mechanisms of brain networks, as well as finding new, more efficacious DBS targets
- First, we briefly describe the underlying techniques and mechanisms for DBS
- We then describe the preliminary results of using DBS and MEG in two patients with chronic pain and cluster headache
- The findings demonstrate the potential of this technique and highlight the mid-anterior orbitofrontal cortex as a potential future candidate for DBS in patients with treatment-resistant chronic pain

Recent developments in deep brain stimulation (DBS) of specific targets in the human brain have been successful in alleviating the symptoms of otherwise treatment-resistant movement and affective disorders (Anderson & Lenz, 2006; Kringelbach et al., 2007b; Perlmutter & Mink, 2006). However, while the treatment and associated neurosurgical methods have shown remarkable promise, the underlying neural mechanisms for DBS are not understood, and in particular it is not at all clear how DBS of specific brain targets changes the neural activity in wider cortical and subcortical regions.

DBS offers a novel and unique possibility for *in vivo* investigation of the functional role of the underlying neural circuitry in humans, by using stimulation parameters which yield different clinical results, and by switching the stimulator on and off. The ensuing changes in whole-brain activity can then be mapped using neuroimaging methods. Yet, some of the most-used neuroimaging technologies—functional magnetic resonance imaging (fMRI) and positron tomography (PET)—are, due to their intrinsic properties, less ideal for this purpose.

In contrast, MEG is of a noninvasive nature, and with its high spatial and temporal resolution holds great promise for elucidating the underlying whole-brain neural mechanisms of DBS by, for example, measuring oscillatory communication between brain regions (Schnitzler & Gross, 2005).

Here, we first provide an introductory overview of the current state-of-art of DBS, and the previous use of neuroimaging techniques with DBS. We then describe the methods and results of using MEG to measure both low- and high-frequency stimulation. We discuss the importance of the findings, as well as potential confounds and future possibilities of combining MEG and DBS.

Deep Brain Stimulation

Direct electrical stimulation of the brain has been in use at least since 1870, when Fritsch and Hirtzig showed that electrical stimulation of the motor cortex of the dog can elicit limb movement (Fritsch & Hitzig, 1870). Direct neuromodulation and recordings have since proved to be very useful for improving human neurosurgical procedures, as first shown in 1884 by Horsley (Gildenberg, 2005). Implantation of DBS pacemaker in select brain regions has become the basis of highly successful therapies for treating otherwise treatment-resistant movement and affective disorders.

Despite the long history of DBS, the underlying principles and mechanisms are still not clear. But it has been proposed that DBS of the normal and diseased brain must fundamentally depend on a number of parameters including, most importantly, (1) the physiological properties of the brain tissue, which may change with disease state; (2) the stimulation parameters, including amplitude and temporal characteristics; and (3) the geometric configuration of the electrode and the surrounding tissue (Kringelbach et al., 2007c). Overall, the weight of the evidence so far suggests that the most likely mode of action for DBS is through stimulation-induced modulation of brain activity, and thus that the similar therapeutic effects of DBS and brain lesions are likely to be achieved through different neural mechanisms.

DBS for Movement Disorders

The most efficacious targets for treating movement disorders with DBS have been the structures in the basal ganglia. The internal globus pallidus (GPi) and subthalamic nucleus (STN) have been demonstrated as safe and efficacious targets for Parkinson's disease (Aziz et al., 1991; Bergman et al., 1990). Long-term benefits of using high-frequency (130-185Hz) DBS for Parkinson's disease are well documented (Bittar et al., 2005a; Krack et al., 2003). Substantial improvements in the symptoms of Parkinson's disease (as measured by motor and daily living scores) (Fahn & Elton, 1987), as well as reductions in the patients' level of medication for Parkinson's disease, have been found in extensive DBS trials for Parkinson's disease (Benabid et al., 1996; Krack et al., 2003; Siegfried & Lippitz, 1994). Recently, translational research has identified the brainstem pedunculopontine nucleus (PPN) as a potential new Parkinson's disease target in monkeys (Jenkinson et al., 2005; Jenkinson et al., 2004; Jenkinson et al., 2006; Nandi et al., 2002) and humans (Mazzone et al., 2005; Plaha & Gill, 2005; Stefani et al., 2007).

The preferred target for dystonia and spasmodic torticollis is the GPi (Bittar et al., 2005c; Kumar et al., 1999). The DBS parameters for dystonia differ from Parkinson's disease, with a broader pulse width (200–400 µs) and higher voltage (typically between 2.2–7V) (Krauss et al., 2004), leading to rapid battery consumption. Blinded, controlled GPi trials have shown 30–50% improvements in patients over 12 months (Vidailhet et al., 2005).

Essential tremor is usually treated with DBS in the ventral intermediate nucleus of the thalamus (VIM) (Hassler, 1955; Lenz et al., 1994), while the DBS target for Parkinson's disease tremor is the STN (Krack et al., 1997). Long-term effects of DBS in VIM have shown an average tremor reduction of over 80% in the majority of patients (Koller et al., 1999; Rehncrona et al., 2003). Thalamic DBS was found to significantly improve tremor compared to thalamotomy, and have fewer adverse effects (Schuurman et al., 2000). A large multicenter study showed continued improvements in tremor ratings in patients with essential tremor after six years of follow-up (Sydow et al., 2003).

DBS for Affective Disorders

DBS for chronic pain has been used for over fifty years since the initial studies using DBS in the hypothalamus (Pool et al., 1956). More recent efficacious targets are in the thalamus (Hosobuchi et al., 1973; Mazars et al., 1973; Mazars et al., 1960) and periventricular-periaqueductal gray region (PVG/PAG) (Hosobuchi et al., 1977; Richardson & Akil, 1977a; b; c). Following two failed clinical trials (Coffey, 2001), FDA approval was not sought by device manufacturers. During the last decade only five centers outside the U.S. have produced case series of more than six patients: (Bittar et al., 2005b; Green et al., 2006; Hamani et al., 2006; Krauss et al., 2002; Marchand et al., 2003; Nandi et al., 2003; Owen et al., 2006a; Owen et al., 2006b; Tronnier, 2003). These studies have shown significant improvements for patients with, primarily, pain after amputation and stroke, and head pain including anaesthesia dolorosa. Patients with cluster headache have been successfully treated with DBS in the hypothalamus (Franzini et al., 2003; Leone et al., 2004).

Other affective disorders that have been successfully treated with DBS include depression, where targets have included inferior thalamic peduncle (Andy and Jurko, 1987; Jimenez et al., 2005) and the subgenual cingulate cortex (Mayberg et al., 2005). DBS for obsessive compulsive disorder have targeted the anterior internal capsule (Nuttin et al., 2003). DBS of the thalamus (Visser-Vandewalle et al., 2003) and GPi (Ackermans et al., 2006) have been reported effective in treating Tourette syndrome.

The Mechanics of DBS: Frames, Targeting and Batteries

The specific methods used for DBS vary among neurosurgical teams. Here, we present the methods adopted in Professor Aziz's lab in Oxford and focus specifically on the procedures used for DBS for pain relief (see Figure 15–1).

A T1-weighted MRI scan of each patient's brain is performed several weeks before surgery. For surgery, a Cosman-Roberts-Wells base ring is applied to the patient's head under local anesthesia. A stereotactic computed tomography (CT) scan is then performed and, using the Radionics Image Fusion® and Stereoplan® (Integra Radionics, Burlington, MA) program, the coordinates for the PVG/PAG and ventro-posterior lateral thalamus (VPL) are calculated. A double-oblique trajectory is used, with an entry point just anterior to the coronal suture, and laterality of approach dictated by ventricular width. The PVG/PAG target is proximally located 2–3 mm lateral to the wall of the third ventricle and 2 mm anterior to the level of the posterior commissure, and distally, the deepest electrode is placed in the superior colliculus. The VPL is located 12 mm lateral and 5–8 mm posterior to the mid-commissural point, at the depth of the anterior/posterior commissure plane. After washing the patient's scalp with alcoholic chlorhexidine, a parasaggital posterior frontal scalp incision 3.0 cm from the midline is made, contralateral to the side of pain.

The VPL is usually implanted with a Medtronic 3387 (Medtronic, Minneapolis, MN) electrode, where stimulation induces parasthesia in the area of pain. The PVG is also implanted with a Medtronic 3387 electrode where stimulation induces relief of pain or a sensation of warmth in the area of pain. The deepest electrode is noted to be in a satisfactory position if eye bobbing is induced at intensity of stimulation at least twice that required for sensory effects. The electrodes are fixed to the skull with a miniplate prior to externalization. In most patients, the electrodes are externalized for a week of trial stimulation.

Pain is assessed before surgery and during stimulation by a self-rated visual analog scale. If the patients are satisfied with the degree of pain relief, full implantation of a Medtronic pulse generator is performed in the following week under general anesthesia.

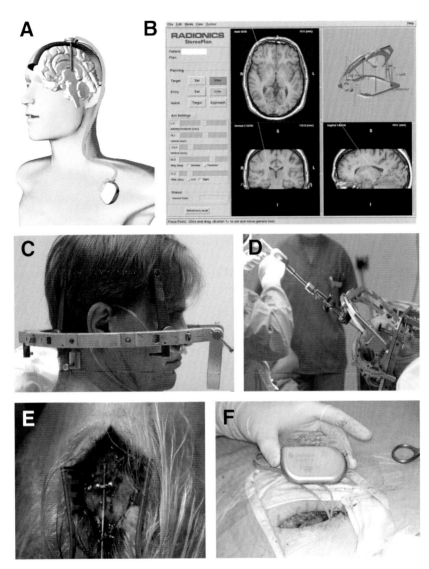

Figure 15-1. The neurosurgical procedures involved in DBS. (A) Schematic of the principles of DBS. (B) Illustration of the process of the neurosurgical pre-planning. (C) Application of the CRW stereotactic head frame on the patient. Note that the base ring is parallel to the orbitomeatal line. (D) The precise positioning of the electrode through perforating the calvarium with a twist drill. (E) Securing the electrode to the skull with a titanium miniplate and screws. (F) Placement of the implantable pulse generator in a subcutaneous pectoral pouch.

Safety and Complications with DBS

The safety of the DBS procedure has been demonstrated in many worldwide trials, and in the longterm follow-up in DBS for the treatment of chronic pain (Hosobuchi, 1986). The long-term efficacy of DBS depends on the generators, where most will last around 3–5 years depending on the current demands of the pulse protocol, although in the case of dystonia, this can be less than one year. Radiofrequency rechargeable pulse generators are available for spinal cord generators, and are being trialed for DBS.

Stereotactic procedures always carry a significant risk, and can lead to intracranial bleeding, usually in around 2.0–2.5% of DBS implants (Benabid et al., 1996; Beric et al., 2001). Other potential risks include hardware-related complications such as dislocation, lead fracture, and infection (6%). The infection rate is equal to that of other surgical procedures, but may necessitate explantation of the stimulator (Hariz, 2002). Stimulation-induced side effects (3%) are also quite common, such as aggression (Bejjani et al., 2002), mirthful laughter (Krack et al., 2001), depression (Bejjani et al., 1999), penile erection (Temel et al., 2004) and mania (Kulisevsky et al., 2002).

Functional Neuroimaging and DBS

In experimental animals, direct neural recordings and measurements of neurotransmitter release have been very useful in mapping the detailed local and monosynaptic effects of DBS. In humans, with the progress in functional neuroimaging, it has become possible to elucidate the whole-brain responses elicited by DBS.

Problems with Using PET and fMRI for DBS

Neuroimaging methods such as PET and fMRI can measure indirect changes of neural activity such as blood flow, blood oxygenation and glucose consumption. It is presently not entirely clear how well these indirect measurements correlate with various aspects of neural activity, but some progress in our understanding has been made under normal physiological conditions (Lauritzen, 2005; Logothetis & Wandell, 2004). In addition, it is important to realize that these methods entail a number of assumptions that may or may not prove to be important for interpreting the subsequent results.

It has become clear that fMRI studies pose a large degree of risk to DBS patients, since the large magnitude of the magnetic fields will interfere with active pulse generators and DBS electrodes. While several studies have been published showing the feasibility of using fMRI of DBS (Rezai et al., 1999; Uitti et al., 2002), there may well be significant problems using the BOLD signal as a measurement, since near-infrared spectroscopy showed considerable variations in blood oxygenation in the frontal cortex, following GPi and thalamic stimulation (Sakatani et al., 1999). Another study has shown that extreme caution must be exercised when studying fMRI with DBS, since strong heating, high induced voltage, and even sparking at defects in the connecting cable have been observed (Georgi et al., 2004). A case report has, however, shown that fMRI can be used to study STN stimulation in a patient with Parkinson's disease, who showed increases in the BOLD signal in primary motor areas, and decreases in supplementary motor areas, during stimulation (Stefurak et al., 2003).

PET is comparably safe, although not without health risks due to the ionized radiation, and has been used for measuring the effects of DBS. Due to the long acquisition periods for PET, usually up to a full minute, investigators have to carefully address the potential movement artifacts when studying movement disorders.

Using PET for Parkinson's disease is therefore rather challenging, and requires careful observation of any movement and removal of potentially confounding scans. One PET study took such precautions while scanning 13 Parkinson's disease patients and showed that STN stimulation led to increased blood flow in the thalamus, GP and midbrain (including STN), and reduced blood flow in frontal parietal and temporal cortices (Hershey et al., 2003). Similarly, a PET study of VIM thalamic stimulation in patients with essential tremor showed increases in blood flow in the thalamus and the cortical targets of thalamic output (Perlmutter et al., 2002). Other studies did not monitor and consider the behavioral effects of patients during the PET scans, and must therefore be cautiously interpreted (Fukuda et al., 2001; Hilker et al., 2004). Taken together, however, these results suggest that STN stimulation increases rather than inhibits the activity of STN output neurons, which in turn leads to increases of inhibition of thalamocortical projections, with subsequent decreases in blood flow in cortical regions.

Using PET to study DBS for affective disorders is less challenging in terms of potential movement artifacts. One PET study investigated the effects of hypothalamic stimulation for cluster headache in 10 patients (May et al., 2006). Stimulation compared with no stimulation elicited significant increases in activity in the ipsilateral hypothalamic gray (at the site of the stimulator tip), as well as in structures in the known pain processing network, including the ipsilateral thalamus, somatosensory cortex and praecuneus, the anterior cingulate cortex, and in the ipsilateral trigeminal nucleus and ganglion. Decreases in activity were found in the posterior cingulate cortex, middle temporal gyrus, and contralateral anterior insula. The results suggest that hypothalamic stimulation for cluster headache functions mainly through modulating the pain processing network.

Another PET study, using stimulation of subgenual cingulate cortex for treatment-resistant depression in four patients, showed marked reduction in activity in cortical and subcortical areas (Mayberg et al., 2005). The results are harder to interpret, given the small numbers of patients and the paucity of knowledge about the brain structures involved in depression, but again suggest that the mode of functioning of DBS would appear to be one of modulating an existing network of interacting brain regions.

Using MEG and DBS

PET and fMRI are not, however, the only neuroimaging techniques currently available. As shown in this book, MEG is noninvasive and without risks to use in patients, and can provide novel spatiotemporal information on the underlying whole-brain activity, with the current density of MEG sensors affording sensitivity such that the spatial resolution is comparable to fMRI (typically around 5 mm^3) but with much better temporal resolution (in milliseconds) (Hillebrand & Barnes, 2002).

The first MEG study of DBS was carried out in a patient with low-frequency PVG/PAG stimulation for severe phantom limb pain (Kringelbach et al., 2006; Kringelbach et al., 2007a) (Figure 15–2). We have since investigated the MEG effects of high-frequency hypothalamic stimulation for cluster headache (Ray et al., 2007) and are in the process of analyzing the results of a whole series of cases. In the following, we provide the details of the two published cases.

Case 1: Phantom Limb Chronic Pain Patient

The 58-year old right-handed male patient, RM, was referred with a 4-year history of severe phantom limb pain in the left leg, stemming from fracturing his leg in May 2001 with subsequent complications including an MRSA infection culminating in an above-the-knee amputation in October 2001. Sympathectomy, spinal cord nerve stimulation, hypnosis and a wide variety of medications had provided little relief. Preoperative testing showed an abnormal neuropsychological profile, with poor performance on all verbally mediated tests and at a level of "caseness" for both anxiety and depression, probably linked to his level of medication, which was repeated prescriptions of Morphine sulphate 380 mgm over 24 hours.

The patient RM was then implanted with a DBS in the right PVG/PAG, and he experienced excellent pain relief. The patient later fell, fracturing the deep-brain electrode, and this caused immediate return of the pain, After surgical revision, pain relief returned. Effective settings for stimulation in RM were 1.5 volts, frequency, 7 Hz and pulse width, 300 μs. This has significantly decreased the level of chronic pain in the patient to a manageable level, reducing the patient's McGill pain score by 74%.

Case 2: Cluster-headache Patient

The second patient was a 56-year old male, YY, with an 11-year history of cluster-headache attacks. The headaches had a seasonal pattern starting in September or October every year, and occurred 3–4 times a day, lasting for 45 minutes on average. The pain originated over the right forehead and radiated to the ipsilateral vertex, and was associated with lacrimation and excess rhinorrhea.

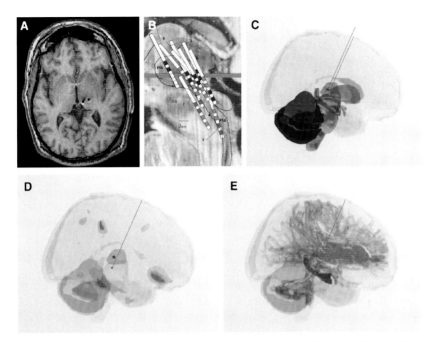

Figure 15–2. DBS for chronic pain. (A) Axial MRI slice showing the implantation of electrodes in PVG/PAG and thalamus in a patient. (B) Schematic illustration of the vertical placement of electrodes in the PVG/PAG in a series of chronic pain patients. (C) Three-dimensional rendering of human brain showing the placement of the two electrodes in the PVG/PAG and thalamus, as well as some of the important subcortical structures. (D) Three-dimensional rendering showing the whole-brain DBS induced activity from stimulation in the PVG/PAG. (E) The connectivity of the PVG/PAG measured with diffusion tensor imaging.

The patient YY was previously tried on carbamazepine, methysergide (2 mg three times daily), cafergot, co-proxamol, verapamil (240 mg twice daily), lithium (800 mg twice daily), amitryptiline and, at the time of referral, was partially controlled on injections of sumatriptan and high-dose prednisolone.

The patient YY was implanted with DBS in the right posterior hypothalamus, and he experienced excellent initial pain relief from his cluster-headaches. Whereas the patient had previously been having 3–4 attacks daily, during the week after the operation he had no further attacks. Given this, the electrodes were internalized and connected to a pacemaker. He was given a patient programmer to turn the stimulator on in the event of an attack, with contacts 1 negative, 2 positive, frequency 180 Hz, pulse width 90 microseconds. No further cluster attacks have occurred following surgery.

Experimental Setup

Patient RM was initially scanned with MEG for 10 minutes, with DBS switched on while resting. He was asked to continuously report his subjective experience of pain using a visual rating scale from 0–9 (where 0 is "not painful" and 9 is "very painful") every 20 seconds. This was then repeated three times with the stimulator switched off, during which his pain scores increased with time.

Patient YY's stimulator was turned off 30 minutes prior to scanning. We attached electrodes to his forearm in order to measure EMG. He was then scanned for 10 minutes. He rated his pain state in the same way as RM.

The patient's stimulator was then turned on and set to the non-effective setting of 7 Hz. After a further 5 minutes we began the second 10-minute scan with the rating task. The protocol was then repeated a final time, with the stimulator set at the effective frequency of 180 Hz.

Data Acquisition

MEG data were collected using a 275-channel CTF Omega system (CTF Systems Inc., Port Coquitlam, Canada) at Aston University. Data were sampled at 2400 Hz with an antialiasing cut-off filter of 200 Hz. The patient directly viewed the visual pain rating scale on a computer monitor.

Before and after surgery the patients were scanned with MRI to get high-resolution T1 volumes with 1x1x1 mm voxel dimensions. Immediately after finishing data acquisition in the MEG laboratory, the head coils were registered to the patients' MRIs using a 3D digitizer (Polhemus Fastrack, Polhemus Corporation, Colchester, VT, U.S.) to digitize the shape of the participant's head relative to the position of the head coils with respect to the nasion, left and right ear on the headset.

Image Analysis

The MEG data were analyzed using Synthetic Aperture Magnetometry (SAM), which is an adaptive beamforming technique for the analysis of EEG and MEG data (Vrba & Robinson, 2001). SAM has been previously used in a variety of studies on the functions of the motor cortex (Taniguchi et al., 2000), the human somatosensory cortex (Hirata et al., 2002), and visual word recognition (Pammer et al., 2004). In addition, SAM has been shown to be able to unveil changes in cortical synchronization that are spatially coincident with the hemodynamic response found with fMRI (Singh et al., 2002).

The SAM analysis links each voxel in the brain to the detection array, using an optimal spatial filter for that particular voxel (Robinson & Vrba, 1999). The data from the MEG sensors is then projected through this spatial filter to give a weighted measure of current density, as a function of time, in the target voxel—which means that the time series for each voxel has the same millisecond time-resolution as the original MEG signals. Fourier analysis was used to calculate the total amount of power in the specified frequency band within each of the *active* and *passive* time epochs of the time series. The jackknife statistical method is used to calculate the difference between the spectral power estimates for the *active* and *passive* states over all epochs to produce a true *t* statistic. A 3-dimensional image of differential cortical activity is produced by repeating this procedure for each voxel in the whole brain.

In this experiment, the SAM analysis created a volume covering the whole brain in the patient, with a voxel size of 5 x 5 x 5 mm. The *passive* state was defined as the time period between -1000 and 0 ms before pain rating; and the *active* state was defined as the time window of from 0 – +1000 ms starting at each rating period. Power changes between the *active* and *passive* states were calculated in the frequency bands of 10–20, 20–30 and 30–60Hz, for DBS on and off. Each t-map was thresholded at $t>2.3$, except for *a priori* predicted regions of interest (e.g., the insula, cingulate, and orbitofrontal cortices).

Results Case 1: Phantom Limb

Subjective Pain Experience

After the stimulator was turned off, RM's subjective reports of pain on the visual rating scale significantly increased with time over the four scans. In the first run with the stimulator on, the ratings were 4.68 ± 0.25 (mean $\pm$ s.e.). With this knowledge, the stimulator was then turned off and in the second, third and fourth runs the ratings were 4.68 ± 0.19, 4.97 ± 0.18 and 5.48 ± 0.20, respectively. Thus, in the fourth run, starting 25 minutes after the stimulator was switched off, the level of reported subjective pain had significantly increased ($p < 0.009$) compared to both when the stimulator was off, and the first and second runs where the stimulator was on. It should be noted that during the short period that the stimulator was turned off, pain levels did not approach pre-implantation levels, and the stimulator was turned on as soon as the fourth run was finished.

Neuroimaging Data

In the *pain* condition when DBS was switched off, and when RM's subjective pain ratings were significantly higher than during the fourth period after the DBS had been switched on, significant activity was found in regions involved in the pain network that have previously been identified using fMRI and PET (see Figure 15–3 and Table 15–1 for list of activations). These regions included the insula, and the primary and secondary somatosensory, lateral orbitofrontal, and anterior cingulate cortices. Activity was also found in the motor networks related to the rating process. In the 10–20 Hz frequency band significant differences in activity were found in somatosensory cortices (SI, SII), intraparietal cortex, motor cortex, premotor area (PMA), middle and posterior insula cortices, occipital lobe, and middle frontal gyrus. In the 20–30Hz band, significant differences were found in motor, parietal, insula, fusiform and motor cingulate cortices, as well as lateral orbitofrontal cortex/anterior insula. In the 30–60Hz band we found significant differences in the parahippocampal, motor and fusiform cortices.

In the *pain relief* condition, during the fourth period after the DBS had been switched on, significant activity was found in brain regions previously identified with fMRI as the pain relief network (see Table 15–1 for list of activations). In the 10–20Hz band, significant differences in activity were found in SI, brainstem, the mid-anterior orbitofrontal cortex and subgenual cingulate cortex. In the 20–30Hz band there were differences in activity in a motor network comprising supplementary motor area (SMA), parietal and

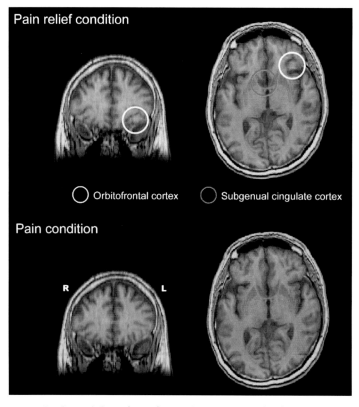

Figure 15–3. Brain activity when the patient reported subjective pain relief (DBS on) and pain (DBS off). Top part of figure shows that in the pain relief condition there was significant activity in the left mid-anterior orbitofrontal cortex and right subgenual cingulate cortex. Activity in these regions was not found in the pain condition (bottom part of figure).

Table 15–1. Active Brain Regions

	Laterality	MNI x	MNI y	MNI z	t score
DBS off (pain)					
10–20 Hz					
Somatosensory cortex (SI, SII)	R	54	−38	56	2.8
Intraparietal cortex	R	4	−82	56	2.7
Motor cortex	R	58	−2	44	2.7
Left posterior insula	L	−38	−34	18	2.7
Occipital lobe	R	36	−94	16	−2.6
Premotor cortex	R	42	22	50	2.4
Middle frontal gyrus	R	6	6	66	2.3
Middle insular cortex	R	46	−10	16	2.0*
20–30 Hz					
Motor cortex	R	58	4	28	3.9
Parietal cortex	R	46	−68	42	3.0
Anterior insula/lateral orbitofrontal cortex	R	48	36	−10	2.6
Occipital lobe	L	−30	−96	−4	−2.6
Fusiform cortex	R	22	−70	-10	−2.4
Anterior insula cortex	R	36	28	4	2.4
Rostral anterior cingulate cortex	R	2	−8	36	2.2*
Motor cingulate cortex	R	12	−6	66	2.1*
30–60 Hz					
Parahippocampal cortex	L	−12	−44	0	2.8
Motor cortex	R	66	−12	24	2.6
Fusiform cortex	R	46	−70	−10	2.4
DBS on (pain relief)					
10–20 Hz					
Somatosensory cortex (SI)	R	56	−36	54	2.4
Brainstem	R	12	−18	−40	2.3
Mid-anterior orbitofrontal cortex	L	−34	26	−10	2.0*
Subgenual cingulate cortex	R	4	6	−8	−1.8*
20–30 Hz					
Supplementary motor cortex	L	−56	12	30	2.8
Parietal cortex	R	28	−78	46	−2.5
Motor cortex	L	−48	−2	54	2.3
30–60 Hz					
Superior temporal gyrus	L	−54	−64	18	3.1
Middle temporal gyrus	L	−52	−40	−18	2.7
Occipital Lobe	L	−18	−102	−10	2.5
Parietal cortex	L	−56	−58	40	2.4
Posterior cingulate cortex	R	8	−60	44	2.3

Activations are significant at t>2.3, uncorrected; unless indicated with * for a priori predicted regions. All brain coordinates are in the standard space of MNI (Montreal Neurological Institute).

motor cortices. In the 30–60Hz band, significant differences were found in the superior and middle temporal gyri, occipital lobe, parietal and posterior cingulate cortices.

Results Case 2: Cluster Headache

The brain regions active in patient YY measured with MEG in all conditions regardless of stimulator activity, which were very similar to those found in patient RM. In all conditions somatosensory and motor cortices were activated in the active (button-press) condition, compared with passive (100ms before the button press). We also found significant activity in the 10–20Hz frequency band in the PAG only when the patient's stimulator was turned off. When the stimulator was turned on, there was activity in frontal brain regions including the orbitofrontal cortex, associated using fMRI with the pain relief network.

Discussion

These studies show that it is feasible to use MEG to map whole-brain changes in neural activity induced by both low- and high-frequency DBS. We found significant changes in brain activity in patient RM with implanted low-frequency DBS in the right PVG/PAG, for severe phantom limb pain in the left leg. This patient reported significantly more pain relatively soon after the DBS was turned off compared to when DBS was switched on.

Similarly, we were able to measure the whole-brain changes during low- and high-frequency stimulation of the posterior hypothalamus for cluster-headache, on MEG recordings. The posterior hypothalamus contains several neurochemically distinct cell groups. One of these is the Hypocr/Orx neurons that are activated by nociceptive stimuli and reach structures involved in nociceptive relay and modulation, including the PAG (Baldo et al., 2003). We found activity in the PAG only when patient YY's stimulator was turned off, which may be related to these patterns of connectivity. In an fMRI study it was found that PAG was activated if participants were anticipating a painful stimulus, even before they were subjected to pain (Fairhurst et al., 2007). Patient YY in the present study was aware that his stimulator had been turned off, and thus the activity in his PAG may have been related to the anticipation of his pain returning.

The obtained changes in brain activity related to both pain and pain relief are consistent with previous findings reported with fMRI and PET (Petrovic & Ingvar, 2002). Testifying to the utility of our method, irrespective of DBS we also found activity in brain regions that are part of the motor network, related to the patient using button-presses to rate his pain.

Pain-specific activity was found when DBS was switched off, and the subjective pain scores were significantly higher than in the pain relief condition (with DBS on). Significant activity was found in the well-documented extended pain network, including insular, SI, SII, lateral orbitofrontal and anterior cingulate cortices (Petrovic & Ingvar, 2002).

Importantly, in the pain-relief condition with effective stimulation parameters in both patients, we found activity in the mid-anterior orbitofrontal cortex, which is a region previously implicated in pain relief. The mid-anterior orbitofrontal cortex has been shown to be more active in placebo-responders than in placebo nonresponders (Petrovic et al., 2002), and it has also been shown to correlate with the subjective pleasantness of various primary and secondary reinforcers (Kringelbach, 2005; Kringelbach et al., 2003). This finding opens up the possibility that the mid-anterior orbitofrontal cortex may be a potential future candidate for DBS in patients with chronic pain.

Potential Problems

The MEG artifacts induced by both unilateral low-frequency stimulation of the right PVG/PAG and high-frequency stimulation of the posterior hypothalamus, would appear to be minimal, although the presence of the magnetic battery can induce long-term data drift (which is present regardless of whether the stimulation is on or off). This long-term drift appears to be linked to the breathing cycle. It should be noted, however, that the reported findings are preliminary and will need further confirmation in more subjects.

Other sources of MEG artifacts include high-amplitude artifacts originating from the percutaneous extension wire, which are locked to the heart beat. Careful experimentation has shown that beamforming is capable of suppressing these artifacts and have quantified the optimal regularization required (Litvak et al. 2010). It is also important to realize that the brain of a patient may not be entirely normal, which is why it is important to also carefully investigate the anatomical structure and connectivity of the patient's brain using high-resolution MRI, CT and DTI. This information can then be used to constrain the MEG analysis.

Future Possibilities

While the MEG results presented here have been obtained from DBS electrodes with both low- and high-frequency stimulation, the experiments were conducted in patients who did not move in the scanner. It would be of great interest to extend these studies to movement disorders such as Parkinson's disease, dystonia and essential tremor—but as mentioned above, great care will have to be taken to minimize head movements in these patients. Another exciting possibility will be to use the recordings from DBS electrodes (while still externalized) as an EEG channel, which can then be used in the subsequent analysis together with the MEG signals.

Conclusion

The results of these studies have demonstrated the feasibility of using MEG to map changes in whole-brain activity induced by both low- and high-frequency DBS. The findings have highlighted the mid-anterior orbitofrontal cortex as potential future candidate for DBS in patients with chronic pain. From a systems neuroscience point of view, the combination of the causal, interventional nature of DBS with the high temporal resolution of MEG, has the makings of a powerful and sophisticated tool for unraveling the fundamental mechanisms of normal human brain function.

References

Ackermans, L., Temel, Y., Cath, D., van der Linden, C., Bruggeman, R., Kleijer, M., et al. (2006). Deep brain stimulation in Tourette's syndrome: two targets? *Mov Disor*, *21*, 709–713.

Anderson, W. S., & Lenz, F. A. (2006). Surgery insight: Deep brain stimulation for movement disorders. *Nat Clin Pract Neurol*, *2*, 310–320.

Andy, O. J., & Jurko, F. (1987). Thalamic stimulation effects on reactive depression. *Appl Neurophysiol*, *50*, 324–329.

Aziz, T. Z., Peggs, D., Sambrook, M. A., & Crossman, A. R. (1991). Lesion of the subthalamic nucleus for the alleviation of 1-methyl-4-phenyl-1,2,3,6-tetrahydropyridine (MPTP)-induced parkinsonism in the primate. *Mov Disord*, *6*, 288–292.

Baldo, B. A., Daniel, R. A., Berridge, C. W., & Kelley, A. E. (2003). Overlapping distributions of orexin/hypocretin- and dopamine-beta-hydroxylase immunoreactive fibers in rat brain regions mediating arousal, motivation, and stress. *J Comp Neurol*, *464*, 220–237.

Bejjani, B. P., Damier, P., Arnulf, I., Thivard, L., Bonnet, A. M., Dormont, D., et al. (1999). Transient acute depression induced by high-frequency deep-brain stimulation. *N Engl J Med*, *340*, 1476–1480.

Bejjani, B. P., Houeto, J. L., Hariz, M., Yelnik, J., Mesnage, V., Bonnet, A. M., et al. (2002). Aggressive behavior induced by intraoperative stimulation in the triangle of Sano. *Neurology*, *59*, 1425–1427.

Benabid, A. L., Pollak, P., Gao, D., Hoffmann, D., Limousin, P., Gay, E., et al. (1996). Chronic electrical stimulation of the ventralis intermedius nucleus of the thalamus as a treatment of movement disorders. *J Neurosurg*, *84*, 203–214.

Bergman, H., Wichmann, T., & DeLong, M. R. (1990). Reversal of experimental parkinsonism by lesions of the subthalamic nucleus. *Science*, *249*, 1436–1438.

Beric, A., Kelly, P. J., Rezai, A., Sterio, D., Mogilner, A., Zonenshayn, M., et al. (2001). Complications of deep brain stimulation surgery. *Stereotact Funct Neurosurg*, *77*, 73–78.

Bittar, R. G., Burn, S. C., Bain, P. G., Owen, S. L., Joint, C., Shlugman, D., et al. (2005a). Deep brain stimulation for movement disorders and pain. *J Clin Neurosci*, *12*, 457–463.

Bittar, R. G., Otero, S., Carter, H., & Aziz, T. Z. (2005b). Deep brain stimulation for phantom limb pain. *J Clin Neurosci*, *12*, 399–404.

Bittar, R. G., Yianni, J., Wang, S., Liu, X., Nandi, D., Joint, C., et al. (2005c). Deep brain stimulation for generalised dystonia and spasmodic torticollis. *J Clin Neurosci*, *12*, 12–16.

Coffey, R. J. (2001). Deep brain stimulation for chronic pain: results of two multicenter trials and a structured review. *Pain Med*, *2*, 183–192.

Fahn, S., & Elton, R. L. (1987). Members of the UPDRS Development Committee. Unified Parkinson's disease rating scale. In: Fahn, S., Marsden, C. D., Goldstein, M., & Calne, D. B. (eds.). *Recent developments in Parkinson's disease. Vol. 2.* (p. 153). Florham Park, New York: MacMillan.

Fairhurst, M., Wiech, K., Dunckley, P., & Tracey, I. (2007). Anticipatory brainstem activity predicts neural processing of pain in humans. *Pain*, *128*, 101–110.

Franzini, A., Ferroli, P., Leone, M., & Broggi, G. (2003). Stimulation of the posterior hypothalamus for treatment of chronic intractable cluster headaches: first reported series. *Neurosurgery*, *52*, 1095–1099; discussion 1099–1101.

Fritsch, G., & Hitzig, E. (1870). Über die elektrische Erregbarkeit des Grosshirns. *Arch. Anat. Physiol*, *37*, 300–332.

Fukuda, M., Mentis, M. J., Ma, Y., Dhawan, V., Antonini, A., Lang, A. E., et al. (2001). Networks mediating the clinical effects of pallidal brain stimulation for Parkinson's disease: a PET study of resting-state glucose metabolism. *Brain*, *124*, 1601–1609.

Georgi, J. C., Stippich, C., Tronnier, V. M., & Heiland, S. (2004). Active deep brain stimulation during MRI: a feasibility study. *Magn Reson Med*, *51*, 380–388.

Gildenberg, P. L. (2005). Evolution of neuromodulation. *Stereotact Funct Neurosurg*, *83*, 71–79.

Green, A. L., Owen, S. L., Davies, P., Moir, L., & Aziz, T. Z. (2006). Deep brain stimulation for neuropathic cephalgia. *Cephalalgia*, *26*, 561–567.

Hamani, C., Schwalb, J. M., Rezai, A. R., Dostrovsky, J. O., Davis, K. D., & Lozano, A. M. (2006). Deep brain stimulation for chronic neuropathic pain: Long-term outcome and the incidence of insertional effect. *Pain*, *125*, 188–196.

Hariz, M. I. (2002). Complications of deep brain stimulation surgery. *Mov Disord 17*, S162–6.

Hassler, R. (1955). The influence of stimulations and coagulations in the human thalamus on the tremor at rest and its physiopathologic mechanism. *Proceedings of the Second International Congress of Neuropathology*, *2*, 637–642.

Hershey, T., Revilla, F. J., Wernle, A. R., McGee-Minnich, L., Antenor, J. V., Videen, T. O., et al. (2003). Cortical and subcortical blood flow effects of subthalamic nucleus stimulation in PD. *Neurology*, *61*, 816–821.

Hilker, R., Voges, J., Weisenbach, S., Kalbe, E., Burghaus, L., Ghaemi, M., et al. (2004). Subthalamic nucleus stimulation restores glucose metabolism in associative and limbic cortices and in cerebellum: evidence from a FDG-PET study in advanced Parkinson's disease. *J Cereb Blood Flow Metab*, *24*, 7–16.

Hillebrand, A., & Barnes, G. R. (2002). A quantitative assessment of the sensitivity of whole-head MEG to activity in the adult human cortex. *Neuroimage*, *16*, 638–650.

Hirata, M., Kato, A., Taniguchi, M., Ninomiya, H., Cheyne, D., Robinson, S. E., et al. (2002). Frequency-dependent spatial distribution of human somatosensory evoked neuromagnetic fields. *Neurosci Lett*, *318*, 73–76.

Hosobuchi, Y. (1986). Subcortical electrical stimulation for control of intractable pain in humans. Report of 122 cases (1970–1984). *J Neurosurg*, *64*, 543–553.

Hosobuchi, Y., Adams, J. E., & Linchitz, R. (1977). Pain relief by electrical stimulation of the central gray matter in humans and its reversal by naloxone. *Science*, *197*, 183–186.

Hosobuchi, Y., Adams, J. E., & Rutkin, B. (1973). Chronic thalamic stimulation for the control of facial anesthesia dolorosa. *Arch Neurol, 29*, 158–161.

Jenkinson, N., Nandi, D., Aziz, T. Z., & Stein, J. F. (2005). Pedunculopontine nucleus: a new target for deep brain stimulation for akinesia. *Neuroreport, 16*, 1875–1876.

Jenkinson, N., Nandi, D., Miall, R. C., Stein, J. F., & Aziz, T. Z. (2004). Pedunculo-pontine nucleus stimulation improves akinesia in a Parkinsonian monkey. *Neuro-report, 15*, 2621–2624.

Jenkinson, N., Nandi, D., Oram, R., Stein, J. F., & Aziz, T. Z. (2006). Pedunculopon-tine nucleus electric stimulation alleviates akinesia independently of dopaminergic mechanisms. *Neuroreport, 17*, 639–641.

Jimenez, F., Velasco, F., Salin-Pascual, R., Hernandez, J. A., Velasco, M., Criales, J. L., et al. (2005). A patient with a resistant major depression disorder treated with deep brain stimulation in the inferior thalamic peduncle. *Neurosurgery, 57*, 585–93; discussion 585–593.

Koller, W. C., Lyons, K. E., Wilkinson, S. B., & Pahwa, R. (1999). Efficacy of unilate-ral deep brain stimulation of the VIM nucleus of the thalamus for essential head tremor. *Mov Disord, 14*, 847–850.

Krack, P., Batir, A., Van Blercom, N., Chabardes, S., Fraix, V., Ardouin, C., et al. (2003). Five-year follow-up of bilateral stimulation of the subthalamic nucleus in advanced Parkinson's disease. *N Engl J Med, 349*, 1925–1934.

Krack, P., Kumar, R., Ardouin, C., Dowsey, P. L., McVicker, J. M., Benabid, A. L., et al. (2001). Mirthful laughter induced by subthalamic nucleus stimulation. *Mov Disord, 16*, 867–875.

Krack, P., Pollak, P., Limousin, P., Benazzouz, A., & Benabid, A. L. (1997). Stimulation of subthalamic nucleus alleviates tremor in Parkinson's disease. *Lancet, 350*, 1675.

Krauss, J. K., Pohle, T., Weigel, R., & Burgunder, J. M. (2002). Deep brain stimulation of the centre median-parafascicular complex in patients with movement disorders. *J Neurol Neurosurg Psychiatry, 72*, 546–548.

Krauss, J. K., Yianni, J., Loher, T. J., & Aziz, T. Z. (2004). Deep brain stimulation for dystonia. *J Clin Neurophysiol, 21*, 18–30.

Kringelbach, M. L. (2005). The orbitofrontal cortex: linking reward to hedonic expe-rience. *Nature Reviews Neuroscience, 6*, 691–702.

Kringelbach, M. L., Jenkinson, N., Green, A., Hansen, P. C., Cornelissen, P. L., Holliday, I. E., et al. (2006). Deep brain stimulation and chronic pain mapped with MEG. *Society for Neuroscience, 782*.1.

Kringelbach, M. L., Jenkinson, N., Green, A. L., Owen, S. L. F., Hansen, P. C., Cornelissen, P. L., et al. (2007a). Deep brain stimulation for chronic pain investigated with magnetoencephalography. *Neuroreport, 18*, 223–228.

Kringelbach, M. L., Jenkinson, N., Owen, S. L. F., & Aziz, T. Z. (2007b). Translational principles of deep brain stimulation. *Nature Reviews Neuroscience, 8*, 623–635.

Kringelbach, M. L., O'Doherty, J., Rolls, E. T., & Andrews, C. (2003). Activation of the human orbitofrontal cortex to a liquid food stimulus is correlated with its subjective pleasantness. *Cerebral Cortex 13*, 1064–1071.

Kringelbach, M. L., Owen, S. L. F., & Aziz, T. Z. (2007c). Deep brain stimulation. *Future Neurology, 2*, 633–646.

Kulisevsky, J., Berthier, M. L., Gironell, A., Pascual-Sedano, B., Molet, J., & Pares, P. (2002). Mania following deep brain stimulation for Parkinson's disease. *Neurology, 59*, 1421–1424.

Kumar, R., Dagher, A., Hutchison, W. D., Lang, A. E., & Lozano, A. M. (1999). Globus pallidus deep brain stimulation for generalized dystonia: clinical and PET investigation. *Neurology, 53*, 871–874.

Lauritzen, M. (2005). Reading vascular changes in brain imaging: is dendritic calcium the key? *Nat Rev Neurosci, 6*, 77–85.

Lenz, F. A., Kwan, H. C., Martin, R. L., Tasker, R. R., Dostrovsky, J. O., & Lenz, Y. E. (1994). Single unit analysis of the human ventral thalamic nuclear group. Tremor-related activity in functionally identified cells. *Brain, 117*, 531–543.

Leone, M., Franzini, A., Broggi, G., May, A., & Bussone, G. (2004). Long-term follow-up of bilateral hypothalamic stimulation for intractable cluster headache. *Brain, 127*, 2259–2264.

Litvak, V., Eusebio, A., Jha, A., Oostenveld, R., Barnes, G. R., Penny, W. D., et al. (2010). Optimized beamforming for simultaneous MEG and intracranial local field potential recordings in deep brain stimulation patients. *Neuroimage*, in press.

Logothetis, N. K., & Wandell, B. A. (2004). Interpreting the BOLD signal. *Annu Rev Physiol, 66*, 735–769.

Marchand, S., Kupers, R. C., Bushnell, M. C., & Duncan, G. H. (2003). Analgesic and placebo effects of thalamic stimulation. *Pain, 105*, 481–488.

May, A., Leone, M., Boecker, H., Sprenger, T., Juergens, T., Bussone, G., et al. (2006). Hypothalamic deep brain stimulation in positron emission tomography. *J Neurosci, 26*, 3589–3593.

Mayberg, H. S., Lozano, A. M., Voon, V., McNeely, H. E., Seminowicz, D., Hamani, C., et al. (2005). Deep brain stimulation for treatment-resistant depression. *Neuron, 45*, 651–660.

Mazars, G., Merienne, L., & Ciolocca, C. (1973). Intermittent analgesic thalamic stimulation. [Preliminary note]. *Rev Neurol (Paris) 128*, 273–279.

Mazars, G., Roge, R., & Mazars, Y. (1960). Results of the stimulation of the spinothalamic fasciculus and their bearing on the physiopathology of pain. *Rev Prat, 103*, 136–138.

Mazzone, P., Lozano, A. M., Stanzione, P., Galati, S., Scanati, E., Peppe, A., et al. (2005). Implantation of human pedunculopontine nucleus: a safe and clinically relevant target in Parkinson's disease. *Neuroreport, 16*, 1877–1881.

Nandi, D., Aziz, T., Carter, H., & Stein, J. (2003). Thalamic field potentials in chronic central pain treated by periventricular gray stimulation — a series of eight cases. *Pain, 101*, 97–107.

Nandi, D., Liu, X., Winter, J. L., Aziz, T. Z., & Stein, J. F. (2002). Deep brain stimulation of the pedunculopontine region in the normal non-human primate. *J Clin Neurosci, 9*, 170–174.

Nuttin, B. J., Gabriels, L. A., Cosyns, P. R., Meyerson, B. A., Andreewitch, S., Sunaert, S. G., et al. (2003). Long-term electrical capsular stimulation in patients with obsessive-compulsive disorder. *Neurosurgery, 52*, 1263–1272.

Owen, S. L., Green, A. L., Stein, J. F., & Aziz, T. Z. (2006a). Deep brain stimulation for the alleviation of post-stroke neuropathic pain. *Pain, 120*, 202–206.

Owen, S. L. F., Green, A. L., Nandi, D., Bittar, R. G., Wang, S., & Aziz, T. Z. (2006b). Deep brain stimulation for neuropathic pain. *Neuromodulation, 9*, 100–106.

Pammer, K., Hansen, P. C., Kringelbach, M. L., Holliday, I., Barnes, G., Hillebrand, A., et al. (2004). Visual word recognition: the first half second. *Neuroimage, 22*, 1819–1825.

Perlmutter, J. S., & Mink, J. W. (2006). Deep brain stimulation. *Annu Rev Neurosci*, *29*, 229–257.

Perlmutter, J. S., Mink, J. W., Bastian, A. J., Zackowski, K., Hershey, T., Miyawaki, E., et al. (2002). Blood flow responses to deep brain stimulation of thalamus. *Neurology*, *58*, 1388–1394.

Petrovic, P., & Ingvar, M. (2002). Imaging cognitive modulation of pain processing. *Pain*, *95*, 1–5.

Petrovic, P., Kalso, E., Petersson, K. M., & Ingvar, M. (2002). Placebo and opioid analgesia—imaging a shared neuronal network. *Science*, *295*, 1737–1740.

Plaha, P., & Gill, S. G. (2005). Bilateral deep brain stimulation of the pedunculopontine nucleus for idiopathic Parkinson's disease. *Neuroreport*, *16*, 1883–1887.

Pool, J. L., Clark, W. D., Hudson, P., & Lombardo, M. (1956). Steroid hormonal response to stimulation of electrodes implanted in the subfrontal parts of the brain. In: Fields, W. S., Guillemin, R., & Carton, C. A. (eds.). *Hypothalamic-Hypophysial Interrelationships* (pp. 114–124). Springfield, IL: Charles C. Thomas.

Ray, N. J., Kringelbach, M. L., Jenkinson, N., Owen, S. L. F., Davies, P., Wang, S., et al. (2007). Using magnetoencephalography to investigate deep brain stimulation for cluster headache. *Biomedical Imaging and Intervention Journal*, *3*, e25.

Rehncrona, S., Johnels, B., Widner, H., Tornqvist, A. L., Hariz, M., & Sydow, O. (2003). Long-term efficacy of thalamic deep brain stimulation for tremor: double-blind assessments. *Mov Disord*, *18*, 163–170.

Rezai, A. R., Lozano, A. M., Crawley, A. P., Joy, M. L., Davis, K. D., Kwan, C. L., et al. (1999). Thalamic stimulation and functional magnetic resonance imaging: localization of cortical and subcortical activation with implanted electrodes. Technical note. *J Neurosurg*, *90*, 583–590.

Richardson, D. E., & Akil, H. (1977a). Long term results of periventricular gray self-stimulation. *Neurosurgery*, *1*, 199–202.

Richardson, D. E., & Akil, H. (1977b). Pain reduction by electrical brain stimulation in man. Part 1: Acute administration in periaqueductal and periventricular sites. *J Neurosurg*, *47*, 178–183.

Richardson, D. E., & Akil, H. (1977c). Pain reduction by electrical brain stimulation in man. Part 2: Chronic self-administration in the periventricular gray matter. *J Neurosurg*, *47*, 184–194.

Robinson, S. E., & Vrba, J. (1999). Functional neuroimaging by synthetic aperture magnetometry (SAM). In: Yoshimoto, T., Kotani, M. Kuriki, S., Karibe, H., & N. Nakasato. (eds.). *Recent Advances in Biomagnetism*. (pp. 302–305). Sendai: Tohoku University Press.

Sakatani, K., Katayama, Y., Yamamoto, T., & Suzuki, S. (1999). Changes in cerebral blood oxygenation of the frontal lobe induced by direct electrical stimulation of thalamus and globus pallidus: a near infrared spectroscopy study. *J Neurol Neurosurg, Psychiatry 67*, 769 773.

Schnitzler, A., & Gross, J. (2005). Normal and pathological oscillatory communication in the brain. *Nat Rev Neurosci*, *6*, 285–296.

Schuurman, P. R., Bosch, D. A., Bossuyt, P. M., Bonsel, G. J., van Someren, E. J., de Bie, R. M., et al. (2000). A comparison of continuous thalamic stimulation and thalamotomy for suppression of severe tremor. *N Engl J Med*, *342*, 461–468.

Siegfried, J., & Lippitz, B. (1994). Bilateral chronic electrostimulation of ventroposterolateral pallidum: a new therapeutic approach for alleviating all parkinsonian symptoms. *Neurosurgery*, *35*, 1126–1129.

Singh, K. D., Barnes, G. R., Hillebrand, A., Forde, E. M., & Williams, A. L. (2002). Task-related changes in cortical synchronization are spatially coincident with the hemodynamic response. *Neuroimage, 16*, 103–114.

Stefani, A., Lozano, A. M., Peppe, A., Stanzione, P., Galati, S., Tropepi, D., et al. (2007). Bilateral deep brain stimulation of the pedunculopontine and subthalamic nuclei in severe Parkinson's disease. *Brain, 130*, 1596–1607.

Stefurak, T., Mikulis, D., Mayberg, H., Lang, A. E., Hevenor, S., Pahapill, P., et al. (2003). Deep brain stimulation for Parkinson's disease dissociates mood and motor circuits: a functional MRI case study. *Mov Disord, 18*, 1508–1516.

Sydow, O., Thobois, S., Alesch, F., & Speelman, J. D. (2003). Multicentre European study of thalamic stimulation in essential tremor: a six year follow up. *J Neurol Neurosurg Psychiatry, 74*, 1387–1391.

Taniguchi, M., Kato, A., Fujita, N., Hirata, M., Tanaka, H., Kihara, T., et al. (2000). Movement-related desynchronization of the cerebral cortex studied with spatially filtered magnetoencephalography. *Neuroimage, 12*, 298–306.

Temel, Y., van Lankveld, J. J., Boon, P., Spincemaille, G. H., van der Linden, C., & Visser-Vandewalle, V. (2004). Deep brain stimulation of the thalamus can influence penile erection. *Int J Impot Res, 16*, 91–94.

Tronnier, V. M. (2003). *Deep brain stimulation*. Amsterdam, London: Elsevier.

Uitti, R. J., Tsuboi, Y., Pooley, R. A., Putzke, J. D., Turk, M. F., Wszolek, Z. K., et al. (2002). Magnetic resonance imaging and deep brain stimulation. *Neurosurgery, 51*, 1423–1428.

Vidailhet, M., Vercueil, L., Houeto, J. L., Krystkowiak, P., Benabid, A. L., Cornu, P., et al. (2005). Bilateral deep-brain stimulation of the globus pallidus in primary generalized dystonia. *N Engl J Med, 352*, 459–467.

Visser-Vandewalle, V., Temel, Y., Boon, P., Vreeling, F., Colle, H., Hoogland, G., et al. (2003). Chronic bilateral thalamic stimulation: a new therapeutic approach in intractable Tourette syndrome. Report of three cases. *J Neurosurg, 99*, 1094–1100.

Vrba, J., & Robinson, S. E. (2001). Signal processing in magnetoencephalography. *Methods, 25*, 249–271.

Author Index

Subject Index

Note: Page number followed by "*f*" and "*t*" refers to figures and tables, respectively.